Practical Approaches to Peripheral Nerve Surgery

AANS Publications Committee
Edward C. Benzel, MD, Editor

Neurosurgical Topics

American Association of Neurological Surgeons
Park Ridge, Illinois

ISBN: 1-879284-03-0

Neurosurgical Topics ISBN: 0-9624246-6-8

Copyright © 1992 by American Association of Neurological Surgeons

Printed in U.S.A.

Robert H. Wilkins, MD, Chairman
AANS Publications Committee

Linda S. Miller, AANS Staff Editor

AANS1.3M392

Forthcoming Books in the *Neurosurgical Topics* Series

1992

Cerebrovascular Occlusive Disease and Brain Ischemia
  Edited by Issam A. Awad, MD

Neurosurgery for the Third Millennium
  Edited by Michael L.J. Apuzzo, MD

Degenerative Disease of the Cervical Spine
  Edited by Paul R. Cooper, MD

Contents

PART IV   **SURGICAL ANATOMY AND EXPOSURE**

PART V   **SPECIAL CONSIDERATIONS**

List of Contributors

Deepak Awasthi, MD
Department of Neurosurgery
Louisiana State University Medical Center
Charity and Ochsner Hospitals
New Orleans, Louisiana

Edward C. Benzel, MD, FACS
Professor and Chief
Division of Neurosurgery
University of New Mexico School of
   Medicine
Albuquerque, New Mexico

Charles L. Branch, Jr, MD
Department of Neurosurgery
Bowman Gray School of Medicine
   of Wake Forest University
Winston-Salem, North Carolina

James N. Campbell, MD
Department of Neurosurgery
Johns Hopkins University
Baltimore, Maryland

Thomas B. Ducker, MD
Associate Professor of Neurosurgery
Johns Hopkins Medical Center
Baltimore, Maryland

Stephen R. Freidberg, MD
Department of Neurosurgery
Lahey Clinic Medical Center
Burlington, Massachusetts

Allan H. Friedman, MD
Assistant Professor, Neurosurgery
Duke University Medical Center
Durham, North Carolina

Earl R. Hackett, MD
Clinical Professor of Neurology
University of Missouri, Columbia
Emeritus Professor and Head, Neurology
Louisiana State University School of
   Medicine
New Orleans, Louisiana

Alan R. Hudson, MD
Department of Surgery
The Toronto Hospital
University of Toronto
Toronto, Ontario, Canada

Lee Kesterson, MD
Neurological Surgery
Modesto, California

David G. Kline, MD
Professor and Head
Department of Neurosurgery
Louisiana State University Medical Center
New Orleans, Louisiana

George E. Omer, Jr, MD, MS, FACS
Professor Emeritus
Department of Orthopedic Surgery
University of New Mexico School of
   Medicine
Albuquerque, New Mexico

Miguel A. Pirela-Cruz, MD, FAAOS, FACS
Assistant Professor
Department of Orthopedic Surgery
University of New Mexico School of
   Medicine
Albuquerque, New Mexico

Steven S. Weinshel, MD
Staff Neurosurgeon
David Grant USAF Medical Center
Travis Air Force Base, California

Brian K. Willis, MD
Chief, Neurosurgery Section, Surgical
  Service
New Mexico Regional Federal Medical
  Center;
Assistant Professor
Division of Neurosurgery
University of New Mexico School of
  Medicine
Albuquerque, New Mexico

Eric L. Zager, MD
Division of Neurosurgery
Hospital of the University of Pennsylvania
Philadelphia, Pennsylvania

AANS Publications Committee

Preface

In the pages that follow, it is hoped that the reader will find a collection of treatises that will allow for the establishment of a practical approach to the surgical management of peripheral nerve injury and entrapment. Collectively, the authors of this text represent decades of experience in the management of complex peripheral nerve disorders. The information offered in this text is, therefore, based on a solid foundation of research and clinical experience.

This text is designed to offer to the clinician who deals with peripheral nerve problems: **(1)** an understanding of the fundamentals pertinent to peripheral nerve injury management schemes, **(2)** an understanding of the etiopathogenesis of the variety of entrapment neuropathies and of the complexities of traumatic peripheral nerve injuries, **(3)** an understanding of the anatomy as it relates to the surgical exposure of peripheral nerves, and **(4)** an appreciation of several special considerations, such as pain, peripheral nerve tumors, and the restoration of extremity function.

In Part I, the morphology, physiology, and electrophysiology of the normal peripheral nerve, as well as the degenerative and regenerative processes that proceed after peripheral nerve injury, are outlined. Strategies for the treatment and repair of the injured peripheral nerve subsequently are addressed.

In Part II, common entrapment syndromes are described and illustrated. Chapter 4 discusses common entrapment syndromes of the upper extremity, excluding carpal tunnel syndrome and cubital tunnel syndrome. These are discussed separately in Chapters 5 and 6 respectively. Special consideration is offered to the latter two syndromes due to their high incidence of occurrence as well as the associated need for surgical intervention. Finally, in Chapter 7, entrapment syndromes of the lower extremity are outlined.

In Part III, traumatic peripheral nerve injuries as well as treatment and rehabilitation strategies are discussed in Chapter 8. Special consideration is given to the variety of modes of injury that exist.

The surgical exposure of the peripheral nerves of the extremities are presented on a regional basis in Part IV. In Chapter 9, the surgical exposure of the brachial plexus is outlined. Exposure of the peripheral nerves of the upper extremity is discussed in Chapter 10, followed by discussion of the surgical exposure of the lumbosacral plexus and proximal sciatic nerve in Chapter 11, and the surgical exposure of the peripheral nerves of the lower extremity in Chapter 12.

In Part V, three unique areas of concern to surgeons dealing with peripheral nerve injuries are discussed. In Chapter 13, pain of peripheral nerve origin is outlined from physiologic, pathophysiologic, and management points of view. In Chapter 14, the complexities of peripheral nerve surgery for tumors are reviewed—from fundamentals to surgical techniques. Finally, in Chapter 15, a dissertation of the restoration of extremity function following irreversible peripheral nerve injury is presented.

It is hoped that *Practical Approaches to Peripheral Nerve Surgery* may function not only as a textbook, but that it also might serve as a practical reference to peripheral nerve surgery.

Edward C. Benzel, MD
Editor

PART I

FUNDAMENTALS

CHAPTER 1

Anatomy, Physiology, and Clinical Electrophysiology of the Normal Peripheral Nerve

Earl R. Hackett, MD

An improved understanding of the structure and physiology of peripheral nerves has led to great advances in the assessment and management of peripheral nerve injuries over the past few decades. This knowledge has been accumulated over the past 150 years, starting with Schwann's descriptions of the cells named after him in 1839 up to the sophisticated ultrastructural studies of recent years.

Peripheral nerves are unique structures that travel over long distances from the spine to the skin, muscles, and viscera. Because of the elongated course of these structures, they are more susceptible to trauma in many areas along their courses. Nerves anatomically and physiologically have evolved to minimize disruption of their function (i.e. to conduct an impulse to or from the neuron in the spinal cord or nerve root ganglion).

This chapter reviews the normal anatomy, physiology, and electrophysiology of peripheral nerves. Emphasis will be placed on features that lead to a better understanding of changes associated with nerve injury and repair. This is not meant to be an exhaustive survey of these subjects. More detailed descriptions may be obtained from standard texts of these disciplines.[1,2,5,11,12,14,16–18]

Anatomy

Gross Anatomy

The cranial nerves and spinal nerves leave the central nervous system in pairs at specific levels of the nervous system, usually in relation to specific anatomic bony structures. The cranial nerves traverse bony foramina in the base of the skull before emerging peripherally. The spinal nerves go through intervertebral foramina. The nerves within the dura are termed *nerve roots* and vary in structure somewhat from the more peripheral nerve. The spinal roots are divided into an anterior motor root and a dorsal sensory root. These coalesce near the point where the root exits through the dura. The roots differ from the more peripheral portions of nerves in that they are not invested with the large amount of connective tissue that is present distally.

After leaving the dura mater, the spinal roots in the cervical and lumbosacral regions join together into plexuses, which rearrange the course of many of the nerve fibers into identifiable peripheral nerves. These nerves then follow well-known anatomic pathways into the extremities. The cranial and thoracic nerves generally do not involve themselves in plexus formation and can be traced from the skull or the spine to their destinations.

The roots, plexuses, and peripheral nerves branch at various levels, sending fibers to specific muscles along their course and receiving sensory fibers from sensory endings in the skin, muscle, and viscera. These branches generally follow a fairly consistent pattern on joining the nerve trunk. The careful observations of Sunderland have shown that this can be variable.[21] This pattern of branching has been helpful to clinicians assessing nerve function following injury and is one of the anatomic bases for electromyographic evaluation of nerve injuries.

The long course of the peripheral nerves makes them susceptible to damage from movements of the limbs. Areas of greater susceptibility exist in most peripheral nerves, and these areas of entrapment are well known clinically but will be enumerated here.

In the upper extremity, the median nerve is entrapped as it traverses the wrist underneath the transverse carpal ligament. Less known but equally damaging is *compression* of the nerve at the ligament of Struthers at the distal extent of the humerus. The anterior interosseous branch may be caught in the pronator teres or in the fascia of the flexor muscles in the forearm. The ulnar nerve may be entrapped at the cubital tunnel or in the groove in the elbow, where it is also susceptible to trauma. Another area of entrapment is found at the wrist in Guyon's canal. The radial nerve is most susceptible to injury in the spiral groove of the humerus, where it is in close apposition to the bone. It also may be bound down as it makes a sharply angled dive to become the posterior interosseous nerve just below the elbow.

In the lower extremity, the peroneal nerve lies very close to the head of the fibula in a superficial position, allowing it to be traumatized quite easily. It also is bound with fibrous tissue to some extent at this point. The nerve also is bound at the ankle. This is probably of little clinical importance, however. The posterior tibial nerve enters the arch of the foot through the tarsal canal, made up of ligaments of the arch and underlying bone, and is subject to trauma in this region. The sciatic nerve can be fixed in the sciatic notch, especially with marked flexion of the hips when squatting (hunkering). The sciatic nerve also pierces the piriformis muscle in a significant number of persons and may be compressed at that point. The femoral nerve is most susceptible as it enters the femoral triangle in the groin area.

Anatomy of the Nerve Trunk

Nerve trunks are made up of axons, Schwann cells, fibrous tissue, and vascular components. The ratio of neural tissue to supportive tissue is variable. Generally, connective tissue predominates, more so in areas where the nerve is in apposition to bone or joints, in areas of potential entrapment, or where the extremities are most movable.

The axons and their associated Schwann cells are coalesced into fascicles within the connective tissue matrix. The fascicles may be numerous or sparse in a nerve and are arranged variably from one area of the nerve to the next. In addition, the pattern of fascicular arrangement varies from nerve to nerve and also between individuals. Nerve fibers may change from one fascicle to another throughout the length of the nerve trunk.[22]

The connective tissue matrix in which the fascicles lie has been divided into an *epineurium* and *perineurium*. Within the fascicles, connective tissue is less obvious and is termed the *endoneurium*.

The epineurium is a loosely organized sheath of connective tissue surrounding the nerve that also separates the fascicles within the nerve itself (interfascicular epineurium) (Figure 1A, B, C). The collagen associated with this connective tissue is generally arranged longitudinally, though the interfascicular epineurium may have some collagen fibers that traverse the nerve. This tissue provides protection, tensile strength, and supports the blood supply to the nerve. The outer portion of the sheath is relatively dense compared to the more inner regions, allowing for greater structural support (this is most useful in suturing cut nerves). The major blood vessels supplying the nerve lie in the epineurium.

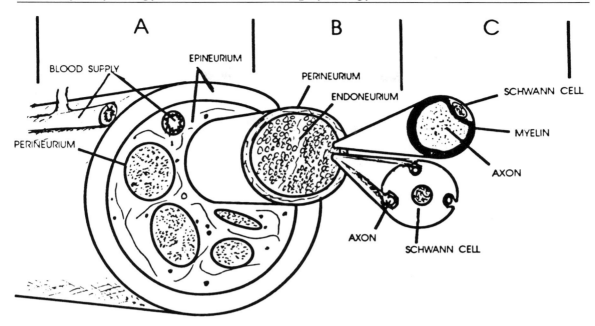

Figure 1A. Cartoon of cross-section of nerve trunk showing epineurium, longitudinally oriented blood supply, fascicles, and perineurium. B. Cross-section of one fascicle showing nerve fibers, perineurium, and endonerium. C. Cross-section of endoneurial tubes with Schwann cells and their relation to the nerve fibers (axons), myelinated and nonmyelinated.

The perineurium is a thin but dense layer of connective tissue arranged circularly about the nerve fiber fascicles. The cells lie in layers bounded by basal lamina on each side. Cells within the same layer have tight junctions between them and connections between various layers of cells are observed.[19] The perineurium extends to the nerve endings. In the nerve root, the pia-arachnoid invests the fascicles. In this region, it is analogous to the perineurium. The tight junctions and layered structure of the perineurium serve, in part, as a blood-nerve barrier, resisting the penetration of substances through the perineurium.

The endoneurium consists of fibroblasts with processes that disseminate through the fascicles between nerve fibers and Schwann cells. The collagen fibers observed in the endoneurium tend to be longitudinal and often are closely apposed to the Schwann cells. This close relationship of endoneurium and Schwann cells helps form the tube through which regenerating nerve may pass following nerve injury.

These connective tissue structures serve to support and protect the underlying nerve tissue. They provide resistance to stretching, have some elastic properties, provide protection from penetration, and help dissipate compressive forces on the nerve. A nerve may, therefore, be stretched without impairment of axon integrity. Tolerance to stretching may vary, in part due to nerves tested, relationship to points of entrapment, and the condition of nerves studied. Generally, the nerves may be stretched up to about 25% to 30% before the axon is damaged.

Anatomy of the Nerve Fibers

The nerve fibers (*axons*) are contained in the fascicles, surrounded by the endoneurium and processes of the Schwann cells. Nerve fiber diameters vary from 20 μm down to under 1.5 μm. Fiber diameter diminishes as the nerve proceeds distally and also is variable from point to point along its course. The larger fibers are myelinated, whereas the smallest fibers are embedded in the Schwann cell walls (Figure 1C).

When viewed longitudinally, myelinated fibers have indentations in the myelin (nodes of Ranvier), which are the borders between adjacent Schwann cells. The axon is exposed in this area for a very short distance, but the exposed area is most critical for propagation of a nerve impulse. Schwann cell nuclei and cell bodies cover the myelin and, in turn, are covered by endoneurium. The axon is narrowed at the nodes and occasionally at other areas, such as under Schwann cell nuclei or other intracellular material within the Schwann cell. Unmyelinated fibers do not show the nodal pattern and are invested by Schwann cell processes. One Schwann cell may incorporate one or more small nerve fibers within its endoneurial tube.

Axons may branch along the course of the nerve, usually distally. This allows one neuron to innervate widely separated regions. Axon reflexes, such as the triple-flare response, may be explained by such branching, as might referred pain, though there is also evidence that referred pain may be a more central phenomenon.

Nerve fibers lie very loosely within the fascicle. This allows some movement within the fascicle but also allows the nerve trunk to be moved or stretched without stretching the axons significantly. The connective tissue structures also tend to be lax, allowing much of the same protection against stretch injury.

Blood Supply of Nerves

The blood supply of a nerve trunk consists of a network of longitudinally oriented arteries within the epineurium and over the nerve sheath. These arteries periodically receive branches from arteries in the surrounding tissues, forming an arborization similar to that observed in the mesentery of the bowel. If one of these nutrient arteries is damaged, as happens in surgical mobilization of the nerve, there is still an adequate blood supply in the nerve through these longitudinal anastomoses. Mobilization of a nerve up to 12 cm has not shown significant impairment of circulation.[13]

Some interconnections between the longitudinal arteries then branch to deeper structures, pierce the perineurium in an oblique manner, and enter the endoneurial space. The capillaries in the endoneurium have tight junctions and form the blood-nerve barrier similar to the type of barrier seen within the brain. This blood-nerve barrier is of importance in some of the metabolic neuropathies, and the breakdown of this barrier in nerve injuries may be of some importance during repair. Although the basic metabolic support of an axon comes from the cell body, there is considerable evidence that the endoneurial blood supply is very important to maintain axonal function. In clinical situations where the blood supply to a nerve has been restricted, symptoms have occurred.

The Schwann Cell

The Schwann cells have an intimate relationship with the axons. They probably have a trophic effect on the axons, help nourish the axon, and help form the "tube" through which the axon travels. The origin of these cells is disputed, but most feel that they migrate from the neural crests along with the axons. The Schwann cells are the source of the myelin in peripheral nerves, analogous with the oligodendroglial cells of the central nervous system. Myelinated axons are invested in myelin by a spiralling of a Schwann cell process about them. Nonmyelinated fibers lie embedded within a Schwann cell. Often such a cell may be surrounding several such axons (Figure 1C).

With axonal death, myelin is destroyed, but the Schwann cells survive and frequently increase in numbers. If the axon regenerates, the Schwann cell reinvests the axon, and forms myelin if needed.

Physiology

Transmission of a nerve action potential is dependent on the integrity of the axonal membrane. Damage to this membrane will interfere with normal neural function. In the steady state, this membrane has a transmembrane electrical potential of about -70 to -90 mV with the inside of the axon being negative.

The reason for this potential difference lies in both the structure of the membrane and the distribution of the solutes in the intracellular and extracellular spaces. The cell membrane is composed of a double layer of phospholipids with protein molecules scattered over the surface but also forming transmembrane channels for ions to cross the membrane. The membrane acts as a semipermeable membrane that allows some molecules to cross it while restricting others. Nerve membrane is quite permeable to K^+ ions, Cl^- ions, and less so to Na^+ and other larger ions. Intracellular K^+ concentration is markedly higher than that found outside the cell. If the K^+ were free to diffuse across the membrane, there would be an efflux of the ion. The high extracellular Na^+ would tend to try to get into the cell, where Na^+ is low. The membrane is less permeable to this ion, so less of a flow is present. The negative potential resists these flows and maintains the stability of the membrane. Other ions also participate in various gradients across the membrane and add their electrotonic forces to the equation, producing the final resting membrane potential. The transmembrane potential of K^+ is very close to the actual resting membrane potential. In addition, an energy-dependent Na^+-K^+ "pump" moves Na^+ ions out of the cell and K^+ into the cell,[9] maintaining the relative concentrations within the cell.

When a chemical or electrical stimulus is applied to this system, a series of events occurs that terminates in the generation of a nerve action potential. Such a stimulus needs to reverse (or depolarize) the negative polarization of the membrane in order to develop the action potential. When a critical level of depolarization is reached, there is a sudden reversal of polarity of the membrane to about $^+30$–$^+40$ mV and an action potential is formed. Each time that threshold is exceeded, the same amplitude of reversal occurs (the "all or none response"). Associated with this event is a sudden, brief change in membrane permeability of Na^+ that flows into the cell. About 1 millisecond later, a

similar but longer-duration change occurs in the K^+ permeability, which acts to end the action potential and repolarizes the membrane.[8] During these brief periods of increased permeability, very few Na^+ ions actually enter the cell, but the Na^+-K^+ pump will work to remove those few ions from the internal milieu.

When the action potential is generated, a current flows into the active areas of the membrane of the axon from the extracellular space. This flow then goes down the axon and exits the axon across the normal surrounding areas of the membrane into the extracellular space, completing the circuit. If the electrical changes in these normal regions exceed the threshold levels, then a new action potential is generated and the action potential is propagated down the axons by way of these local circuits. In unmyelinated fibers this process is relatively slow; however, the addition of myelin speeds up this process considerably. With the insulation provided by the myelin sheath not allowing the exit of electrical current except where it is absent (nodes of Ranvier), the flow of electrical current leaves the axon at some distance from the action potential (one to three nodes away). A new action potential is thus generated much farther down the nerve, allowing it to propagate down the nerve at a much faster rate (saltatory conduction). The longer the internode distance, the more rapidly the axon will conduct the action potential.

It should be noted that the metabolism in an axon is greater in the nodal regions. Mitochondria are grouped in these regions, providing for the energy needed to sustain the Na^+-K^+ pump. The propagation of an action potential requires no energy, but maintenance of the resting membrane potential does.

Axon metabolism, in part, depends on substances produced in the cell body, which are conveyed distally by axoplasmic flow. Both a slow and a fast transport system occur down the axons,[3] and, in addition, there seems to be a flow in the opposite direction.[4] There probably are some Schwann cell[20] and endoneurium contributions to axonal metabolism. Certainly, oxygen and carbon dioxide gaseous exchange occurs in the nodal areas, as vascular occlusion of the vasa nervorum will cause malfunction of the axon.

Clinical Electrodiagnosis

Electrodiagnostic tests are an extension of the bedside examination of the peripheral nervous system. They add objective data about the function of the peripheral nerve and should provide accurate localizing information if a nerve is damaged. These tests are useful when minor changes are unable to be identified clinically or when the functions tested are in locations that are difficult to examine clinically. They shed light on pathophysiologic mechanisms that otherwise would be difficult to delineate at the bedside (e.g. differentiating neuropraxia from a more severe injury to the axon, or delineating sensory nerve root involvement from a plexus injury).

Clinical electrophysiologists have to be well versed in neuroanatomy, topographic anatomy, and nerve physiology to make meaningful assessments of nerve function. The procedures require discrete placements of the recording electrodes, needles, and stimulating probes to be accurate. Inaccurate placement of either the stimulating or recording electrodes greatly diminishes the value of the studies. In addition, knowledge of the disease processes affecting peripheral nerves is of great importance to the examiner in order for him or her to interpret the test findings in the proper context of the nerve dysfunction.

Clinical electrophysiologic testing of the peripheral nervous system can be divided into two broad categories: **(1)** nerve conduction studies with their related studies, somatosensory evoked reponses, and long latency reflexes (H-reflex, F wave); and **(2)** electromyography (EMG). These studies will be dealt with separately.

Nerve Conduction Studies

The function of the peripheral nerve is to transmit an electrical impulse from one point to another. The electrical stimulus normally comes from the nerve cell body or from receptor structures. In nerve conduction studies, however, the nerve is stimulated by an external electrical source. When the nerve is near the surface of the body, skin electrodes may deliver the shock. Deeper nerves require needle electrodes. With nerves exposed at surgery, stimulating electrodes may be applied directly to the nerves. Stimulation is made with supermaximal shocks to make sure that all nerve fibers are stimulated and that a maximal response is obtained. Less than maximal stimulation may give spurious results.

Recording electrodes may also be surface, needle, or directly applied types. They may be placed over muscle to record the evoked muscle action potential, or they may be applied directly over a nerve to record a nerve action potential. In sensory nerves, the potential is purely a sensory nerve action potential (SNAP), but over a nerve trunk, elements of both motor and sensory nerve action potentials are present (mixed nerve action potential). Conduction velocities measure the fastest conducting fibers of the nerve.

Motor nerve conduction studies are done by stimulating the nerve at two or more points along the course of the nerve and measuring the evoked motor responses from an appropriate muscle. If the nerve length can be measured between the stimulus sites, conduction velocities can be calculated. Various segments along the nerve may be tested, allowing for greater precision in identifying an area of dysfunction.

Motor nerve conduction velocities vary from nerve to nerve but generally are comparable from side to side; therefore, it is most helpful to have information from the "normal" nerve on the opposite side to compare with the target nerve being evaluated. Exact normal velocities expressed in meters per second vary somewhat from lab to lab but generally are similar.

Sensory nerve conduction studies may be performed in two ways. A stimulus may be applied distally to a pure sensory nerve and recorded proximally (orthodromic) or to a nerve trunk and recorded distally off of the pure sensory branch (antidromic). Both methods achieve comparable results, though antidromic stimulation may elicit motor responses that may obscure the smaller sensory response. Like motor conduction studies, comparison with the other side is often helpful.

Conduction velocities are only part of the information that can be obtained from the test. The amplitude of the response, whether motor or sensory, is a reflection of the numbers of axons that are conducting an impulse. Low-amplitude responses suggest problems with or loss of axons between the nerve cell body and the site of recording. The presence of normal sensory nerve action potentials in the presence of severe sensory loss points to a lesion proximal to the dorsal root ganglion, suggesting an avulsion of a nerve root.

Somatosensory evoked potentials (SEPs) are most helpful in evaluating the proximal segments of a peripheral nerve that normally are inaccessible to conventional nerve conduction studies. A stimulus is usually applied to a nerve peripherally, and recordings of potentials are made from proximal nerve sites, areas of entry into the spinal cord, sites on the spinal cord, and more proximal areas within the brain. SEPs, therefore, allow evaluation of the entire sensory system. Proximal nerve segments, therefore, can be compared with the more peripheral segments. SEPs should be performed unilaterally and also simultaneously for comparison between the two sides.

The H-reflex, first described by Hoffmann,[10] is the electrical evocation of the spinal monosynaptic reflex. It therefore allows for the assessment of both proximal sensory and proximal motor nerve pathways. It is best elicited from the calf muscles but also is seen in the flexor carpi radialis. The stimulus in the leg is applied to the posterior tibial nerve, allowing evaluation of conduction in the sciatic nerve and in the S1 root. In the arm, the median nerve, the lateral cord and upper trunk of the brachial plexus, along with the C6 and C7 root, may be assessed with the H-reflex.

F waves measure the motor conductions along the proximal portions of the nerve. The stimulus impulse travels toward the cord in the motor axon (antidromic). Upon reaching the motor neuron in the anterior horn, it reverses itself and goes peripherally along the same axon to the muscle (orthodromic).[15] Unlike the H-reflex, which can be elicited only in a few nerves, the F wave response may be obtained from any accessible motor nerve.

Nerve conduction studies may be affected by numerous factors. Nerve conduction velocities are faster in larger nerves and those nerves that are myelinated. They tend to be faster in the proximal segments than distally.[7] Higher temperatures may increase conduction velocities. This, in part, may account for the above observation. Conversely, cool temperatures slow conductions, giving the impression that nerve conduction velocities are slower in wintertime when the extremities tend to be colder. Constant temperature conditions in the examining room minimize these effects. Age affects conduction velocities, with infant velocities being low and speeding up to adult levels at about 3 years of age.[6,23] Ischemia within a limb also may slow conduction.

The greatest slowing in conduction velocities occurs with demyelinization or compression of the nerve, or both. Neuropraxia and nerve lacerations abolish nerve conduction across the lesion; however, after a neuropraxic lesion, the distal segment remains excitable and conduction remains normal. After a transection, the distal nerve may remain excitable for 4–7 days after the injury and then stop functioning.

Reports of nerve conduction studies should include (1) distal latency (the time required to elicit a response in the distal most studied segment of a nerve); (2) amplitude of the elicited response (as noted previously, this gives some idea of the numbers of functioning axons within the nerve); (3) conduction velocities (this is the rate of transmission of an impulse between two points on a nerve. The segment being tested should be indicated in the report); and (4) normal ranges for the lab performing the test (standard textbooks of electrodiagnosis[12,16] often contain tables of normal values for reference where the norms are not otherwise available).

Electromyography

EMG tests the electrical activity of muscles and indirectly the function of both the upper motor neuron system and the lower motor neuron. Defects anywhere in this pathway will alter the EMG findings. The basic unit of muscle activity is the *motor unit*. This consists of a variable number of muscle fibers innervated by one neuron. When the neuron transmits its impulses, all of its component muscle fibers are activated and an electrical potential is generated. This potential represents the summation of electrical events in the individual muscle fibers within the motor unit and can be recorded by an electrode placed nearby. Needle electrodes are used and multiple locations must be sampled within each muscle in order to assess the numbers of motor units in the target muscle.

When a needle is inserted into a normal muscle, a brief burst of electrical activity occurs that subsides immediately. This "insertional activity" may be altered by both denervation and muscle disease. It may be helpful in differentiating between them. The muscle should be observed next in the relaxed state. In normal muscle, no electrical activity occurs at rest. Denervated muscle will demonstrate fibrillations and positive sharp waves as individual muscle fibers become hyperexcitable and discharge spontaneously. The muscle is examined next during increasing volitional movement. Motor unit potentials appear with minimal activity. As strength increases, new motor units will be recruited until, ultimately, individual motor units cannot be identified (interference pattern). Denervation decreases the numbers of motor units available for recruitment or, if complete, will show no motor unit activity. There also may be changes in the form, amplitude, and duration of individual motor units as the result of denervation. Muscle disease also may alter these parameters of motor unit potentials that are observed. Reports generated by the EMG should reflect information from observations in all four of the preceding areas of assessment.

The EMG requires knowledge of derivation of nerve fibers going to each muscle. Nerve fibers in the nerve roots pass through plexuses and may go to a large number of muscles through various peripheral nerves. When evaluating injury to the peripheral nervous system, muscle should be tested in a logical sequence

in order to determine the location of the lesion. Evaluation of a nerve root lesion should include EMG of the paraspinous muscles, as these muscles are innervated by the posterior ramus of the spinal nerve that branches at the nerve root.

Following nerve injury, the EMG changes of denervation will not be present until 2–3 weeks have elapsed. With this in mind, EMG investigation should not be attempted until 3 weeks after an injury if one is to obtain full benefit from the examination. This wait also allows soft tissue changes to resolve in order to better appreciate the location of muscles and the nerves to be tested. EMG should be done with great care in anticoagulated patients and probably should not be done in patients with infections in areas through which the needle electrodes might traverse. No other contraindications to this procedure exist.

References

1. Asbury AK. Peripheral nerves. In: Haymaker W, Adams RD, eds. *Histology and Histopathology of the Nervous System*. Springfield, Ill: Charles C Thomas; 1982;2:1566–1610.
2. Barchi RL. Excitation and conduction in nerve. In: Sumner AJ, ed. *The Physiology of Peripheral Nerve Disease*. Philadelphia, Pa: WB Saunders;1980:1–40.
3. Barondes SH. Axoplasmic transport. *Neurosci Res Program Bull*. 1967;5:307–415.
4. Burdwood WO. Rapid bidirectional particle movement in neurons. *J Cell Biol*. 1965;27:A115
5. Dyck PJ, Thomas PK, Lambert EH, et al. *Peripheral Neuropathy*. 2nd ed. Philadelphia, Pa: WB Saunders; 1984:1.
6. Gamstorp I. Normal conduction velocity of ulnar, median and peroneal nerves in infancy, childhood and adolescence. *Acta Paediatr Scand Suppl*. 1963: 146:68–76.
7. Gilliatt RW, Thomas PK. Changes in nerve conduction with ulnar lesions at the elbow. *J Neurol Neurosurg Psychiatry*. 1960;23:312–320.
8. Hodgkin AL, Huxley AF. Movement of sodium and potassium ions during nervous activity. *Cold Spring Harb Symp Quant Biol*. 1952;17:43–52.
9. Hodgkin AL, Keynes RD. Active transport of cations in giant axons from *Sepia* and *Loligo*. *J Physiol (Lond)*. 1955;128:28–60.
10. Hoffmann J. Ueber chronische spinale muskelatrophie im kindesalter, auf familiärer basis. *Dtschl Nervenheilkunde*. 1893;3:427–470.
11. Katz B. *Nerve, Muscle and Synapse*. New York, NY: McGraw Hill; 1966.
12. Kimura J. *Electrodiagnosis in Diseases of Nerve and Muscle: Principles and Practice*. 2nd ed. Philadelphia, Pa: FA Davis; 1989.

13. Kline DG, Hackett ER, Davis GD, et al. Effects of mobilization on the blood supply and regeneration of injured nerves. *J Surg Res.* 1972;12:254–266.

14. Landon DN. *The Peripheral Nerve.* New York, NY: John Wiley & Sons; 1976.

15. Mayer RF, Feldman RG. Observations on the nature of the F wave in man. *Neurology.* 1967;17:147–156.

16. Oh SJ. *Clinical Electromyography: Nerve Conduction Studies.* Baltimore, Md: University Park Press; 1984.

17. Schadé JP. *The Peripheral Nervous System.* Amsterdam, NY: Elsevier; 1966.

18. Schmidt RF. *Fundamentals of Neurophysiology.* 3rd rev ed. New York, NY: Springer-Verlag; 1985.

19. Shanthaveerappa TR, Bourne GH. The perineurial epithelium—a new concept. In: Bourne GH, ed. *The Structure and Function of Nervous Tissue.* New York, NY: Academic Press; 1968:379–459.

20. Singer M, Saltpeter MM. The transport of ^{3}H-l-histidine through the Schwann and myelin sheath into the axon, including a reevaluation of myelin function. *J Morphol.* 1966;120:281–316.

21. Sunderland S. *Nerves and Nerve Injuries.* 2nd ed. New York, NY: Churchill Livingstone; 1978.

22. Sunderland S, Bradley KC. The cross-sectional area of peripheral nerve trunks devoted to nerve fibres. *Brain.* 1949;72:428–449.

23. Thomas JE, Lambert EH. Ulnar nerve conduction velocity and H-reflex in infants and children. *J Appl Physiol.* 1960;15:1–9.

CHAPTER 2

Morphology, Physiology, and Electrophysiology of Peripheral Nerve Degeneration and Regeneration

Eric L. Zager, MD

An understanding of the morphology, physiology, and electrophysiology of peripheral nerve regeneration is fundamental to clinical decision-making by the peripheral nerve surgeon. Questions regarding the type and timing of nerve repair can be addressed logically only if the underlying condition of the injured nerve can be ascertained.

After nerve injury, a detailed history of the mechanism of injury along with a directed physical examination and electrophysiologic studies are obtained by the surgeon. The clinical course is followed carefully in terms of improvement, stabilization, or deterioration. These data should then be transformed into mental images of the histology and physiology within the nerve fascicles at the injury site, and in the nerve segments proximal and distal to that site. Appropriate decisions can then be made regarding the clinical options of further observation, exploration, and neurolysis with or without nerve grafting, or reconstructive procedures such as tendon transfers.

The morphology, physiology, and electrophysiology of peripheral nerve regeneration cannot be analyzed in isolation. These regenerative processes are a continuum of the entire response to nerve injury, including concomitant degenerative processes.

Just as degenerative and regenerative processes are simultaneous and interdependent, so are the structural and physiological aspects of the responses to nerve injury. They cannot be discussed in isolation, either.

In this chapter, the clinically relevant fundamentals of the anatomic, physiologic, and electrophysiologic changes observed in injured and regenerating nerves are reviewed. The discussion is broad enough to apply to most major mechanisms of nerve injury-traction or stretch, contusion, laceration, missile injury, injection, entrapment, and compression.

Classification of Nerve Injuries

Figure 1 reviews briefly the major categories of nerve injury. The two most widely used classification schemes are those of Seddon[16] and Sunderland.[20] Seddon described three basic types of nerve injury: neurapraxia, axonotmesis, and neurotmesis. These categories are encompassed within Sunderland's expanded classification: Neurapraxia (conduction block) is equivalent to Sunderland's first-degree injury; axonotmesis is synonymous with Sunderland's second-degree injury; and neurotmesis is Sunderland's fifth-degree or most severe injury. All of these injuries initially produce complete loss of neurologic function. The clinical importance for the peripheral nerve surgeon of classification schemes lies in its predictive value—i.e. its prognostic significance.

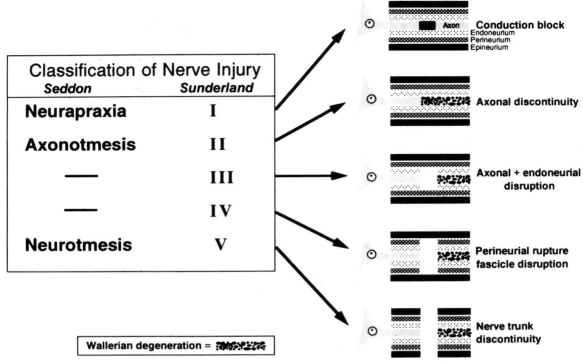

Figure 1. *Classification of nerve injury according to Seddon and Sunderland.* [16,19]

First-Degree Injury (Neurapraxia)

In terms of nerve regeneration, first-degree injuries are not strictly relevant in that no true regeneration occurs. A first-degree injury involves interruption of signal conduction across the injured site, usually due to compression or ischemia, with full and relatively rapid recovery of function. The axon is preserved, there is no Wallerian degeneration, and pathological changes are mild and fully reversible.

For unknown reasons, motor fibers are more susceptible to this type of injury than are sensory or sympathetic fibers. Susceptibility by modality, in descending order, is: motor, proprioception, light touch, temperature sensation, pain sensation, and sympathetic function. Recovery generally occurs in a reverse sequence, and is usually complete within days to a few months. Any residual deficit indicates a more severe degree of injury involving loss of axonal continuity.

Second-Degree Injury (Axonotmesis)

Second-degree injury is defined pathologically by loss of axonal continuity and subsequent Wallerian degeneration. The endoneurial sheath is preserved, however, and each regenerating axon is confined to its original sheath. This ensures faithful reinnervation of the appropriate end organ, and full functional recovery inevitably results. In clinical terms, the initial deficit involves complete motor, sensory, and sympathetic function. Nerve conduction distal to the injury site disappears within 24–72 hours after the injury, and fibrillation potentials (see "Electrophysiology") are present within the denervated muscles.

Recovery of motor function in second-degree injury follows sequentially from proximal to distal muscles. The timing of recovery follows quite predictably the rate of axonal growth—approximately 1 mm per day or 1 inch per month, although the growth rate is more complex when carefully studied as described in the next section. The progression of regeneration can be followed along sensory fibers by tracing the progress of Tinel's sign. The delay in recovery of function exceeds that observed after first-degree injury, and is usually measured in months rather than days or weeks.

Third-Degree Injury

Third-degree injuries are intrafascicular injuries that involve disruption of axons as well as their endoneurial tubes (basal lamina of Schwann cells), with subsequent Wallerian degeneration. The perineurium is spared and, therefore, the fascicular architecture of the nerve is preserved. Retrograde degeneration is severe, and some neuronal cell bodies are lost, reducing the number of axons available for regeneration.

Intrafascicular fibrosis (scar), which results from the associated hemorrhage, edema, and ischemia, presents an impediment to axonal regeneration. Recovery is, therefore, incomplete. Regenerating axons are confined within their original fasciculi, but are no longer confined within their original endoneurial tubes. Therefore, misdirected regrowth can occur—e.g. sensory axons may regenerate along original motor tubes. This constitutes wasteful regeneration. More proximal injuries are more likely to result in neuronal cell death and in a significant proportion of misdirected axons.

Recovery after third-degree injury is considerably delayed. The Tinel's sign is not a reliable marker of functional recovery after third-degree injury because sensory axons may be descending along a "dead-end" motor endoneurial tube. The external appearance of such a nerve will not accurately reflect the severe degree of intrafascicular disruption and disorganization present—an important point for the peripheral nerve surgeon to remember.

Fourth-Degree Injury

This severe injury involves rupture of the perineurium and, thus, disrupted fasciculi. The nerve trunk is still in continuity, but is con-

verted at the injury site into a solid scar containing Schwann cells and regenerating axons, which enlarge to form a neuroma. Retrograde neuronal effects are more severe than in third-degree injuries; therefore, even fewer axons survive to regenerate. Those axons that do regenerate are no longer confined within fascicles, and many stray into surrounding interfascicular tissue to end blindly. Few axons reach their appropriate targets. Functional recovery, if any, is usually quite limited. Fourth-degree injuries require surgical excision of the involved segment and an appropriate type of nerve repair.

Fifth-Degree Injury (Neurotmesis)

This most severe degree of nerve injury involves complete loss of nerve trunk continuity. The severed nerve ends may remain separated, or they may be joined by a scar-tissue bridge composed of fibroblasts, Schwann cells, and regenerating axons. The extent of scar tissue varies, but often there is a proximal neuroma and distal bulb that form either a dumbbell-shaped structure or an amorphous mass of scar tissue. Regeneration across this formidable barrier is severely limited, at best, and is functionally negligible. Even with resection and nerve repair, significant barriers to full recovery remain. These include loss of axons due to retrograde effects of the injury, and misdirected axons. The chances of useful recovery are markedly enhanced by an appropriate surgical repair.

Morphologic and Physiologic Changes after Nerve Injury/Repair

Degenerative Changes

Before regeneration of nerve fibers can occur, a series of degenerative processes must take place. Many of these are direct preludes to regeneration. The success of regeneration depends to a large extent upon the severity of the initial injury and the resultant degenerative changes. Pathologic changes are mild or absent in first-degree injuries in which conduction block alone occurs, and no true degeneration or regeneration occurs.

In second-degree injuries (axonotmesis), there is little histologic change at the site of the injury or proximal to it. The major changes occur distal to the injured segment in what is well-known as Wallerian, or anterograde degeneration.

The primary histologic change in this process involves physical fragmentation of both axons and myelin, which begins to appear within hours of the injury. Ultrastructurally, both neurotubules and neurofilaments become disarrayed, and axonal contour becomes irregular, due to varicose swellings. By 48–96 hours postinjury, axonal continuity is lost and conduction of impulses is no longer possible. Myelin disintegration lags slightly behind that of axons, but is well advanced by 36–48 hours.

Axonal and myelin debris is removed by the phagocytic action of macrophages and Schwann cells, a process which can take from 1 week to several months. Schwann cells become active within 24 hours of the injury, exhibiting nuclear and cytoplasmic enlargement as well as an increased mitotic rate. Schwann cells appear to ingest axonal and myelin debris, and then pass this on to macrophages. The latter migrate into the traumatized region, primarily through a hematogenous route, passing through the walls of capillaries, which have become permeable in the injury zone.

Endoneurial mast cells play a pivotal role in this process, proliferating markedly within the first 2 weeks. They release histamine and serotonin, which enhance capillary permeability and allow macrophage migration. During the initial stages the endoneurial tubes swell in response to the trauma, but after the first 2 weeks these tubes become smaller in diameter. By 5–8 weeks, the degenerative process is usually complete, and the nerve fiber is composed of Schwann cells within an endoneurial sheath.[12,19]

In third-degree injuries, a more severe local reaction to the trauma occurs. These intrafas-

cicular injuries involve retraction of the severed nerve fiber ends due to the elastic endoneurium. Local vascular trauma leads to hemorrhage and edema, which results in a vigorous inflammatory response. Fibroblasts proliferate, and a dense fibrous scar results in a fusiform swelling of the injured segment. Interfascicular scar tissue also develops so that the entire nerve trunk, which is left in continuity, is permanently enlarged. Often, it is adherent to perineural scar tissue as well.

Distal to the injured segment, Wallerian degeneration follows a sequence very similar to that observed in second-degree injuries. One important difference is that intrafascicular injury impairs axonal regeneration and, therefore, the endoneurial tubes remain denervated for prolonged periods. Shrinkage of the endoneurial tubes (diameter 2–4 μm) reaches a maximum at approximately 4 months postinjury. The endoneurial sheath progressively thickens due to collagen deposition along the outer surface of the Schwann cell basement membrane. If the endoneurial tube does not receive a regenerating axon, progressive fibrosis ultimately obliterates the tube.

The stacked Schwann cell processes comprising collapsed endoneurial tubes have been labelled "bands of Büngner." Schwann cells appear to contribute to the deposition of collagen, and then revert to a more primitive form indistinguishable from fibroblasts. In addition to these degenerative changes that occur distal to the injured segment, retrograde changes occur proximal to the injury site in third-degree and in more severe injuries (as discussed next).

In fourth- and fifth-degree injuries, local reaction to the severe trauma is pronounced. Endoneurial tubes, as well as fasciculi, are disrupted and Schwann cells and axons are no longer confined. The epineurium is also damaged and reactive epineural fibroblasts are present at the severed nerve ends within 24 hours. These are accompanied by proliferating Schwann cells and perineurial and endoneurial fibroblasts. Vigorous cellular proliferation peaks within the first week and continues for a prolonged period. As in third-degree injuries, capillary permeability increases, probably as a result of mast cell degranulation, and edema and macrophage infiltration follow.

Each nerve end becomes a swollen mass of disorganized Schwann cells, capillaries, fibroblasts, macrophages, and collagen fibers. Regenerating axons reach the swollen bulb of the proximal stump and encounter formidable barriers to further growth. Many axons form whorls within the scar tissue, or are turned back along the proximal segment or out into surrounding tissue. Some of the regenerating axons may reach the distal stump, an accomplishment which is dependent upon multiple factors, including the severity of the original injury, the extent of scar formation, and the delay before axons reach the injury site. As in third-degree injuries, endoneurial tubes left unoccupied for prolonged periods undergo progressive shrinkage and fibrosis, ultimately becoming completely obliterated by collagen fibers.

Changes in neuronal cell bodies and in nerve fibers proximal to the site of injury depend upon the severity of the injury as well as the proximity of the injured segment to the cell body. Schwann cells are lost a few millimeters proximal to the injured segment, and axons and myelin are reduced in diameter. If the cell body actually degenerates, which occurs in severe trauma, the entire proximal segment undergoes Wallerian degeneration. The Wallerian degeneration lags somewhat behind this process in the distal segment.

In the presence of a surviving neuronal cell body the axon is reduced in diameter, particularly if functional connections to appropriate end organs are not re-established. Nerve conduction velocity is accordingly reduced. As regeneration proceeds, the axonal diameters increase, but may never reach normal levels. A definite interdependence exists between the cell body and the axon in terms of recovery: the cell body does not recover fully without the re-establishment of functional peripheral connections, and the final axonal caliber depends to a great extent upon the recovery of the cell body.

The nerve cell body itself reacts in a relatively predictable fashion after axonal injury. Within 6 hours of the injury, the nucleus migrates to the periphery of the cell and Nissl granules break up and disperse. This process is called chromatolysis. Simultaneously, there is a brisk proliferative response of perineuronal glial cells, most likely signalled by the process of chromatolysis. Glial cell processes extend to the affected neuron and interrupt synaptic connections, possibly to isolate the neuron for its recovery phase. Some neurons go on to degenerate and are subsequently phagocytosed by microglia.

More often, recovery begins within 2–3 weeks of the injury and continues for up to several months. The earliest signs of recovery are the return of the nucleus to the cell center and the reappearance of compact Nissl granules. Subcellular metabolic functions are altered during the chromatolytic and recovery phases, including an increase in ribonucleic acid (RNA) synthesis, a decrease in neurotransmitter synthesis, and an increase in production of proteins and lipids needed for axonal regeneration. Both fast and slow components of axoplasmic transport supply materials from the cell body to the sites of axonal regeneration.[19]

Regenerative Changes

In nerve injuries of the first and second degree (neurapraxia and axonotmesis), restoration of function is the rule. This is either early through reversal of conduction block, or late through axonal regeneration. Functional recovery is complete in these milder degrees of injury. Both morphologic and physiologic changes are fully reversible.

In the more severe nerve injuries in which endoneurial tubes are disrupted, regenerating axons are no longer confined to their original sheaths. These axons may meander into surrounding tissue or into inappropriate endoneurial tubes, thus failing to reinnervate their proper end organs. Neurologic recovery is compromised, generally to a degree proportional to the severity of the injury.

Functional recovery after nerve injury involves a complex series of steps, each of which may delay or impair the regenerative process. For any degree of nerve injury, it is useful initially to categorize these regenerative steps anatomically on a gross level. The sequence of regeneration may be divided into zones: **(1)** the neuronal cell body, **(2)** the segment between the cell body and the injury site, **(3)** the injury site itself, **(4)** the distal segment between the injury site and the end organ, and **(5)** the end organ itself. A delay in regeneration or unsuccessful regeneration may be attributed to pathologic changes which impede normal reparative processes at one or more of these zones.[12,19,20]

Neuronal Cell Body

Recovery of the neuronal cell body is marked by a reversal of chromatolysis and its associated depression of protein synthesis. Nucleoproteins reorganize into the characteristic form of Nissl granules. A complex and incompletely understood interaction occurs between the cell body and the regenerating axon tip. Axoplasm, which serves to regenerate the axon tip, appears to arise in the axon segment proximal to the injury site. An intense increase in the rate of protein synthesis in the cell nucleus influences the rate of advance and the final caliber of the regenerating axon. The human peripheral neuron's capacity to initiate a regenerative response appears to persist for at least 12 months after injury; and a robust response can be elicited even after repeated injuries.

Segment Between Cell Body and Injury Site

The length of the segment between the regenerating axon tip and the injury site depends on the severity of the original injury and the consequent retrograde degeneration. The first signs of axon regrowth in this segment may be seen as early as 24 hours after injury, they may be delayed for weeks in more severe degrees of injury. The rate of axonal regrowth is determined by changes within the cell body, the activity of the specialized growth cone at the tip of each axon sprout, and the resistance of the injured tissue between cell body and end organ.

There may be multiple axon sprouts within each endoneurial sheath, even in milder injuries, which do not involve destruction of the sheath itself. The fate of these multiple sprouts is not clear even in experimental paradigms. The timing of degenerative and regenerative processes is such that there must be a significant overlap between these in certain segments (Figure 2). For example, in milder injuries in which there is no significant delay in regeneration across the injury site, the advancing axon tip must encounter the debris of Wallerian degeneration in the distal segment. This debris does not appear to impose a barrier to regeneration.

However, in very proximal injuries in which there is a considerable delay before the advancing axon tip reaches the distal segment, the empty endoneurial tubes distally have decreased in diameter. This factor may be responsible, in part, for a terminal slowing in axonal regrowth. Surgical intervention that interrupts entering nutrient arteries does not appear to impair axonal regeneration, provided that longitudinal arteries within the nerve itself are not disrupted.

Injury Site

In severe nerve injuries that disrupt the endoneurial tubes, nerve fascicles, or trunks, formidable obstacles face the regenerating axons that reach the injury site. There may be a gap between the disrupted nerve ends, allowing regenerating axon sprouts to wander into surrounding tissue. Scarring is inevitably present at the site of severe injury; the extent depends upon multiple factors, including the timing of arrival of the regenerating sprouts after injury.

It has been well documented that regenerating axons may at times successfully traverse long gaps spontaneously, despite the presence of substantial scar tissue. However, there is no

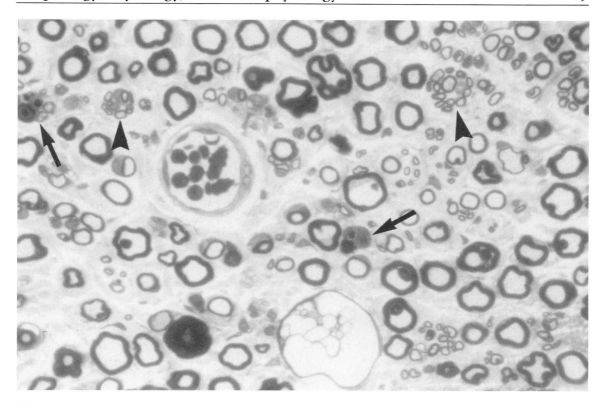

Figure 2. *Cross-section of rat sciatic nerve 15 weeks after exposure to a neurotoxin. The myelinated fiber density is reduced. There is myelin debris (arrows), indicating recent myelin breakdown. Coexisting clusters of small diameter axons (arrow heads) are regenerating myelinated fibers. Reproduced courtesy of Mark J. Brown, MD with permission.*

question that an appropriate surgical repair can eliminate the gap and reduce the amount of intervening scar tissue. This procedure provides no guarantee of proper fascicle orientation, of course, and regenerating axons may grow into functionally inappropriate endoneurial tubes or even may fail to re-enter an endoneurial tube. Either circumstance results in wasted axons.

Previously nonmyelinated axons may regenerate into endoneurial sheaths which formerly contained myelinated axons (and vice versa). This regeneration will not be wasteful. The resistance that an axon meets at the injury site results in the formation of multiple smaller axon sprouts. These daughter axons do not all find their way into the distal segment. No specific neurotropism is known to enhance the growth of a regenerating axon into its original

endoneurial tube, but some form of neurotropic influence has been demonstrated in experimental paradigms. Scarring within the bridging tissue impedes regeneration and misdirects axon sprouts into functionally unrelated endoneurial tubes. Residual scar tissue also interferes with the maturational processes of axons that do negotiate the injury site.

Segment Between Injury and End Organ

Axons that successfully enter endoneurial tubes in the segment distal to the injury site stand a good chance of reaching the end organ, given reasonable growth conditions. The distal regeneration rate is slower if the endoneurial tubes have been disrupted. The specialized growth cone at the tip of each axon sprout contains multiple filopodia, which adhere to the basal lamina of the Schwann cell. Several small axon sprouts may enter the same endoneurial tube. Hence, a regenerated nerve fiber may contain more axons than the original nerve.

If a functionally unrelated end organ is reached, further development of the axon and remyelination do not occur. Similarly, axonal development and maturation are aborted if the end organ, due to prolonged denervation, has undergone degenerative changes that do not allow the establishment of functional connections. If the entry of regenerating axons into the distal segment is delayed more than approximately 4 months, the axons are entering endoneurial tubes of small diameter, generally 3 μm or less. This shrinkage does not appear to impede regeneration or to impair functional recovery, most likely due to the elastic properties of the endoneurium.

The return of function does not require absolutely faithful recovery of nerve fiber architecture. The effects of prolonged denervation, which do appear to impair functional recovery, are at the level of the injury site—i.e. preventing the regenerating axons from entering appropriate endoneurial tubes—or at the end organ.

End Organs

End organs undergo characteristic histologic changes with nerve degeneration and subsequent reinnervation. Muscle fibers atrophy quite rapidly (70% average reduction of cross-sectional area by 2 months) and cell nuclei assume a central rather than the normal peripheral position. The synaptic folds of motor end plates are preserved for at least a year after denervation.

Tremendous proliferation of fibroblasts also characterizes the histologic picture of denervation. New collagen is deposited in both the endomysium and perimysium. In general, muscle fibers are not replaced by connective tissue, but rather atrophied fibers are separated by thickened connective tissue, so that the overall internal pattern of muscle architecture is preserved. Occasional dropout of muscle fibers does occur. This is a relatively late phenomenon, generally observed between 6–12 months after denervation.

Regenerating axonal sprouts follow the original Schwann cells to the denervated motor end plates to reform neuromuscular junctions. Collateral sprouting also occurs, resulting in groups of reinnervated muscle fibers, all of the same fast or slow types. This is a characteristic finding in reinnervated muscle, contrasting sharply with the random pattern observed in normal muscle.

Unfortunately, incomplete motor recovery is a common occurrence after moderate-to-severe nerve injuries. This is due to a number of factors, within the muscle itself and in the regenerating nerve. Intramuscular fibrosis may limit the efficiency of the contraction produced by a nerve impulse. Appropriate physical therapy can be an important intervention that maintains the denervated muscles in an optimal condition to receive the regenerating axon terminals.

The role of electrical stimulation of denervated muscle or of regenerating nerve remains controversial. Motor recovery is obviously impaired if a significant number of axons do not successfully reform functional connections with the muscle. Even if the numbers are adequate, erroneous cross-reinnervation may produce a suboptimal functional result: an originally "fast" muscle may be reinnervated by axons previously innervating a "slow" muscle, and the result may be a mixed form with inefficient contraction.

Concomitant sensory deficits, particularly in proprioception, further impede functional motor recovery. A variety of explanations have been proposed for the generally poor recovery of intrinsic hand muscles after a severe, proximal upper extremity nerve injury with or without nerve repair. One of the explanations most commonly proffered is a loss of motor end plates in the denervated muscles due to the long delay before reinnervation occurs. While this factor may well play a role, Sunderland seriously questioned its overall significance and cited instead a number of primarily neurogenic factors for the disappointing recovery of hand function.[19]

studies of practical utility have dealt with techniques and timing of nerve repair, as well as the appropriate selection of patients for surgery.[6,8-10] Future studies will likely involve the development of methods for enhancing axonal regeneration, including transport systems, growth factors, specific neurotropic factors, and possibly the use of nerve allografts or synthetic bioabsorbable conduits.

Axonal transport systems play an important role in the normal maintenance of nerve processes and in regenerative efforts-conveying structural proteins, enzymes, and organelles to and from the advancing axon tip. Adjustments in fast and slow transport systems are to be expected during regeneration, and have been measured in various experimental paradigms. The literature to date contains conflicting reports regarding the nature of these changes. A greater understanding of the regulatory mechanisms controlling these transport systems may allow manipulation of axonal transport to effect more efficient regeneration. New techniques are being developed to study transport mechanisms.[4]

Neurite growth-promoting factors have recently been revived as subjects of intense investigation. Levi-Montalcini and colleagues initiated this field with pioneering studies of nerve growth factor (NGF) in the 1950s.[11] This polypeptide induces sprouting of sympathetic and sensory neurons in tissue culture; it plays an important role in vivo in the regulation of growth and the development and maintenance of these neurons in sympathetic and dorsal root ganglia. The nature of its role in axonal regeneration after nerve injury and repair is poorly understood. It is presumably produced by Schwann cells (among others), and is transported in a retrograde manner to neuronal cell bodies. In situ hybridization studies of NGF receptor mRNA suggest a role for NGF in motor neuron regeneration.[15]

Other neurite growth-promoting factors have captured the spotlight in nerve regeneration research. Acidic fibroblast growth factor (aFGF) is the first highly purified protein since NGF that has been shown to enhance nerve regeneration in vivo. A collagen-aFGF mixture inside a polyethylene guide tube increases axonal growth across a gap in a transected rat sciatic nerve.[2] Whether this is a direct effect on neurons, on angiogenesis, or on non-neuronal cells has not been determined. Components of the extracellular matrix and basement membranes have been examined for their potential neurotropic effects.

The glycoprotein laminin, the major noncollagenous protein of basement membranes, has received considerable attention because of its ability to enhance neurite outgrowth both in vitro[5] and in vivo.[13,14,21,22] A novel homologue of laminin, s-laminin, has been identified in association with the basal lamina of the synaptic cleft.[7] This glycoprotein may be responsible, in part, for the striking topographic specificity of synapse formation demonstrated by regenerating motor axons on denervated muscle fibers. P30, a heparin-binding protein with cell adhesive properties, promotes neurite outgrowth in developing rat central nervous system and appears to play a role in interactions between neurons and Schwann cells in regenerating péripheral nerves.[3]

Gangliosides have also been proposed as neurite growth promoters in both in vitro[17] and in vivo[18] studies. Electromagnetic field and direct current stimulation of regenerating axons has received a great deal of investigative attention, analogous to the orthopedic studies of these modalities in bone healing. While the latter studies demonstrated a beneficial effect on fracture healing related to increased collagen deposition, the nerve regeneration studies have not been conclusive. A variety of biological and synthetic nerve conduits have been proposed as replacements for nerve autografts in nerve repair; these include prepared skeletal muscle, collagen membrane, arterial and nerve allografts, polyglycolic acid, and Silastic. Proposed replacements for traditional suture repair techniques include fibrin glue and laser welding. Although none of these techniques has demonstrated convincing advantages in the clinical setting over the "gold standard" of the nerve autograft and careful microsurgical suture repair, there are promising theoretical arguments for pursuing them.

References

1. Adams RD, Victor M. *Principles of Neurology.* 4th ed. New York, NY: McGraw-Hill; 1989.

2. Cordeiro PG, Seckel BR, Lipton SA, et al. Acidic fibroblast growth factor enhances peripheral nerve regeneration in vivo. *Plast Reconstr Surg.* 1989; 83:1013–1019.

3. Daston MM, Ratner N. Expression of P30, a protein with adhesive properties, in Schwann cells and neurons of the developing and regenerating peripheral nerve. *J Cell Biol.* 1991;112:1229–1239.

4. Davey DF, Ansselin AD. Labelling of restricted numbers of axons by solid rhodamine implantation into nerve trunks. *Neurosci Lett.* 1991;121:83–87.

5. Hammarback JA, Palm SL, Furcht LT, et al. Guidance of neuritic outgrowth by pathways of substratum-adsorbed laminin. *J Neurosci Res.* 1985;13:213–220.

6. Hudson AR, Hunter D. Timing of peripheral nerve repair: important local neuropathological factors. *Clin Neurosurg.* 1977;24:391–405.

7. Hunter DD, Shah V, Merlie JP, et al. A laminin-like adhesive protein concentrated in the synaptic cleft of the neuromuscular junction. *Nature.* 1989;338:229–234.

8. Kline DG. Physiological and clinical factors contributing to the timing of nerve repair. *Clin Neurosurg.* 1977;24:425–455.

9. Kline DG, Hackett ER. Reappraisal of timing for exploration of civilian peripheral nerve injuries. *Surgery.* 1975;78:54–65.

10. Kline DG, Hackett ER, Happel LH. Surgery for lesions of the brachial plexus. *Arch Neurol.* 1986;43:170–181.

11. Levi-Montalcini R, Angeletti PU. Nerve growth factor. *Physiol Rev.* 1968;48:534–569.

12. Mackinnon SE, Dellon AL. *Surgery of the Peripheral Nerve.* New York, NY: Thieme; 1988.

13. Madison RD, Da Silva C, Dikkes P, et al. Peripheral nerve regeneration with entubulation repair: comparison of biodegradable nerve guides versus polyethylene tubes and the effects of a laminin-containing gel. *Exp Neurol.* 1987;95:378–390.

14. Politis MJ. Exogenous laminin induces regenerative changes in traumatized sciatic and optic nerve. *Plast Reconstr Surg.* 1989;83:228–235.

15. Saika T, Senba E, Noguchi K, et al. Effects of nerve crush and transection on mRNA levels for nerve growth factor receptor in the rat facial motoneurons. *Brain Res Mol Brain Res.* 1991;9:157–160.

16. Seddon H. *Surgical Disorders of the Peripheral Nerves.* 2nd ed. New York, NY: Churchill Livingstone; 1975.

17. Skaper SD, Katoh-Semba R, Varon S. GM1 ganglioside accelerates neurite outgrowth from primary peripheral and central neurons under selected culture conditions. *Brain Res.* 1985;355:19–26.

18. Sparrow JR, Grafstein B. Sciatic nerve regeneration in ganglioside-treated rats. *Exp Neurol.* 1982;77:230–235.

19. Sunderland S. *Nerve Injuries and their Repair: A Critical Appraisal.* New York, NY: Churchill Livingstone; 1991.

20. Sunderland S. *Nerves and Nerve Injuries,* 2nd ed. New York, NY: Churchill Livingstone; 1978.

21. Toyota B, Carbonetto S, David S. A dual laminin/collagen receptor acts in peripheral nerve regeneration. *Proc Natl Acad Sci USA.* 1990;87:1319–1322.

22. Woolley AL, Hollowell JP, Rich KM. Fibronectin-laminin combination enhances peripheral nerve regeneration across long gaps. *Otolaryngol Head Neck Surg.* 1990;103:509–518.

CHAPTER 3

Treatment Strategies for the Patient Suffering from Peripheral Nerve Injury

Deepak Awasthi, MD, Alan R. Hudson, MD, and David G. Kline, MD

The management of a patient suffering from an injured peripheral nerve requires an understanding of the mechanics of injury, the pathological response, and subsequent regenerative capacity. Decisions concerning whether to operate, when to operate, and what to do once the lesion is exposed must be based upon not only a firm understanding of the pathology of the repair but also some acceptance of the limitations for neural regeneration in terms of practical functional recovery. Clinical examination, electrodiagnostic studies, and radiologic studies are helpful in making such decisions. Patient selection for operation as well as timing, type(s) of operation, and the value of operation persist as controversial issues.

Guidelines for Injury Evaluation

The major determinants for deciding whether or not to operate on injured nerves are **(1)** the mechanism of injury, **(2)** the severity of the neurological loss, and **(3)** the presence of severe pain. Sharp or blunt lacerations involving soft tissues and nerve(s) with severe distal loss will require operation. Blunt injuries associated with stretch, fracture, contusion, compression, and even gunshot wound (GSW) are more likely to preserve some physical continuity of the involved nerve and may or may not improve without operation (Figure 1).

If loss is complete distal to the injury, complete improvement with time is less likely but can, on occasion, still occur. When loss is incomplete and continuity of the nerve is likely because of the mechanism of injury, function will usually improve with time. There are, of course, exceptions: **(1)** when the partially injured nerve, although in continuity, is compressed by a pseudoaneurysm or expanding clot (Figure 2A,B), and **(2)** when the site of nerve injury is close to an area of potential entrapment—e.g. ulnar nerve at the olecranon notch, median nerve at the wrist, posterior interosseous nerve in the region of the supinator, or peroneal nerve at the head of the fibula.

Although regeneration following proximal nerve lesions is faster than that which follows distal injury, axons must traverse great distances to reach distal target sites. Thus, in most cases, gaining good results is more difficult following proximal lesions than distal ones and delays in their repair should be avoided.

Axonal Regeneration Considerations

The injured peripheral nerve has characteristic neuronal and axonal responses which have been discussed in other chapters. The severity of injury will partly determine the degree of axonal regeneration. Although the rate of axonal growth and maturation of motor function is slow, the rate of regeneration is predictable. Re-

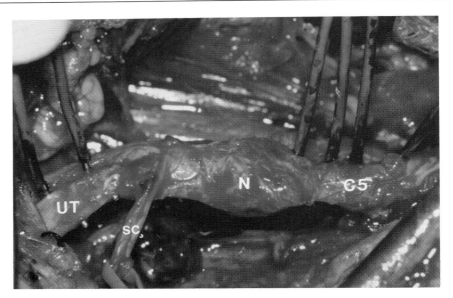

Figure 1. Intraoperative photograph shows stimulation and recording across an upper trunk (UT) injury caused by a .44 caliber magnum gunshot wound to the left supraclavicular area sustained about 2 months previously. Clinical and electrical studies showed that the patient had complete C5 and C6 to UT functional loss. Intraoperative nerve action potential (NAP) studies were done using a three-pronged stimulating electrode (seen here on the C5 spinal nerve) and a two-pronged recording electrode (seen here on the anterior division of the UT). No NAP could be evoked through the lesion by stimulating C5 and recording from the anterior or posterior divisions of the UT or the suprascapular nerve (SC). Stimulating the C6 spinal nerve evoked only a small NAP from the anterior division of the UT, but no NAP from the posterior division or the SC. Sural interfascicular graft repair from C5 to the anterior and posterior divisions as well as the SC was performed on this patient. There were no viable fascicles from C6 for grafting. N = neuroma in continuity.

generation proceeds at the rate of 1 mm per day or 1 inch per month. This helps the physician establish approximate deadlines in relationship to time of injury or previous repair in expecting clinical signs of reinnervation.

If the first target muscle begins to show function at the expected time and power improves over the next 1–2 months, the decision against surgery is clear. If the expected time schedule is not met, or the subsequent early quantitative extent of motor activity in the first target muscle does not match the expectancy after repair, operative intervention is indicated.[19] Unfortunately, too much time is required for many nerve lesions to reach even early regenerative milestones. Under these circumstances, if repair is delayed until after these deadlines are met, results are not as good as with earlier repair.

The time required for regeneration involves the following considerations:

1. There is a delay before regenerating axons reach the nerve distal to either injury or suture repair. The segment of retrograde degeneration proximal to the injury must first be overcome, and then there is usually a delay of 1-2 weeks before axons penetrate the injury or repair site and reach the distal stump.[19] This period of delay may be 2–4 weeks.

2. Once the fibers have reached the distal stump, the rate of axonal growth decreases as the distance of the injury from the neuron increases.

3. A terminal delay of weeks to several months takes place between the time when axons reach their distal targets and when suf-

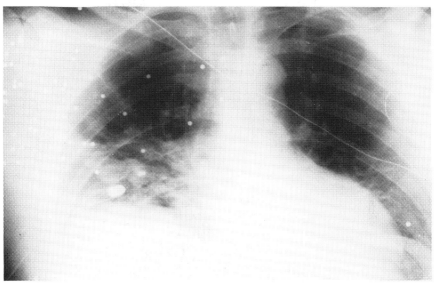

Figure 2A. Chest radiograph of a patient who had a .22 caliber gunshot and shotgun wound to the right shoulder. Patient presented with a pneumothorax (note the right-sided chest tube), pain in the right shoulder, and no function in his right hand or forearm. Numerous shotgun pellet fragments can be seen in the right shoulder/axillary region. Right brachial arteriogram performed on the day of the injury did not reveal any vascular injury or pseudoaneurysm. Clinical and electrical studies continued to demonstrate a complete middle/lower trunk to cord level functional loss at 5 months postinjury.

ficient maturation of the axons and their receptors occurs to allow maximal function. Thus, it is not enough for axons to reach their distal targets; they must do so in sufficient number and with enough caliber and myelination to produce acceptable function.[7,10,19]

Evidence of regeneration, as gauged by return of nerve function, can help guide the initial management of such lesions. Positive evidence for some significant nerve function, either initially or within 6 weeks postinjury, implies a favorable result. When a significant proportion of axons have escaped initial dysfunction or have suffered only a minor degree of nerve fiber injury, regeneration occurs, exceeding the best that nerve repair could yield.

The more frequent clinical situation is that of total nerve dysfunction in which the lesion has not been operatively inspected, or in which exposure at surgery has revealed a neuroma in continuity. If a nerve repair has been performed elsewhere under uncertain circum-

stances, a similar management dilemma arises. In these cases, delayed surgical exploration with intraoperative nerve action potential recordings is invaluable in making the final decision regarding resection and repair of the damaged nerve.

Clinical Evaluation

Motor Examination

A point to stress regarding clinical moter examination for specific nerve injuries is that the single most important step in management of any nerve injury is a detailed examination of the limb, with careful grading of *all* motor and sensory function. The examination must then determine whether loss is complete or incomplete distal to the injury site. Only in this fashion can one can tell on subsequent examinations whether or not function has changed.

Motor examination is sufficient by itself as proof of regeneration when recovery is obvious. Clinically observed voluntary motor func-

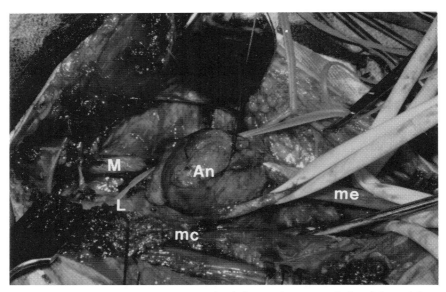

Figure 2B. *Intraoperative photograph of this patient revealed a 6.5 × 4.5 × 3 cm pseudoaneurysm (An) of the axillary artery compressing and stretching the cords of the brachial plexus and their distal outflow. The pseudoaneurysm was resected and the artery repaired with a piece of muscle fascia. Stimulation of the medial (M) and posterior cords did not evoke a nerve action potential (NAP) from the median (me)/ulnar nerves and the radial nerve, respectively. A NAP could be evoked from the musculocutaneous (mc), median (me), and axillary nerves upon stimulation of their respective cord contributions (lateral [L] to mc, lateral to me, posterior to axillary). Sural interfascicular grafts (2.5–3 inches in length) were performed from the medial cord to the median and ulnar nerves and from the posterior cord to the radial nerve.*

tion can also be confirmed by motor response to nerve stimulation.[37] Nerve stimulation is especially helpful in early recognition of adequate peroneal recovery and avoidance of a needless operation.[19]

Patients with injury to the peroneal nerve are unable to initiate voluntary action in the peroneus and anterior tibial muscles (eversion and dorsiflexion of the foot). This may continue for several weeks after electrophysiologic recovery has been demonstrated by strong muscle contraction on peroneal nerve stimulation: **(1)** just behind the head of the fibula or, **(2)** just inside the lateral hamstring, where the nerve trunk is readily palpated.[19] Importantly, one must be certain that the muscle observed to contract is in the distribution of the nerve presumed to be stimulated.

Tinel's Sign

If paresthesias are obtained by percussion of nerve distal to the injury, there is a suggestion that some sensory axons are continuous from the point percussed through the lesion to the central nervous system. If the response moves further distally with time, and especially if this is associated with diminished paresthesias in response to tapping over the injury site, evidence of continued sensory fiber regeneration down the distal stump is present (positive Tinel's sign). A positive Tinel's sign, however, implies only fine fiber regeneration and tells the examiner nothing about the quantity and eventual quality of the new fibers.

On the other hand, total neural interruption is strongly suggested by an absence of distal sensory response (negative Tinel's sign) after adequate time has elapsed for fine fiber regeneration to occur (4–6 weeks).[19] A negative Tinel's sign is more valuable in clinical evaluation than a positive Tinel's sign.

Sweating

Return of sweating in an autonomous zone signifies sympathetic nerve fiber regeneration. This return may antedate sensory or motor return by weeks or months, since autonomic fibers regenerate rapidly. Return of sweating does not necessarily mean that sensory or motor function will follow.

Sensory Recovery

True sensory recovery is a useful sign, especially when it occurs in autonomous zones where overlap from adjacent nerves is minimal.[21,28,29] Autonomous zones for the median nerve include the volar and dorsal surfaces of the forefinger and volar surface of the thumb. The radial nerve does not have a reliable autonomous zone. If there is any sensory loss in its distribution, it will usually involve the region of the anatomic snuff box. The autonomous zone for the ulnar nerve includes the palmar surface of the distal 1 1/2 phalanges of the little finger. Autonomous zones for the tibial nerve include the heel and a portion of the sole of the foot, while for the peroneal nerve it includes mid-dorsum of the foot. Unfortunately, sensory recovery, even in an autonomous zone, does not ensure subsequent motor recovery.

Electrophysiologic Studies

Electromyography

A thorough baseline electromyographic (EMG) study (Figure 3A) 2–3 weeks following the injury will document the extent of denervation and will confirm the pattern or distribution of the injury.[5,9,16,36,37] EMG studies should be done serially to search for signs of reinnervation or persistence of denervation. With re-

generation, insertional activity will begin to return and the fibrillation and denervation potentials will decrease in number and sometimes be replaced with occasional nascent motor action potentials. Such changes indicate that some regenerating fibers have reached muscle and that some axon-to-motor end plate connections have been reconstructed.[19]

These signs tell nothing, however, of the eventual extent or quality of regeneration. Nonetheless, when decreased numbers of fibrillations as well as nascent potentials are found in muscles in the distribution of an injured nerve, a short interval of further conservative management is suggested. The EMG is important because it can give evidence of regeneration weeks or months before voluntary motor function is detectable.[5] It can also detect retained motor units to indicate a partial lesion early after injury.[12]

The EMG is particularly helpful in defining the level of injury in a brachial plexus lesion and thus in selecting patients for operation as well as the type of operation to be used.[15,20,24] Paraspinal muscle denervation suggests a proximal lesion(s) to one or more roots and thus is a negative finding.[15,16,20,24] Proximal damage to the lower three roots can result in extensive paraspinal denervation while the C5 and even the C6 roots may be more laterally injured and are, thus, repairable. The electromyographer has difficulty sampling distinct spinal levels within the paraspinal muscle because there is so much overlap.

An operation is usually indicated in brachial plexus lesions if complete loss in the distribution of one or more upper roots (C5,C6,C7) and their distal outflows does not begin to reverse clinically or electrically in the early months postinjury.[15,24]

The presence of EMG changes suggesting reinnervation does not guarantee recovery of function, and the test must be weighed in conjunction with clinical findings and other electrical data.[19] Because the EMG can continue to show quite severe denervational changes even though the muscle contracts voluntarily, the EMG should never be substituted for a careful

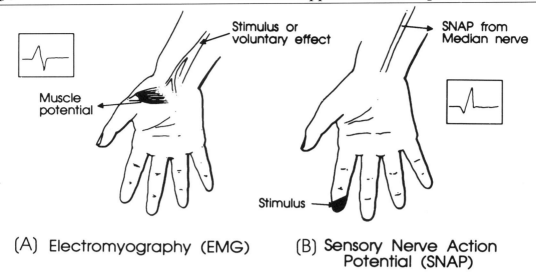

(A) Electromyography (EMG)   (B) Sensory Nerve Action
                                       Potential (SNAP)

*Figure 3A, B. (A) Electromyography (EMG). A thorough baseline EMG study 2–3 weeks following the injury documents the extent of denervation and confirms the pattern or distribution of the injury. This study is particularly helpful in defining the level of injury in a brachial plexus lesion. **(B)** Sensory nerve action potentials (SNAP) studies are performed by stimulating fingers in the C6 (thumb and index finger), C6–7 (long finger), and C8–T1 (little and ring fingers) distributions and recording from the median, radial, and ulnar nerve proximally. SNAP studies can be helpful in evaluating the level of brachial plexus stretch injuries (pre- vs. postganglionic injury). There is retention of sensory conduction from an anesthetic area in injuries restricted to the preganglionic region because sensory fibers between dorsal root ganglion and spinal cord do not degenerate. Detailed evaluation of upper roots, however, is not possible with SNAP recordings.*

clinical examination. Rather, it should supplement the clinical examination. EMG is especially valuable in identifying anomalous innervation, such as occurs frequently in the forearm and hand.[19,34]

Sensory Nerve Action Potential (SNAP)

SNAP studies (Figure 3B) can be helpful in evaluating the level of brachial plexus stretch injuries. Lesions at a root level that are restricted to the preganglionic region and do not extend into the postganglionic region produce complete distal sensory loss and preservation of distal sensory conduction. The latter is preserved because sensory fibers damaged distal to the dorsal root ganglion do not degenerate.

This retention of sensory conduction from an anesthetic area can be tested by stimulating fingers in the C6 (thumb and index finger), C6–7–8 (long finger), and C8–T1 (little and ring fin-

gers) distributions and recording from the median, radial, and ulnar nerves proximally. The presence of a compound sensory nerve action potential substantiates a preganglionic injury in the distribution of one or more roots.[16] Since even distal sensory distributions of roots overlap with one or more other roots, it is difficult to be certain by these studies that one root, C6 for example, has a preganglionic injury.

Stimulation of an anesthetic forefinger (or even thumb) can produce a SNAP in the median nerve distribution if either C6 or C7, or C6 and C7 roots, are damaged at a preganglionic level. This makes it difficult to determine by SNAP studies whether or not the C6 root has incurred a preganglionic injury. The situation is even less favorable for the C5 root since there are no specific noninvasive stimulation or recording sites for this outflow: Detailed evaluation of upper roots by SNAP recordings is not possible at this level.

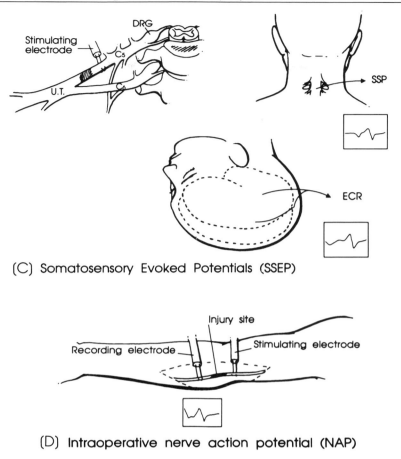

(C) Somatosensory Evoked Potentials (SSEP)

(D) Intraoperative nerve action potential (NAP)

Figure 3C, D. (C) Somatosensory-evoked potential (SSEP) studies can be used intraoperatively for stretch/ contusion brachial plexus injuries. If the injury is postganglionic, stimulation of the root proximal to the level of the injury (as shown in the illustration) should evoke a somatosensory potential over the cervical spine (SSP) and an evoked cortical response over the contralateral cranium (ECR). If the injury is preganglionic or pre- and postganglionic, stimulation of the root, even within or close to the intervertebral foramen, will evoke no such response and then repair of at least that element is unlikely to be successful. DRG = dorsal root ganglion, UT = upper trunk. (D) Intraoperative nerve action potential (NAP) recording involves operative exposure of the nerve trunk on either side of the injury site. It becomes an important definitive test when gross appearance of a neuroma in continuity is equivocal and the first target muscle is more than 3 inches downstream. At surgery, the critical observation is whether or not there is a recordable response and not its form or even its velocity.

Somatosensory-Evoked Potential (SSEP)

SSEP study (Figure 3C) has been used in evaluating the level of injury—i.e. preganglionic versus postganglionic—in brachial plexus lesions.[15,16] In the authors' experience, somatosensory studies have limited value in the early months following injury.

Somatosensory studies can, however, be used at the time of surgery for stretch/ contusion brachial plexus injuries. If the injury is postganglionic, stimulation of the root proximal to the level of the injury should evoke a somatosensory potential over the cervical spine (SSP) and an evoked cortical response over the contralateral cranium (ECR). If the injury is preganglionic or pre- and postganglionic, stimulation of the root, even within or close to the intervertebral foramen, will evoke no such responses. Repair of at least that element is unlikely to be successful.[16]

Unfortunately, production of an SSP or ECR probably requires only a few hundred or so intact fibers between site stimulated and site recorded, so a positive response only ensures minimal continuity of spinal nerve or root. A negative ECR is of more importance than a positive ECR.

Intraoperative Nerve Action Potential (NAP)

NAP study (Figure 3D) involves operative exposure of the nerve trunk on either side of the lesion (Figure 4). Since one ideally seeks to decide whether to repair a nerve by 8 weeks after injury, NAP becomes an important definitive test when gross appearance of a neuroma in continuity is equivocal and the first target muscle is more than 3 inches downstream (Figure 1).[15,16,19]

The important considerations with NAP recordings are:

1. The gross appearance of a neuroma in continuity does not necessarily correlate with the internal architecture.

2. If axons have been given an opportunity to traverse the lesion, their presence may be recorded by the NAP long before those axons have had an opportunity to reach their end target.

3. This technique is particularly useful in lower-extremity nerve lesions in which the first target muscle may lie 6–8 inches below the lesion. Thus, neither nerve stimulation nor EMG can settle the issue for 6–8 months or more, but it is important that decisions regarding resection be made before that time.

4. NAP recordings are also very helpful in defining the extent of brachial plexus lesions and provide a useful index of how much of the proximal stump of the lesion in continuity to resect. Most brachial plexus injuries selected for operation will have one or more elements in continuity, but with a variable amount of intraneural damage.[15] Intraoperative NAP recording helps sort out the need for resection.

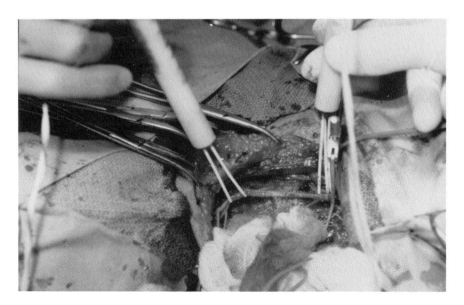

Figure 4. Intraoperative photograph of an accessory nerve exploration shows the intraoperative nerve action potential (NAP) recording technique. The stimulating electrode (proximal to the injury site on the accessory nerve) is three-pronged and the recording electrode (distal to the injury site on the accessory nerve) is two-pronged.

At surgery, the critical observation is whether or not there is a recordable response, and not its form or even its velocity. Regenerative NAP responses are small and usually slow, while those due to partial sparing may be small but are usually faster or have conduction in a normal range. Where there has been preganglionic without postganglionic injury, more distal recording will show a rapid conducting, large NAP, which is just as diagnostic as absence of an SSP or ECR when the root is stimulated at that level.

Radiologic Studies

Cervical Spine and Other X-rays

Cervical spine fractures are frequently associated with severe proximal, irreparable stretch injuries, at least at the root levels associated with those vertebrae.[8,16,20,24] Fractures of other bones such as the humerus, clavicle, scapula, and/or ribs, when observed, give rough estimates of the forces brought to bear on the shoulder, arm, and neck, but do not necessarily help localize the level or document the extent of the injury.[8,16] Damage to the plexus is usually more proximal than the fracture site would indicate, frequently at the root level.

Midhumeral fractures are especially associated with radial nerve injuries. Comminuted fractures of the radius and ulna at midforearm level can also be associated with combined median and ulnar nerve injuries, and on occasion with posterior interosseous nerve palsy.[19] The peroneal component of the sciatic nerve is often, but not always, selectively involved in hip dislocation or fracture. Lower femur fractures as well as tibial and fibular fractures may involve the peroneal and/or tibial nerves. Once again, the nerve injury may be more proximal than the fracture(s) site(s) may suggest. A midshaft femur fracture may be associated with a more proximal sciatic stretch injury at the buttock level.

Chest radiographs may reveal elevation of a nonfunctioning diaphragm, which denotes phrenic nerve paralysis. This is a relatively poor prognostic sign for repairability of the C5 nerve root following closed injuries, because it usually implies proximal damage at that level of the neck.

Myelography

Myelography may be an important part of the work-up in a patient with severe brachial plexus stretch injury. It is usually not indicated for infraclavicular or axillary level plexus lesions (most gunshot wounds to the plexus), unless there is radiologic evidence of damage to the cervical spine or a medial supraclavicular trajectory.[15,18] A meningocele at a given level indicates that enough force was applied at a proximal root level to tear the arachnoid and produce a leakage of contrast agent. It does not necessarily mean that the root is avulsed out of the spinal cord.[18] More commonly, the presence of a meningocele implies that, although the root may still be in gross continuity, it has significant internal damage at a very proximal level.[15,18,20]

A number of patients have had successful repair of roots at levels where meningoceles were absent (usually upper root levels), despite meningoceles on other roots (usually lower levels).[18] Nonetheless, if a meningocele is present, it is most likely that the root has proximal and thus irreparable damage.[18] This finding also makes it more likely that damage at other levels without meningoceles is very proximal. Modern myelography with water-soluble contrast agents may delineate the rootlets in the subarachnoid space, and comparison of the affected and unaffected sides may delineate sites of root disruption. Myelography is still a useful adjunct in the decision-making process concerning plexus injuries.

Computed Tomography (CT) and Magnetic Resonance Imaging (MRI)

Computed tomography (CT) scanning with intrathecal contrast is of interest in stretch injuries, although an abnormality may still be missed[16,18] because slices are usually not thin enough to cover all of the root regions at each level. As a result, myelography still remains the preferred radiologic study.

Magnetic resonance imaging (MRI) may help visualize the nerve root. Such studies should only supplement the myelogram and not replace it.[18] Cerebrospinal fluid (CSF) within meningoceles can be seen on MRI, but usually with less clarity than it is visualized by conventional myelography.

Guidelines for Timing of Repair

General Considerations

In deciding when to repair, the surgeon must define: **(1)** when the time for useful recovery by spontaneous regeneration has passed, and **(2)** the elapsed time when a nerve repair has little to offer. When the duration of total muscle denervation exceeds 24 months ("24-month rule"),[19] most muscles are subject to relatively severe time limitations for the return of useful function. This is less likely to be so for large bulky muscles, such as biceps and gastrocnemius-soleus, than for smaller muscles, such as those of the forearm and hand. An exception to this guideline are the facial muscles which, although relatively small, may benefit from late reinnervation by facial nerve repair or neurotization procedures.

Other exceptions to the "24-month rule" may occur in a few lesions that have maintained some nerve fiber continuity. If some fibers traverse the lesion, even though their number is insufficient to produce useful function distally, they may promote distal stump architecture preservation. Very late repair after resection of the lesion in continuity can occasionally produce function.[19]

Distance from the site of nerve injury to the desired muscle influences the timing of surgery. When the site of injury is a long distance from an important muscle, it is essential to perform the repair within a few months postinjury.[19] This is especially so with sciatic nerve and brachial plexus injuries.

Relatively early repair of other nerve injuries also is beneficial. For example, when the radial nerve is injured in association with a closed midhumeral fracture, the probability for good spontaneous recovery is high. Exploration should be undertaken if there is no recovery by 4 months. By this time, a midhumeral axonotemetic injury of the radial nerve should have regenerated to the next muscle downstream, the brachioradialis. If the radial nerve is seriously damaged between the fracture fragments, repairing it much later would begin to yield less satisfactory results for return of motor function.

In contrast, there exist cases when the distance between the nerve injury and the muscle to be reinnervated is such that repair, early or late, will not accomplish a useful degree of motor recovery. For example, repair of the ulnar nerve near the axilla or peroneal nerve above the midthigh may accomplish little in the way of function to important distal muscles. Other high repairs may be indicated, however, either because there are useful proximal muscles (such as the triceps and proximal forearm extensors in case of radial nerve) or because sensory recovery is valuable (such as that in the distribution of the median nerve).

Time limitation is less severe in sensory recovery than in motor recovery. This is an important consideration in favor of median nerve repair as high as the axillary level, even though it may only contribute minimal motor function at the hand level. A high median nerve repair is especially important if a mechanically useful hand can be provided by substituting or transferring some of the ulnar and radial motor function that does exist.

Similarly, repair of the tibial component of the sciatic nerve at a level as high as the sciatic notch may be indicated. Protection to weight-bearing plantar areas can be given by even a low-grade recovery of sensory function.[19] Thus, restoration of protective sensation to the sole of the foot is important enough to warrant a proximal repair. Some degree of useful plantar flexion will usually come about as well.

Finally, motor recovery from spontaneous regeneration (without nerve repair) also has limitations in time. High nerve lesions will usually result in lack of useful distal motor function if the muscle is over 24 inches distal to the lesion and is totally denervated by the injury. Relatively early evidence for some recovery of motor function, even if only detectable by EMG, will greatly improve the prognosis. These findings must be evident by 2–3 months postinjury. Therefore, in some high lesions, measures to compensate for lost motor function can be taken quite early. Tendon transfers can be performed without awaiting the effect of possible late regeneration from a high or proximal ulnar nerve lesion.

Early (Primary) versus Delayed (Secondary) Repair

Early operative intervention is infrequently needed in most peripheral nerve stretch injuries. There are notable exceptions.[19] An enlarging hematoma or aneurysmal sac will convert a partial in-continuity nerve injury into a complete and, with time, irreversible lesion unless the mass is removed as early as possible (Figure 2). A severely contused forearm or a distal humeral fracture associated with brachial artery injury predisposing to Volkmann's ischemic contracture are other exceptions regarding delay of an operation. In this instance, early fasciotomy, treatment of the vascular injury, and in many cases neurolysis of one or more nerves are necessary.

A similar syndrome can involve the anterior compartment of the lower leg, requiring urgent intervention if irreversible neural as well as muscular changes are to be avoided. A severe noncausalgic pain syndrome secondary to a missile embedded in nerve also can benefit from an early operation and removal of the missile fragment.[15] Injury to nerve in areas of potential entrapment may also require early release of the nerve and section of the connective tissue structures likely to cause entrapment. This is done to avoid potentially irreversible changes in the nerve.[19,23]

Early (primary) repair is a valid option for the repair of simple, clean lacerating injuries such as those caused by glass and knives.[11,13,23,33,34] In civilian injuries, primary repair is best for sharply transected supraclavicular and axillary level brachial plexus and sciatic nerve injuries; immediate exploration provides the best op-

portunity for both accurate identification and end-to-end repair without need for grafts.[13]

This is especially so with sharp plexus injuries in which there is vascular damage that must be repaired at once.[19] If such a wound site is explored some weeks later, one is usually confronted by heavy scar that makes dissection and identification of involved neural elements difficult. At the time of exploration, one must make sure that the transection is sharp and clean before a primary repair is done. When confronted with a transected nerve, the following factors favor primary repair:[19]

1. Nerve stumps are easy to locate and their relationships to other injured structures usually are preserved.
2. Nerve stumps are minimally retracted.
3. A single operative procedure is definitive and may be the only operation necessary to repair soft tissue as well as nerve injury.

Primary repair should only be undertaken by surgeons who have total mastery of the anatomy of the injured region and who have been trained in macro- and microperipheral nerve surgical techniques.

Not all transecting injuries lend themselves to primary repair. If the ends are ragged or contused, a delayed repair is preferable. In this case, the surgeon cannot know how much of either stump to resect in order to get back to healthy neural tissue. Even with injuries caused by sharp objects, a contused rather than transected nerve can result, and delayed repair then becomes mandatory. If clinical or substantial EMG recovery does not occur in the first 2–3 months, reoperation to evaluate the lesion in continuity and to make a decision for or against resection and repair is indicated.

In summary, the arguments favoring delayed or secondary repair include:

1. Damage to the proximal and distal stumps has had time to be defined by visible intraneural scarring on cross-section. The surgeon can then be certain that resection back to normal neural tissue is accomplished.
2. Associated injuries have had a chance to heal, infection has been minimized, and the

patient has learned to use the extremity before being subjected to operation and sometimes to immobilization and its attendant discomfort.

3. The epineurium has thickened so as to allow easier placement of epineural sutures.

4. Operation is elective and can be performed accurately.

5. The distal stump is cleared of degenerating axoplasm and myelin.

6. Approximately 15% to 20% of lacerations have not transected the nerve or nerves in a limb with associated complete loss of function in the distribution of one or more nerves. It is impossible to decide immediately postinjury whether or not to resect such a lesion in continuity.[19]

When the nerve is not known to be transected (closed injury) but is without function, especially following high-velocity missile wounding as shown in Figure 1, delayed (secondary) repair is indicated. The majority of closed injuries to the nerve are due to stretch/contusion. The nerve is not divided and there is a variable degree of intraneural damage. This may be a mixture of axonotmesis, neurotemesis and neuropraxia, or may be due to complete neurotemesis. Thus, a delay of several months is necessary, since this will permit **(1)** any element of neuropraxia to resolve, **(2)** associated injuries to heal, and **(3)** most importantly, physiologic evaluation of the lesion at the operating table.[17] If adequate regeneration is occurring, spontaneous activity can be detected by means of intraoperative NAP recording techniques by 8–10 weeks postinjury.

If a NAP is present, the nerve will fare well with simple neurolysis. Most often, external neurolysis is performed. This consists of freeing the nerve from surrounding tissue, including scar, and exposing the entire circumference of the nerve.[17] Internal neurolysis, involving resection of scar tissue away from the nerve fascicles, is usually reserved for certain partial nerve lesions requiring split repair and management of refractory neuritic pain.[1,17] Figure 5 shows a high peroneal division split repair.

Neurolysis may or may not assist in continued regeneration and hasten recovery. Some authors believe that adhesions and scar tissue can obstruct or delay the growth of regenerating axons and even block conduction in nerve fibers.[1,35] Other investigators say that recovery under these circumstances would have occurred even if neurolysis had not been done.[31]

Neurolysis may also relieve or ameliorate noncausalgic neuralgic pain by removing adhesions or constricting scar that fix and at times deform the nerve (Figure 6).[17,35] Neurolysis or nerve repair is less likely to ameliorate pain in nonfocal injuries, such as stretch-contusion, particularly of the plexus.[19] A daily regimen of carbamazepine and amitriptyline may help relieve pain. Vigorous physical therapy is essential in pain management. Early mobilization of the involved limb should be stressed to the patient and family. Reassurance of the temporary nature of the pain, at least in patients with acute nerve injury, is also helpful. Occasionally, patients may benefit from transcutaneous peripheral nerve stimulation devices.[4,22]

If a NAP is not present and 8 weeks have elapsed, recovery will not occur unless resection back to healthy neural tissue and repair are performed.[13] An end-to-end repair is preferred. Use of autologous grafts, usually using the sural nerve, is the method of choice for bridging a gap that cannot be closed without tension by an end-to-end union (Figure 7A,B). The success of nerve grafting declines as the length of the graft increases, usually because the lengthier injuries requiring longer grafts are more severe.[27,35]

Grafting very long defects under unfavorable conditions is not worthwhile in some nerves, because the chances of obtaining any useful function are remote. In such cases, alternative methods such as neurotization procedures should be considered. These include use of the cervical plexus, accessory nerve, or intercostal nerves as proximal outflow to attach to sural grafts.[3,6,38] Such procedures have sometimes provided either shoulder abduction or biceps/brachialis contraction. Neurotization has difficulty substituting for loss of more than one

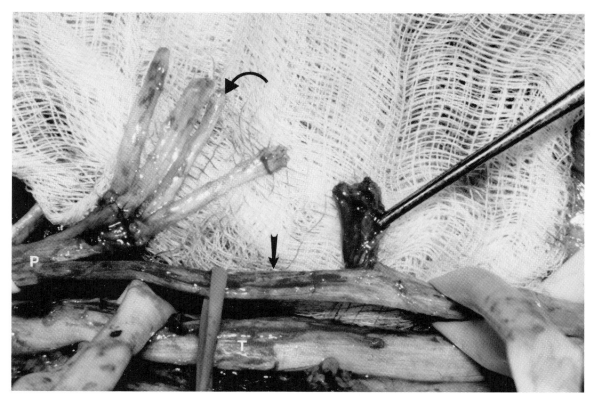

Figure 5. *Intraoperative photograph of the peroneal division (P) of the sciatic nerve at the thigh level of a patient who sustained a .22 caliber handgun wound to the proximal lateral thigh. Clinical and electrical studies showed that the patient had complete right peroneal loss with no improvement 4 months postinjury (time of exploration). No intraoperative nerve action potential (NAP) could be evoked across a neuroma in continuity on the peroneal division of the sciatic nerve at the upper thigh level. A good NAP response was evoked across the tibial (T) division. Internal neurolysis and split repair using interfascicular sural nerve grafts (curved arrow) was performed on the peroneal division. Note the two fascicular bundles (arrow) of the peroneal division not involved in the neuroma and thus spared (NAPs could be elicited across these fascicles).*

function, although a recent report in a small number of patients suggests that this may still be a possibility.[38]

After it is clear that recovery is unlikely, an injured nerve should be repaired with the least possible delay. This minimizes distal nerve trunk and fascicular atrophy which will lead to poor results. According to Sunderland, such atrophy is evident by the end of the first month postinjury, reaches a peak somewhere between the third and fourth months, and then levels out.[35] As a general guideline, focal lesions in continuity (those associated with fracture, soft tissue contusion, and some gunshot wounds) can be accurately evaluated intraoperatively at 2–3 months postinjury.[17]

Stretch or severe contusion injuries (those associated with vehicular and skiing accidents, falls, crush injuries, and shotgun pellets) produce lengthier lesions and need to be followed longer to assess full regenerative capacity. These lesions can usually be accurately evaluated intraoperatively by electrical recordings at 3–5 months postoperatively.[17] Delay in referral, healing of associated injuries, and management of infection may alter the timing of operation.

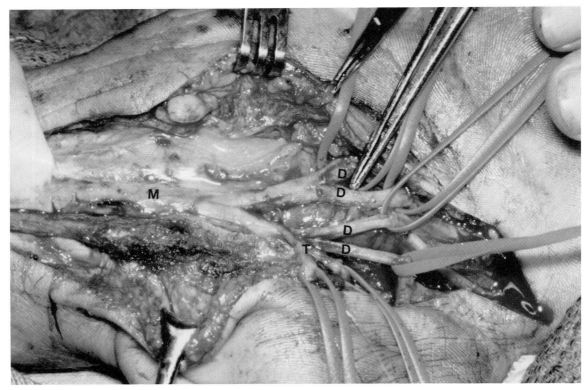

Figure 6. Intraoperative photograph of the median nerve (M) at the wrist level as well as its palmar branches. This patient suffered a crushing-type injury of his right hand while lifting a 2 × 12 end of timber. He had two prior operations with "nerve" section to relieve severe thumb pain and palmar hyperesthesia. At this operation (20 months after the injury) a 2 cm neuroma was found in a digital sensory branch (forefinger) of the median nerve (M). The neuroma along with the sensory nerve was resected. Internal and external neurolysis of the thenar (T) and digital (D) branches was performed with good postoperative pain relief. The importance of adequate exposure and mobilization of the injured peripheral nerve is emphasized in this case.

Despite these guidelines for lesions in continuity, when one is in doubt about the direction of recovery, it is better to assess the nerve directly. Excessive delay in nerve repair leads to poor results.[2,35] Table 1 summarizes these guidelines for lesions in continuity.[17]

Selection of Patients for Surgery

Despite the guidelines outlined above, controversy concerning the value and timing of

surgery as well as patient selection continues to exist. This is especially evident in the management of brachial plexus stretch/contusion injuries. Some authors consider few or none of these injuries suitable for surgery, while others believe that all stretch injuries should be explored.[18] This brings one to the question: How does one select patients with brachial plexus stretch lesions for surgery? Table 2 summarizes some of the criteria currently used for selection.

Very proximal injury involving the roots

TABLE 1
Management of the Neuroma in Continuity*

Incomplete loss with significant distal sparing
1. Most cases will improve with conservative treatment. They are followed by serial clinical and EMG examinations.
   Physical therapy is important.
2. Operation may still be required:
   a. Partial lesions associated with expanding masses due to hematoma, aneurysm, or A-V fistula usually require urgent operation.
   b. Partial lesions close to or in areas of potential entrapment may require relatively early operation.
   c. Lesions where distal loss, although partial, is significant may require later operation.
   d. Neural pain not amenable to medications and physical therapy may require later operation.

Complete or near complete loss with little or no distal sparing
1. Relatively focal lesions in continuity due to fracture or gunshot wound.
   a. Follow by clinical and EMG examinations for 2-3 months.
   b. If no significant clinical or electrical improvement, explore.
   c. Intraoperative stimulation and NAP studies used to decide for or against resection.
2. Relatively lengthy lesions in continuity due to stretch/contusion or shotgun
   a. Follow by clinical and EMG examinations for 4-5 months.
   b. If no significant clinical or electrical improvement, explore.
   c. If no response to stimulation and no NAP across lesion, resection and repair by suture or graft are necessary.
   d. Intraoperative evoked cortical or somatosensory studies may be necessary to evaluate repairability of proximal spinal nerves. (See Table 2).

*Reference 17

close to the spinal cord and/or the cord itself is the most frequent reason for not attempting direct repair on these injuries.[18,24] However, most patients requiring surgical treatment have **(1)** proximal lesions close to and, in some cases, involving the spinal cord, and **(2)** lengthy lesions requiring long grafts for repair.[17,30] If the sensory root has evidence of a very proximal (preganglionic) injury, successful repair of the motor root at such a proximal level is technically difficult, although not impossible. Direct repair is impossible if the roots are avulsed from the spinal cord, or if secondary cord damage makes regeneration through the grafts unlikely. Some of these patients may be candidates for neurotization procedures.

Also not candidates for operation are stretch lesions confined to the lower plexus elements, such as C8 and T1 nerve roots, or the lower trunk to the medial cord. Results with repair of these lesions are poor, except in children.[18] Adults seen 1 year or later after injury do not usually benefit from direct neural repair, and thus are not good operative candidates for such an approach.

Other relative contraindications ("stops") to surgery include flail arm, Horner's syndrome, and meningoceles and other myelographic abnormalities (Table 2).[18] Patients with total arm paralysis due to severe brachial plexus stretch injury are very difficult to salvage by direct repair. It is especially difficult to recover distal forearm and hand function in patients with flail arms. In these patients, every attempt is made to regain significant shoulder abduction and flexion of the forearm. Presence of Horner's syndrome, although an indication of proximal T1 and/or C8 root injury, does not necessarily mean that roots at higher levels are damaged at such a proximal level.[18]

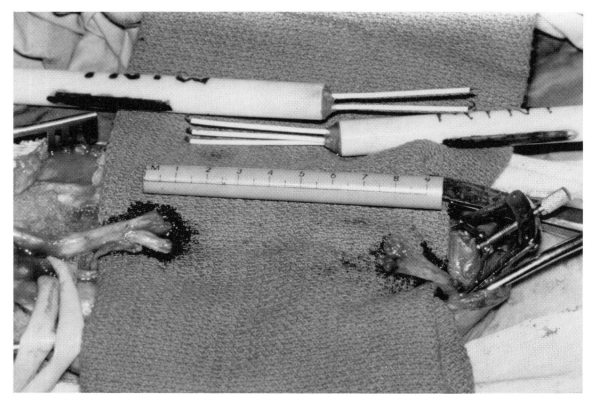

Figure 7A. *Intraoperative photograph of a left posterior tibial nerve repair at the ankle level. This patient lacerated his tibial nerve while kicking his left foot through a glass door. The patient underwent an immediate exploration of his left ankle at which time his Achilles' tendon was repaired and the posterior tibial nerve was noted to be transected. The two ends could not be identified at that time. Pain in the left foot as well as numbness of the sole continued over the subsequent 3 months (time of re-exploration). The distal and proximal stumps of the lacerated nerve were identified and resected back to healthy neural tissue. There was a 2.5-inch gap between the two ends.*

Informed Consent

Once the data derived from the clinical examination and the electrophysiologic and radiologic studies are assembled, the managing physician should sit down with the patient and the family to explain the sites and nature of the nerve injuries. Most patients will be familiar with electrical cables, and this may serve as a good analogy, as long as they understand that restoration of continuity does not, alone, produce function. It is useful to explain to the patient that the delay following injury is according to plan, and has allowed distinction of those elements which show evidence of re-

covery from those nerve elements which do not.

The patient and the family should also understand that the patient will be under the care of the managing physician for 2–6 years, during which time spontaneous recovery and recovery following surgery is observed and further management decisions are made. By 2–3 years after repair, sufficient return will have occurred so as to allow the experienced evaluator to give a prognosis regarding the ultimate function. This sets the stage for appropriate reconstructive operations, such as muscle transfers and joint fusions, which will further facilitate functional recovery of the limb.

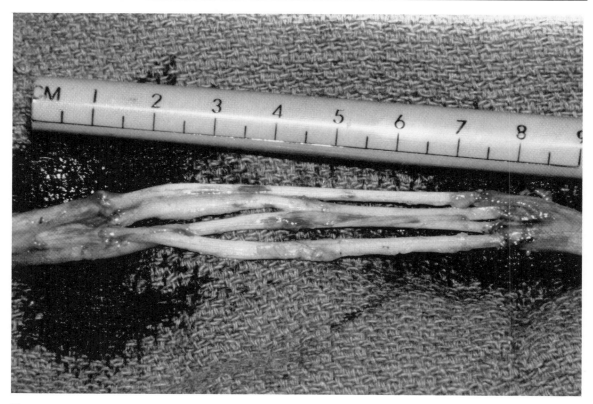

Figure 7B. Four interfascicular 2³/₄-inch sural nerve grafts were used to bridge the gap in the patient seen in 7A. Note the lack of tension between the two ends of the repair.

The patient must understand that a personal quest for recovery is an absolute prerequisite for a successful outcome. Initially the patient may receive direction from a physical therapist, but very rapidly the patient should receive the physical therapy program at home. Victims of nerve injury should be forewarned that they may experience uncomfortable sensations during the regeneration phase, and that it is essential for them to be vigorous in their exercise program or these uncomfortable sensations will assume an overwhelmingly negative context. If the patient is not prepared to actively strive for recovery with diligence for 2 years, there is scarcely any reason to attempt intricate nerve surgery as the patient's lack of compliance will ensure a poor result.

The experienced clinician should, relatively speaking, be able to predict the functional status of the patient several years following nerve repair. Appropriate vocational and educational goals may then be outlined for the patient. If it is immediately apparent that an individual will never be able to resume an occupation involving heavy physical labor, appropriate vocational retraining should be instituted at the beginning rather than at the end of the management program.

Patients with devastating neurologic injuries may require considerable psychological support initially. This support should be withdrawn by 6 months after the repair. The patient should be totally independent in the performance of exercise programs, visiting physical therapy departments with checks in progress, application of splints, etc. The coincidence of severe head injury with major peripheral nerve injury may carry a relatively poor prognosis.

TABLE 2
Selection of Plexus Stretch Injuries for Operation*

Clinical questions:
1. Is lesion complete or incomplete in distribution of one or more elements?
2. Does significant motor (not sensory) improvement occur in first 4 months?
3. If injury is at a nerve root level, how proximal?

Relative "stops" (contraindications to direct neural repair):
1. Winging of the scapula—long thoracic nerve
2. Rhomboid paralysis—dorsal scapular nerve
3. Diaphragm paralysis—phrenic nerve
4. Extensive paraspinal denervation by EMG—posterior branch of anterior root (more distal and, thus, repairable injury to some roots may still be present)
5. Positive sensory potentials can suggest preganglionic injury at C8, T1, and sometimes C7; higher roots may still be operable
6. Myelopathy and/or fracture/dislocation of spine

Less certain "stops":
1. Total flail arm
2. Sensory improvement without motor improvement
3. Horner's syndrome
4. Meningoceles at some (usually lower) but not all levels
   a. False positive and negative rates are significant.
   b. Meningoceles strongly suggest but do not prove proximal root damage.
   c. Meningoceles at one or more levels suggest but do not prove proximal damage at other root levels without meningoceles.
   d. Absence of meningoceles does not prove lateral damage nor does presence of a meningocele always mean proximal damage or any damage at all.

*References 18,20

Patients lacking in motivation following head injury will usually not have the drive to successfully complete the entire course of rehabilitation during the period of nerve regeneration.

Technical Considerations

Peripheral nerve operations should only be performed in operating rooms with appropriate facilities that include excellent illumination and the provision of magnification during surgery. A range of instruments is required from conventional forceps and scissors to delicate microinstruments. An appropriate range of sutures from 10-0 through 1-0 is required. Cases vary in duration, and the duration of the operation is often unpredictable as the final decisions for and against grafting are only made during the operation itself.

Because of the uncertainty of the nature of the surgery, these operations should be under-

taken by surgeons who have the ability to perform external neurolysis, nerve suture, nerve grafting, and neurotization procedures. Facility with vein and arterial repair is also essential. Operating rooms must have appropriate electrophysiologic equipment and personnel so that intraoperative NAP and SEP studies can be repeatedly conducted during the course of an operation.

Failure to achieve useful regeneration to the extent that is expected after nerve repair may be due in part to excessive conservatism on the part of the surgeon, who may be reluctant to resect scarred nerve ends back to normal nerve segments when this creates an extensive gap to be bridged (Figure 8).[19,25] Incisions for exposure of the lesion should be large enough to fully mobilize the injured neural element(s) (Figure 9). Mobilization of the nerve is necessary to overcome the gap that results from retraction of the stumps and resection of the

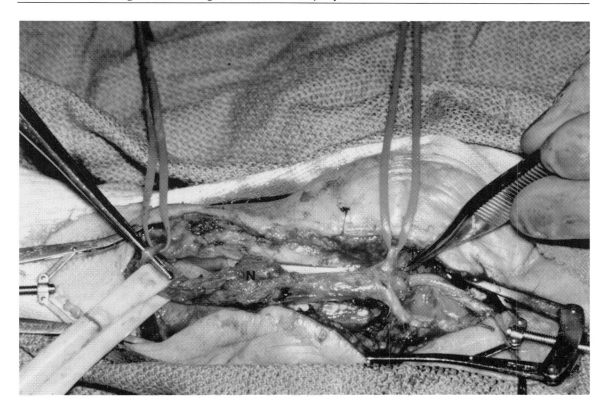

Figure 8. Intraoperative photograph of a median nerve neuroma (N) in continuity at the wrist level. This patient presented with left median nerve palsy 3 weeks after a left carpal tunnel release at another medical center. During the earlier procedure, extensive scarring around the median nerve was noted. The surgeon did not attempt to fully resect the scar tissue. The patient continued to have numbness, tingling, and pain in her hand as well as weakness in the median innervated hand muscles. The patient gave a history of injury to the left wrist about 4 months before this procedure and an old laceration injury to the same wrist years before. Intraoperative recordings evoked only a small nerve action potential (NAP) across the neuroma. Internal neurolysis was initially performed. Several sutures were found embedded in the neuroma/scar tissue. Eventually, the neuroma had to be resected back to healthy neural tissue and sural interfascicular grafting performed (four 1.5-inch grafts). The importance of resecting a scarred nerve back to healthy appearing nerve segments is emphasized in this case.

damaged nerve ends.[19,35] Maximal nerve length is obtained by dissecting to and somewhat beyond the distal and the proximal joints.

Neurophysiologic studies have shown that extensive mobilization does not affect the subsequent function of a normal nerve or the regenerative process in one that is injured.[19] Mobilization allows the surgeon to resect back to healthy-appearing neural tissue, to shorten the gap between resected stumps, and to join separated nerve ends. Nonetheless, grafts are a

useful alternative and most large gaps can be closed by a combination of nerve mobilization and graft repair.

Repair of a nerve will yield the best results when there is no cross-sectional area of scar to block a maximal downgrowth of axons from above or to prevent the maximum availability of receiving tubules distally.[19] The appearance of healthy nerve ends usually coincides with brisk bleeding. Healthy nerve ends facilitate maximum fascicular apposition when the

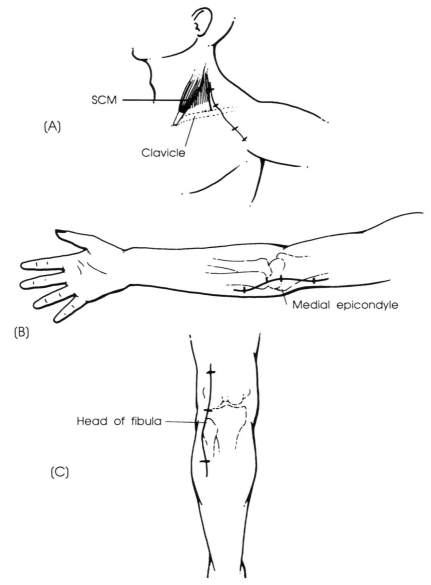

Figure 9. Proposed skin incisions for brachial plexus (A), ulnar nerve at the elbow level (B), and peroneal nerve at the knee level (C) explorations. Exposure of the lesion should be large enough to fully mobilize the injured neural element(s). Mobilization of the nerve is necessary to overcome the gap that results from retraction of the stumps and resection of the damaged nerve ends. SCM = sternocleidomastoid muscle. Skin incisions are depicted as solid lines with cross-hatches.

nerve ends are brought together end-to-end or are joined by multiple interfascicular grafts. This helps to promote the entry of regenerating axons into fasciculi of the distal stump and not into interfascicular epineural tissue.[35]

Distraction in nerve repair should be avoided. This makes mobilization, transposition, and accurate apposition of the nerve stumps all the more important. If the nerve is under too much tension, distraction is likely to occur, particularly if flexion of the extremity is needed to gain an end-to-end apposition. In this case, the surgeon should resort to relatively short interfascicular nerve grafts, using an autologous nerve such as the sural nerve (Figures 5 and 7A,B).[14,25,26,27,32] The importance of tension as a contributing factor for failure of nerve repair has been demonstrated experimentally in the primate model (Kim et al, unpublished data, 1991). Other factors leading to failure of nerve repair include tissue manipulation that is not gentle, sacrifice of longitudinal vessels deep to the epineural level, and intraoperative or postoperative stretch of the nerve.[19]

Patient Follow-up

Prior to discharge from hospital, the patient should have a very clear understanding of what was performed at operation. A simple sketch may assist in explaining. Sutures and staples are conventionally removed between the eighth and tenth postoperative day. Those removing the sutures should understand the required duration of immobilization.

Following simple neurolysis, the managing physician may want the patient to move into a vigorous passive and active physical therapy program without delay. If a direct nerve suture has been performed, immobilization of the joints may be required for 3 or more weeks, with progressive extension of the joints for up to 6 weeks. Premature mobilization may result in suture-line disruption. Those with graft repairs are permitted more motion in the early weeks but should avoid hyperextension or hyperabduction of the joints.

If possible, it is appropriate to reassess the patient at approximately 6 weeks following nerve repair. This allows the physician to be certain that the patient understands what is required and that the patient is not adopting an overly passive stance. Third-party insurance agencies should understand the significance of the injury and the likely duration of disability. If the patient can return to the labor force, even in a reduced capacity, this should be encouraged immediately.

The next follow-up visit should coincide with the anticipated time of initial motor recovery of the first downstream muscle. At this stage, the patient should be encouraged to exercise those muscles which have received axonal regrowth. This is also a good time to observe whether or not there is evidence of malingering, medical-legal neurosis, or prolongation of disability by compensation payments. In these cases, evidence of sympathetic dystrophy may become more and more obvious as prolonged overprotection and immobilization of limbs leads to secondary, sympathetically maintained pain syndromes and joint contracture.

Decision-making with regard to patients suffering from peripheral nerve injury is straightforward if there is either clear-cut evidence of progressive improvement or obvious evidence of no improvement. The management of patients demonstrating partial improvement requires considerable experience. On occasion, re-exploration may be judged too risky, as the patient has too much to lose and not enough to gain. On other occasions, reoperation may be indicated.

Conclusions

Treatment strategies for the injured peripheral nerve are guided by an accurate evaluation of the initial injury. A reasonable approach to these injuries is presented as a simplified flow chart in Figure 10.

The level, particularly the proximal extent, of the injury should be determined very carefully, using clinical, electrodiagnostic, and radiologic criteria (Table 2). This assessment is especially critical in selecting patients for direct brachial plexus repair, which provides the best opportunity for some functional recovery.

Signs of regeneration should be sought by using clinical examination and electrophysiologic studies. Initial neural recovery is best demonstrated by return of motor activity. Nerve stimulation may be required to establish with certainty that motor function has returned. Definite sensory recovery in autonomous zones can be important early evidence of regeneration in distal lesions of major sensory nerves. Sensory recovery usually occurs rela-

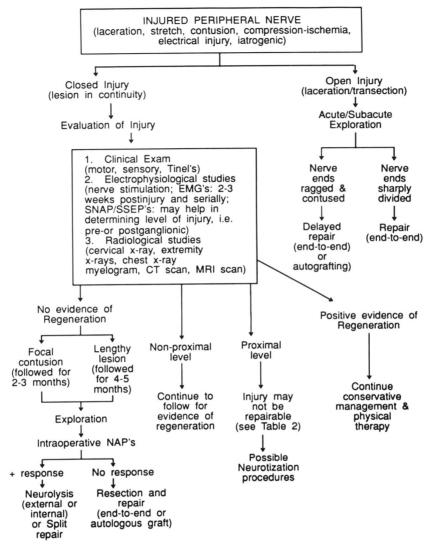

Figure 10. Simplified flow chart for the management of peripheral nerve injuries. Although some nerves and muscles may recover better than others, the figure provides some general guidelines. Overall results with all types of nerve repair may vary with the nerve as well as the level involved.

tively late, however, and this may be misleading, especially in the case of radial and peroneal nerves.

The ability to obtain NAP recordings across the nerve lesion provides additional early evidence for adequate regeneration. This usually requires an operative exposure of the involved nerve. Other qualitative evidence for neural regeneration is provided by Tinel's sign and EMG. If each of these sources fails to give even slight evidence favoring regeneration, and the

deadline for significant reinnervation is many months away, surgical exploration will be necessary. Should a neuroma in continuity be found at exploration, the surgeon is best guided with regard to resection and nerve repair by NAP recordings. If nerve resection and repair is needed, adequate mobilization of the nerve and apposition of healthy nerve ends either end-to-end or with autologous nerve grafts is indicated.

Results with all types of nerve repair are related to the specific nerve involved as well as level involved.[17] Radial repairs fare better than median, and median better than ulnar. In the lower extremity, tibial and femoral nerves fare better than peroneal nerve. The need for rehabilitation and good physical and occupational therapy pre- and postoperatively is very important for useful recovery. Even this will fail unless patients and their families are taught the need for range of motion and exercise many times a day. Significant reinnervation will fail to produce function in a stiff and often painful hand or foot.

References

1. Brown BA. Internal neurolysis in traumatic peripheral nerve lesions in continuity. *Surg Clin North Am.* 1972;52:1167–1175.

2 Brown PW. Factors influencing the success of surgical repair of peripheral nerves. *Surg Clin North Am.* 1972;52:1137–1155.

3. Brunelli G. Neurotization of avulsed roots of the brachial plexus by means of anterior nerves of the cervical plexus. *Int J Microsurg.* 1980;2:55–58.

4. Campbell JN, Long DM. Peripheral nerve stimulation in the treatment of intractable pain. *J Neurosurg.* 1976;45:692–699.

5. Clippinger FW, Goldner JL, Roberts JM. Use of electromyogram in evaluating upper extremity peripheral nerve lesions. *J Bone Joint Surg. Am.* 1962;44A:1047–1060.

6. Friedman AH. Neurotization of elements of the brachial plexus. *Neurosurg Clin North Am.* 1991;2:165–174.

7. Guttmann E, Young JZ. Re-innervation of muscle after various periods of atrophy. *J Anat.* 1944;78:15–43.

8. Hudson AR, Tranmer B. Brachial plexus injuries. In: Wilkins R, Rengachary S, eds. *Neurosurgery.* New York, NY: McGraw Hill Book Co; 1985;2:1817–1832.

9. Kline DG. Perspectives concerning brachial plexus injury and repair. *Neurosurg Clin North Am.* 1991;2:151–164.

10. Kline DG. Selection of brachial plexus cases for operation based on results. In: Samii M, ed. *Peripheral Nerve Lesions.* Berlin, Germany: Springer-Verlag; 1990:396–410.

11. Kline DG. Surgical repair of peripheral nerve injury. *Muscle Nerve.* 1990;13:843–852.

12. Kline DG. Macroscopic and microscopic concomitants of nerve repair. *Clin Neurosurg.* 1979;26:582–606.

13. Kline DG. Physiological and clinical factors contributing to timing of nerve repair. *Clin Neurosurg.* 1977;24:425–455.

14. Kline DG, DeJonge BR. Evoked potentials to evaluate peripheral nerve injuries. *Surg Gynecol Obstet.* 1968;127:1239–1248.

15. Kline DG, Hackett ER. Reappraisal of timing for exploration of civilian peripheral nerve injuries. *Surgery.* 1975;78:54–65.

16. Kline DG, Hackett ER, Happel LH. Surgery for lesions of the brachial plexus. *Arch Neurol.* 1986;43:170–181.

17. Kline DG, Hackett ER, May PR. Evaluation of nerve injuries by evoked potentials and electromyography. *J Neurosurg.* 1969;31:128–136.

18. Kline DG, Hudson AR. Acute injuries of peripheral nerves. In: Youmans JR, ed. *Neurological Surgery.* 3rd ed. Philadelphia, Pa: WB Saunders Co; 1990: 2423–2510.

19. Kline DG, Hudson AR. Surgical repair of acute peripheral nerve injuries: timing and technique. In: Morley T, ed. *Controversies in Neurosurgery.* Philadelphia, Pa: WB Saunders Co; 1976:184–197.

20. Kline DG, Judice DJ. Operative management of selected brachial plexus lesions. *J Neurosurg.* 1983;58:631–649.

21. Livingston WK. Evidence of active invasion of denervated areas by sensory fibers from neighboring nerves in man. *J Neurosurg.* 1947;4:140–145.

22. Long DM. Neuromodulation for the control of chronic pain. *Surg Rounds.* 1982;5:25–34.

23. MacKinnon SE, Dellon AL. *Surgery of the Peripheral Nerve.* New York, NY: Thieme Medical Publishers; 1988.

24. McGillicuddy JE. Clinical decision making in brachial plexus injuries. *Neurosurg Clin North Am.* 1991;2:137–150.

25. Millesi H. Reappraisal of nerve repair. *Surg Clin North Am.* 1981;61:321–340.

26. Millesi H. Surgical management of brachial plexus injuries. *J Hand Surg.* 1977:367–378.

27. Millesi H, Meissl G, Berger A. The interfascicular nerve grafting of the median and ulnar nerves. *J Bone Joint Surg Am..* 1972;54A:727–750.

28. Moberg E. Criticism and study of methods for examining sensibility in the hand. *Neurology.* 1962;12: 8–19.

29. Moberg E. Objective methods for determining the functional value of sensibility in the hand. *J Bone Joint Surg Br.* 1958;40B:454–476.

30. Narakas A. Brachial plexus surgery. *Orthop Clin North Am.* 1981;12:303–323.

31. Nulsen FE, Slade HW. Recovery following injury to the brachial plexus. In: Woodhall B, Beebe GW, eds. *Peripheral Nerve Regeneration: A Follow-up Study of 3656 World War II Injuries.* Washington, DC: U.S. Government Printing Office; 1956:389–408.

32. Samii M. Modern aspects of peripheral and cranial nerve surgery. *Adv Tech Stand Neurosurg.* 1975;2:33–85.

33. Seddon HJ. *Surgical Disorders of the Peripheral Nerves.* Baltimore, Md: Williams & Wilkins Co; 1972.

34. Sunderland S. *Nerve Injuries and Their Repair: A Critical Appraisal.* New York, NY: Churchill-Livingstone; 1991.

35. Sunderland S. *Nerve and Nerve Injuries.* Baltimore, Md: Williams & Wilkins Co.; 1968.

36. Terzis JK, Dykes RW, Hakstian RW. Electrophysiological recordings in peripheral nerve surgery: a review. *J Hand Surg.* 1976;1:52–66.

37. Van Beek A, Hubble B, Kinkead L, et al. Clinical use of nerve stimulation and recording techniques. *Plast Reconstr Surg.* 1983;71:225–238.

38. Yamada S, Peterson GW, Sloniuk DS, et al. Coaptation of anterior rami of C-3 and C-4 to the upper trunk of the brachial plexus for cervical nerve root avulsion. *J Neurosurg.* 1991;74:171–177.

PART II

ENTRAPMENT NEUROPATHIES

CHAPTER 4

Entrapment Neuropathies of the Upper Extremity

Stephen R. Freidberg, MD

This chapter discusses the less common entrapment neuropathies of the upper extremity. The most common entrapment neuropathies are the median nerve at the carpal tunnel and the ulnar nerve at the cubital tunnel, which are discussed in Chapters 5 and 6. This chapter, however, briefly addresses issues covered in other chapters, such as surgical exposure of the nerves of the upper extremity, which is discussed in Chapter 10, and electrophysiologic findings, which are outlined in Chapter 1. An appropriate duplication, therefore, will be used to emphasize important points.

Etiology

Spinner and Spencer[24] discussed basic principles of entrapment neuropathy. They stressed that the compressed segment is in a specific location on the nerve as determined by the local anatomy, i.e. where the nerve traverses a tunnel bound by bone and fibrous tissue or where the nerve passes from one compartment to another. Changes in the tissue consistency that surrounds the nerve can precipitate entrapment. Trauma with direct injury or callus formation after fracture also has been implicated. Systemic diseases that have been associated with entrapment include hypothyroidism, acromegaly, rheumatoid arthritis, osteoarthritis, giant-cell arteritis, and amyloidosis. An anatomic variant, such as an accessory muscle, arterial aneurysm, or congenitally small tunnel,

can precipitate an entrapment neuropathy as well.[9] Compression of the posterior interosseous nerve, for example, has been described with hemihypertrophy[5] and with a lipoma in the region of the elbow.[1] The author has observed compression of the median nerve by a lipoma in the deep palmar space and compression of the ulnar nerve by a schwannoma in the cubital tunnel.

Occupational causes of neuropathy are common. Carpal tunnel syndrome has been reported as an overuse syndrome in persons who employ sign language for the deaf.[4] The carpal tunnel syndrome has been observed in patients with paraparesis who use crutches for walking. Compression of the ulnar nerve in Guyon's canal is seen in cyclists. Compression of the ulnar nerve is legendary in patients who spend long hours leaning their elbows on bars.

The probable cause of entrapment neuropathy is a decrease in the neural blood supply. The nerve receives its blood supply from the mesoneurium, which is flexible and permits continuing perfusion as the extremity moves. Venous obstruction caused by compression increases intrafascicular pressure. This, in turn, decreases perfusion, which leads to edema. A vicious cycle ensues. An ingrowth of fibroblasts and scar ultimately results. This adds to the vicious cycle of worsening hypoxia. Diabetes, which compromises the blood supply, places the nerve at an additional risk of compression and repetitive injury.[16] Compression and atrophy can be so long-standing that end organ fibrosis may result. In this situation, decompression of the nerve will not improve the neurologic symptoms.

The electrodiagnostic findings in any entrapment neuropathy depend on a number of variables including **(1)** the timing of the study, **(2)** the severity of the injury, and particularly **(3)** the relative amounts of demyelination and axonal loss (JA Russell, personal communication, 1991). In the experience of a competent electrodiagnostician, normal findings are rarely identified as abnormal. Conversely, electrodiagnostic evaluations may be inadequate to identify minor injuries to nerves. This situation can occur in proximal demyelinating lesions when conduction studies cannot be obtained above and below the suspected lesion due to technical limitations. In addition, false-negative results or inconclusive results may occur because of premature testing. Complete expression of an abnormality may require up to 7 days for motor nerve conduction, 9–10 days for sensory conduction, and 3 weeks for needle examination of muscle; however, electrodiagnostic studies are useful to diagnose other syndromes, such as proximal lesions, multiple lesions, or lesions that accompany diabetes mellitus.

Differential Diagnosis

Strict criteria should be used to diagnose entrapment neuropathies. The author regularly sees patients with spondylotic myelopathy and radiculopathy who have undergone unnecessary carpal tunnel surgery. The peak age for both conditions is the same, and many of these patients have electrical evidence of carpal tunnel syndrome.

Radiculopathy involving the C8 nerve root can be confused with ulnar neuropathy. When the patient has thenar atrophy as well as involvement of the ulnar nerve, a C8 nerve root lesion should be suspected strongly. Osterman[15] described a double crush syndrome in which cervical or thoracic outlet compression worsens median or ulnar entrapment. It is unusual for a patient to have more than one lesion. A high index of suspicion, the unique

symptoms and physical findings, the results of electrodiagnostic studies, and, when necessary, cervical spine imaging should lead to the correct diagnosis.

Internal Neurolysis

The value of internal neurolysis at the time of decompression has long been debated. Mackinnon and colleagues[13] documented an improved electrical and morphologic recovery with neurolysis compared to decompression alone in a rat model. In a clinical paper, however, Mackinnon and colleagues[12] demonstrated that although neurolysis is a safe procedure, it does not provide clinical benefit in patients who have had carpal tunnel surgery. Gumley[8] stated that neurolysis of a nerve whose diameter is diminished by a circumferentially thickened and scarred epineurium may improve nutrition and permit nerve expansion during healing. Nevertheless, neurolysis is not necessary for all patients undergoing carpal tunnel surgery or with compressed nerves. Phalen[17] stated that performance of internal neurolysis in every carpal tunnel operation courts disaster. Peimer[16], who favors neurolysis, believes that it is important to evaluate the intraneural pathologic findings. The decision on whether or not to perform a neurolysis depends on the observation of the nerve in the operating room. If the nerve remains narrowed after the surgical decompression or if intraneural scarring is present, neurolysis should be done. Patients who present with recurrent symptoms should have neurolysis. After neurolysis, the fascicles, even if atrophic, will be obvious and not hidden in thick epineurium.

Median Nerve

The more proximal median compression syndromes can produce pain, neurologic deficit, or both.[14,24] The compression can occur above the elbow at the ligament of Struthers or below the elbow by the pronator teres muscle (Figure 1A,B,C).

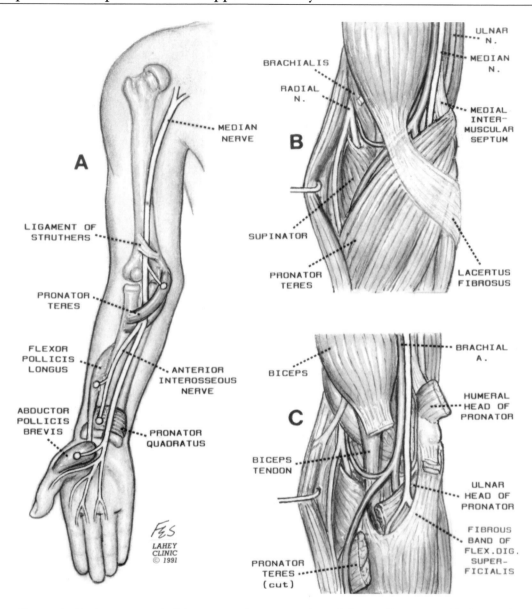

Figure 1. Median nerve. A. Diagrammatic presentation of the median nerve. B. Anatomic presentation of the median nerve in the articulated fossa. C. Anatomic presentation of the median nerve with the pronator teres muscle divided.

Entrapment at Ligament of Struthers

The ligament of Struthers, which should not be confused with the arcade of Struthers (which produces ulnar neuropathy), is located 5 cm proximal to the medial epicondyle. The median nerve and brachial artery both pass be-neath this ligament. Nerve compression at the ligament of Struthers usually produces a syndrome of pain and local tenderness.[25] Stern[25] noted that the anterior interosseous nerve branch of the median nerve can be compressed at the ligament of Struthers, with resultant motor neuropathy (as described later). This phenomenon is unusual. The electrodiagnostic findings demonstrate a reduced or absent median sensory potential (JA Russell, personal communication, 1991). With a predominantly demyelinating lesion, conduction velocity may be slowed across the involved segment with a normal conduction velocity below. Conduction study motor amplitudes will be reduced after axon loss, regardless of the site of stimulation. With demyelination, however, motor amplitudes are abnormal only with stimulation above the site of the lesion. With any amount of axon loss, denervation will be evident in all median innervated muscles of the hand and forearm. Section of the ligament effectively relieves symptoms.

Pronator Syndrome

The pronator syndrome is characterized by mild to moderate pain in the forearm.[14] The pain increases with movement of the elbow, with repeated supination and pronation, and with repeated use of the grip. Loss of dexterity in the hand, mild weakness, and median nerve paresthesia occur. Numbness may be present, not only in the fingers, but also in the thenar region of the palm because of involvement of the palmar cutaneous nerve that branches distal to the site of compression.[9,24] These symptoms resemble carpal tunnel syndrome, but the symptoms of paresthesia while sleeping are absent.[9,24] The pain in the forearm and the local tenderness can be reproduced by resisted pronation. Tinel's sign may be present over the nerve.

The anatomic level of compression is within the substance of the pronator teres muscle. The median nerve with the brachial artery lies between the two heads of the pronator teres and passes deep to the fibrous origin of the flexor digitorum superficialis muscle. Compression may be caused by the thickened lacertus fibrosus, by a hypertrophied pronator muscle, or by a tight fibrous band of the flexor digitorum superficialis muscle. Results of electrodiagnostic studies are often normal. When results are abnormal, they parallel the findings in patients with the ligament of Struthers syndrome except that no denervation is present in the pronator teres muscle (JA Russell, personal communication, 1991).

Treatment of patients with the pronator syndrome is initially conservative with administration of anti-inflammatory medication and use of splints.[9] An attempt is made to eliminate precipitating events. Should these measures be ineffective, surgery should provide good results. The lacertus fibrosus is released and the median nerve is translocated to a subcutaneous position anterior to the pronator teres muscle. The nerve should be exposed from the distal upper arm to the middle forearm. The median nerve and its major branches should be visualized. Care should be taken to preserve the branches of the medial cutaneous nerve of the forearm. Injury to this nerve can produce a painful neuroma.

Anterior Interosseous Nerve Syndrome

The anterior interosseous nerve syndrome originally was described by Kiloh and Nevin[10] who believed that the cause was neuritis. The anterior interosseous nerve separates from the main median nerve approximately 8 cm distal to the lateral epicondyle.[9] It gives off a sensory branch to the wrist joint and provides motor innervation to the flexor pollicis longus muscle, the flexor digitorum profundus muscle of the index and middle fingers, and the pronator quadratus muscles.[24] The site of compression is slightly more distal in the mass of the pronator teres muscle than that for the pronator syndrome. The compression is caused by the tendinous origin of the deep head of the pronator teres muscle, which crosses the anterior interosseous nerve at its origin from the parent median nerve. An enlarged bicipital bursa has also been described as the causative agent. Whereas pain and tenderness are present in the forearm of patients with the anterior interosseous nerve syndrome, the predominant symptoms and objective findings are motor.[9,25] Harter[9] noted that when untreated, the pain often resolves. Motor loss then follows. Characteristically, an abnormal pinch is produced because of the inability to flex the interphalangeal joint of the thumb.

Results of nerve conduction studies typically are normal in patients with the anterior interosseous nerve syndrome (JA Russell, personal communication, 1991). Results of needle electromyography indicate denervation restricted to the three muscles innervated by the nerve. Occasional patients may present clinically with the anterior interosseous nerve syndrome and with electrodiagnostic proof of a more proximal lesion of the median nerve. Presumably, the fascicles destined to become the anterior interosseous nerve are affected more selectively in this situation. The surgical exposure for patients with this syndrome is similar to that described for the pronator syndrome.[9]

Ulnar Nerve

In addition to the ulnar nerve compression found at the cubital tunnel, which is discussed in Chapter 6, ulnar neuropathies can be caused by compression at the arcade of Struthers and in Guyon's canal. Because the sensory symptoms are located on the medial aspect of the hand and arm, it is necessary to be certain that the condition is not caused by a C8 nerve root or lower brachial plexus lesion.

Arcade of Struthers

The arcade of Struthers (Figure 2A) is located where the ulnar nerve passes through the medial intermuscular septum into the posterior compartment.[24] The arcade is a fibrous septum that is located 8 cm proximal to the medial epicondyle. It is present in only 70% of patients. The arcade of Struthers is rarely a site of primary compression. It may, however, become important following an anterior transposition of the nerve as a proximal tether impinging on the nerve. It is important to release the band when transposing the nerve to prevent this secondary compression.

Guyon's Canal

Guyon's canal is found on the medial aspect of the wrist (Figure 2B). The anterior border of Guyon's canal is the volar carpal ligament, whereas the posterior border is the transverse carpal ligament.[9,14] Within the canal, the ulnar nerve runs with the ulnar artery and vein and divides into motor and sensory branches. The distal lesion affects only the motor branch, and the more proximal lesion affects both the motor and the sensory branch.[24] Because the motor branch is deeply placed and tethered as it passes around the hook of the hamate bone, it is prone to compressive lesions (GJ Gumley, personal communication, 1991). Space-occupying lesions, such as ganglia, produce compression as does chronic occupational trauma in cyclists and in persons who use their hands as hammers. Space-occupying lesions may be encountered in patients with fracture of the pisiform bone or hook of the hamate bone.

Pure motor paresis produces a clawhand as a result of intrinsic weakness and separation of the fourth and fifth fingers (Wartenberg's sign). Mixed nerve compression produces paresthesia and sensory loss as well as the typical clawhand.

Electrodiagnostic findings again depend on whether the lesion is predominantly axonal or demyelinating (JA Russell, personal communication, 1991). With demyelinating lesions, slowing of motor and sensory latencies across the wrist may be expected, particularly when sensory studies are performed by the palmar technique, and the motor conductions are performed while recording from the first dorsal interosseous muscle. In axonal lesions, motor and sensory amplitudes are reduced and denervation is found in the ulnar muscles of the hand. Reduced amplitude of the dorsal cutaneous branch of the ulnar nerve or denervation in the ulnar muscles of the forearm implies the existence of a lesion proximal to the wrist.

When the patient's condition does not respond to the use of splints and the administration of anti-inflammatory medications, the canal should be explored. Harter[9] suggested

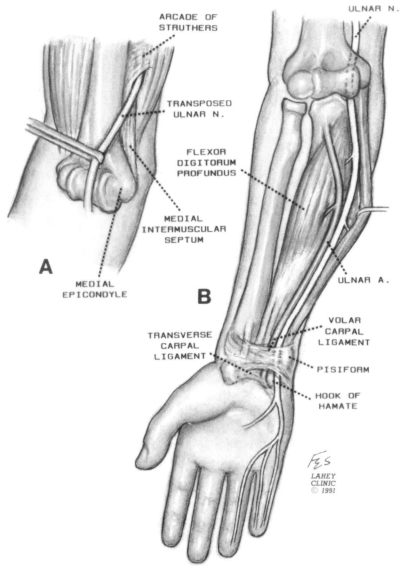

Figure 2. Ulnar nerve. A. Fibrous septum in the arcade of Struthers. B. Anatomic presentation of the ulnar nerve from above the elbow to the hand.

that surgery in this instance usually is indicated earlier than in patients with other compression neuropathies because of the motor involvement. Both superficial and deep branches of the nerve within the canal should be explored carefully. Any mass within the canal, such as a ganglion cyst or a displaced hook of the hamate bone, should be removed.

Radial Nerve

Compression neuropathies of the radial nerve produce clinical syndromes dependent on the level of compression (Figures 3 and 4).[9,14] The lesion in the proximal arm is rarely spontaneous but is associated with trauma, most commonly fracture of the humerus. "Sat-

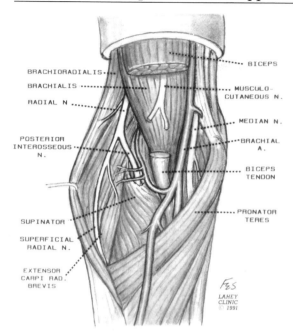

Figure 3. *Radial nerve. Anatomic demonstration of the radial nerve at the articulated fossa.*

urday night palsy" results from compression of the radial nerve when the patient sleeps heavily with the posterior arm resting against a firm edge. The patient presents with wristdrop and an inability to extend the fingers. This condition usually is associated with sensory loss because of the high level of the nerve injury. Of patients who present with radial nerve palsy, 80% recover spontaneously (GJ Gumley, personal communication, 1991); therefore, exploration is not performed early in most instances. If the palsy is associated with fracture of the humerus, however, early surgery may be appropriate. When the nerve is explored, it should be freed from the bone fragments or callus and reanastomosed when divided.

In patients with demyelinating lesions of the radial nerve at the middle to proximal humerus, results of conduction studies distal to the lesion are normal (JA Russell, personal communication, 1991). Studies performed proximal to the lesion will show a reduced or slowed motor response compared with stimulation distal to the lesion. In patients with axonal lesions, radial motor and sensory amplitudes are reduced and denervation is found in all radial muscles inner-

vated distal to the triceps muscle. Changes on electromyography are not observed until 3 weeks after the injury.

The radial nerve curves around the posterior humerus in the spiral groove and enters the anterior aspect of the arm, 10 cm proximal to the lateral epicondyle, by passing through the lateral intermuscular septum[9] (GJ Gumley, personal communication, 1991). The radial nerve passes anterior to the radiohumeral joint where it divides into superficial and deep branches. The superficial branch proceeds distally, deep to the brachioradialis muscle, to provide sensation to the dorsum of the first web space in the hand. The deep branch spirals around the neck of the radius, passing between the two heads of the supinator muscle, to enter the posterior aspect of the arm as the posterior interosseous nerve (Figure 4A). The deep branch supplies the extensor muscles of the wrist, hand, and thumb except for the extensor carpi radialis longus muscle, which is innervated by a branch from the radial nerve before it enters the supinator muscle.[9]

Radial Tunnel Syndrome

The clinical syndrome associated with compression of the deep branch of the radial nerve has been called the radial tunnel syndrome. It may be confused with tennis elbow. The radial tunnel syndrome, however, produces a deep somatic ache in the extensor muscles, usually exacerbated by exercise, without sensory or motor symptoms. Four potential sites of compression exist: **(1)** by fibrous bands anterior to the radial head (Figure 4B), **(2)** by vessels of the leash of Henry that pass over the radial nerve to supply the brachioradialis muscle, **(3)** by the tendinous margin of the extensor carpi radialis brevis muscle, and **(4)** by the arcade of Frohse,[23,24] which is the sharp ligamentous margin of the superficial head of the supinator muscle (Figure 4C). The latter is the most common site of compression.[23] This sharp edge is not present in the fetus. It is fibrotendinous in 30% of limbs. Spinner[23] postulated that the arcade of Frohse forms in response to repeated rotary movements of the arm. Spinner[23] found

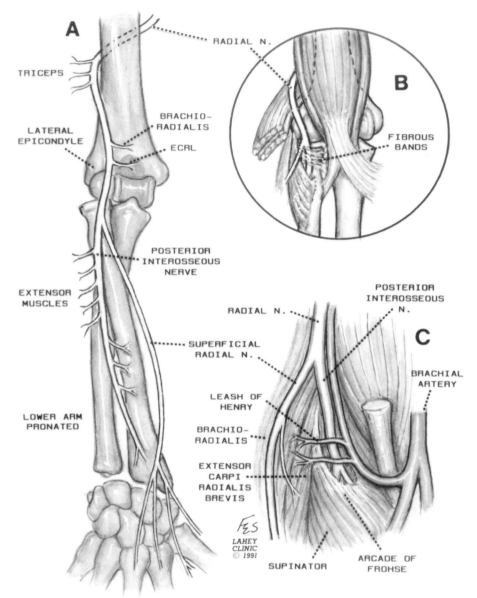

Figure 4. *A. Diagrammatic presentation of the radial nerve. B. Anatomic presentation demonstrates the radial nerve compressed by fibrous bands distal to the lateral epicondyle. C. Anatomic presentation demonstrates the radial nerve compressed at the arcade of Frohse and by vessels of the leash of Henry.*

this syndrome in the dominant arm in 89% of patients. Most patients have a history of repetitive trauma, such as is observed in bricklayers, pipe fitters, machine operators, orchestra conductors, and tennis players. Other causes of compression may be tumor, lipoma, synovial proliferation in rheumatoid arthritis, or fracture of the head of the radius.

Tennis Elbow

In discussing the broad diagnosis of tennis elbow, Roles and Maudsley[21] described a range of disorders from lateral epicondylitis to severe extensor weakness. They included the radial tunnel syndrome. On examination, tenderness is present over the lateral epicondyle of the humerus or just distal to the radial head where the nerve travels into the supinator muscle.[9] A typical increase in pain occurs when extension of the middle finger is resisted. This maneuver will tighten the origins of the extensor carpi radialis brevis muscle and further compress the nerve. Injury to the origin of the extensor carpi radialis brevis tendon at the lateral epicondyle is related to epicondylitis—the classic tennis elbow. Local injection with lidocaine and a corticosteroid provides only temporary relief of symptoms.

Results of electrodiagnostic studies may demonstrate delays in motor latencies from the spiral groove to the medial border of the extensor digitorum communis muscle, but they are frequently normal. For patients whose neuropathy does not respond to avoidance of trauma, use of splints, and administration of anti-inflammatory medications, surgical exploration with decompression of the superficial radial nerve is indicated.[24]

Posterior Interosseous Nerve Syndrome

The syndrome of the posterior interosseous nerve differs from the radial tunnel syndrome in that the predominant symptoms and findings are motor rather than pain or sensory loss.[24] The arcade of Frohse is the major constricting structure. Severe weakness of the radial innervated muscles exists with inability to extend the fingers at the metacarpophalangeal joint. The wrist dorsiflexes in a dorsoradial direction because of paralysis of the extensor carpi ulnaris and the extensor digitorum communis muscles.[24] The brachioradialis, extensor carpi radialis longus, extensor carpi radialis brevis, and supinator muscles are not weak because these muscles are innervated by branches that arise before the point at which the radial nerve enters the arcade of Frohse. In this syndrome, pain and local tenderness are followed by progressive motor loss.[9] When sensory loss is present, a more proximal lesion must be considered.

The electrodiagnostic findings of an axonal injury to the posterior interosseous nerve consist of normal radial sensory studies (JA Russell,

personal communication, 1991). Normal or reduced amplitude of the radial motor response occurs when recording from a distal radial nerve innervated muscle. Denervation will be found in all radial nerve innervated muscles excluding the triceps, brachioradialis, extensor carpi radialis longus, extensor carpi radialis brevis, and anconeus muscles.

For patients with the posterior interosseous nerve syndrome with significant motor findings, surgical exploration is indicated.[9] For patients with a less severe clinical course, rest, the use of splints, and the administration of anti-inflammatory medications are indicated.

Wartenberg's Syndrome

Wartenberg's syndrome is a rare syndrome that results from the compression of the superficial radial nerve in the forearm.[9,24] This syndrome is characterized by pain in the proximal forearm and hypoesthesia over the dorsal thumb. No weakness is present. The compression is usually caused by trauma or wearing a tight band or watch. Electrodiagnostic findings of a superficial radial neuropathy consist solely of a diminished or absent radial nerve sensory response (JA Russell, personal communication, 1991).

Suprascapular Nerve Entrapment Neuropathy

The suprascapular nerve is a mixed peripheral nerve that provides motor innervation to the supraspinatus and infraspinatus muscles (Figure 5).[20] The nerve has no cutaneous distribution but provides sensory supply to the posterior capsule of the shoulder joint. The syndrome of suprascapular nerve compression includes aching in the posterior aspect of the shoulder with weakness and ultimately atrophy of the muscles involved. Weakness and atrophy produce difficulty in lifting the arm overhead and weakness of external rotation. Wasting of the infraspinatus muscle is obvious because less tissue overlies the infraspinatus muscle. The lack of involvement of the deltoid and

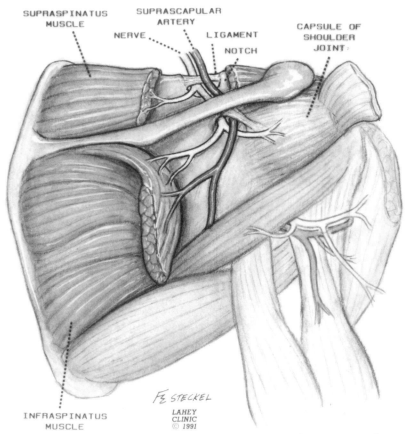

SUPRASPINATUS
MUSCLE

SUPRASCAPULAR
ARTERY

NERVE

LIGAMENT

NOTCH

CAPSULE OF
SHOULDER
JOINT

INFRASPINATUS
MUSCLE

F.E. STECKEL
LAHEY
CLINIC
© 1991

Figure 5. Suprascapular nerve. Anatomic drawing demonstrates the suprascapular nerve passing through the suprascapular notch and then around the spine of the scapula to the infraspinous fossa.

rhomboid muscles differentiates this lesion from a C5 nerve root lesion.

The suprascapular nerve begins as a branch from the upper trunk of the brachial plexus and runs parallel and lies deep to the inferior belly of the omohyoid muscle. It travels deep to the trapezius muscle and through the suprascapular notch into the supraspinous fossa. In the notch the suprascapular ligament compresses the nerve. The suprascapular artery passes superficial to the ligament. In the supraspinous fossa, the remainder of the nerve curves around the lateral margin of the spine to enter the infraspinous fossa. Rengachary and colleagues[19] described the shape of the suprascapular notch as a continuum between a widely patent notch and a bony foramen. The smaller notch is more likely to be involved with

entrapment neuropathy. These authors[19] demonstrated a sling effect in which the nerve is compressed by the sharp inferior edge of the ligament. Plain roentgenography of the scapula, visualizing the notch, may be helpful in establishing the diagnosis.

In a companion article, Rengachary and colleagues[18] provided a comparative study of the suprascapular notch. A suprascapular ligament is present in humans and New World monkeys but is not present in Old World monkeys and subprimates.

Repetitive trauma has been implicated in the origin of this neuropathy, although the author has observed it in patients with isolated trauma. Goldner,[7] in a discussion of the paper by Rengachary and colleagues,[19] described this injury in football players. Shabas and Scheiber[22] described the condition in a person who used poorly fitted crutches with excess shoulder depression and an exaggerated swing. They[22] also associated hammering and throwing a baseball with this palsy.

Conduction studies of the suprascapular nerve are not accomplished readily (JA Russell, personal communication, 1991). Denervation in the supraspinatus and infraspinatus muscles, sparing the cervical paraspinal, deltoid, and rhomboid muscles, is consistent with this diagnosis.

Clein[3] believes that surgical release of the nerve should be performed early. His opinion, which is similar to the author's, is that relief of pain is prompt, but that motor function returns slower.

Thoracic Outlet Syndrome

The thoracic outlet syndrome is a controversial subject. In some institutions, it is diagnosed and treated so often that one would think it constitutes a menace to public health. In other institutions, it is rarely diagnosed. Before the controversy is discussed, the conventionally held views regarding anatomy, symptoms, findings, and treatment are described.

Luoma and Nelems[11] recently reviewed the anatomy and various syndromes categorized under the umbrella of the thoracic outlet syndrome (Figure 6). The brachial neurovascular bundle goes through the thoracic outlet to enter the arm. The thoracic outlet is divided into the intrascalene triangle, the costoclavicular space, and the subcoracoid tunnel. Most cases of neurovascular compression occur in the first portion by an anomalous first rib or by fibromuscular bands running from the tip of an incomplete rib or a prominent C7 transverse process to the scalene tubercle of the first rib. Other acquired conditions that can compress the brachial plexus should be kept in mind, such as fracture with callus formation, aneurysms of the subclavian artery, and tumors (most commonly a Pancoast tumor).

Wilbourn[26] described five clinical syndromes. The first is a major arterial syndrome. This syn-

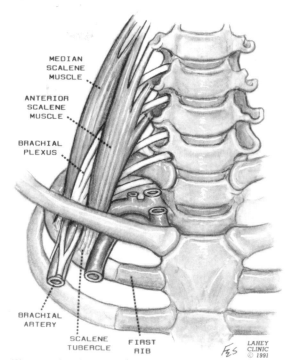

Figure 6. *Thoracic outlet. Anatomic drawing shows the relationship between the brachial artery and the brachial plexus, the anterior and middle scalene muscles, and the first rib and the clavicle.*

drome is associated with a bony anomaly, such as a cervical rib. The arterial wall is damaged and poststenotic dilatation occurs. Thrombus may be found in the vessel, disposing to distal emboli and Raynaud's phenomenon. This condition may constitute a surgical emergency.

The second is a minor arterial syndrome. Eighty percent of adults reduce or obliterate their radial pulse when they elevate, abduct, and externally rotate their arm. Using photoplethysmography during provocative tests in normal subjects, Gergoudis and Barnes[6] found considerable but asymptomatic arterial obstruction in 60% of subjects and bilateral obstruction in 33% of subjects.

The third is the venous obstruction syndrome. Spontaneous thrombosis of the subclavian or axillary vein may be observed in young adults after vigorous repetitive activity of the upper extremity. Cyanosis, swelling, and aching of the limb occur. The brachial plexus is not involved. The classification of this syndrome as a type of a thoracic outlet syndrome may not be correct.

The fourth is the true neurogenic thoracic outlet syndrome. The major component in this syndrome is weakness and wasting of the intrinsic muscles of the hand. This syndrome is also associated with intermittent aching in the medial forearm and is the only widely accepted thoracic outlet syndrome. The pathologic finding is usually the fibrous band from a rudimentary cervical rib to the first rib that compresses the lower trunk of the brachial plexus. In 75% of patients, all of the intrinsic muscles are weak and wasted. The thenar muscles are most severely wasted because the lower trunk plexopathy most severely affects median nerve fibers to the thenar eminence. Rarely will a patient with true neurogenic thoracic outlet syndrome have reduced ulnar sensory amplitude as well as reduced median and ulnar motor amplitude on the affected side (JA Russell, personal communication, 1991). Median, ulnar, and radial nerve innervated muscles, which are also innervated by the lower trunk and medial cord of the brachial plexus, will be denervated. Treatment is surgical removal of the offending band. The prognosis for the wasted muscle of the hand is poor.

The last group is termed by Wilbourn[26] as the "disputed neurogenic thoracic outlet syndrome." Most operations are performed for this group. Wilbourn[26] believes that the criteria for surgery are usually broad and poorly defined. This pain syndrome is without anatomic or physiologic changes. No objective clinical or laboratory findings exist. Results of electrodiagnostic studies are normal. No evidence is present to suggest that serious neural compression will occur if the condition is not treated. The incidence of documented neurosis and litigation is high in this group of patients. Wilbourn's[26] skepticism is echoed by Cherington[2] who believes that a moratorium should be placed on surgery for patients with the disputed thoracic outlet syndrome. Cherington[2] cited a significant complication rate associated with the operation. Postoperative evaluations by an independent neurologist reported persistence of symptoms in the face of the surgeon's report of excellent results.

In the thoracic outlet syndrome, as well as in the other entrapment neuropathies, careful evaluation of the history and physical examination and results of electrodiagnostic studies should permit proper selection of patients for treatment and performance of the appropriate surgical procedures.

References

1. Bieber EJ, Moore JR, Weiland AJ. Lipomas compressing the radial nerve at the elbow. *J Hand Surg Am.* 1986;11A:533–535.
2. Cherington M. Surgery for thoracic outlet syndrome? *N Engl J Med.* 1986;314:322.
3. Clein LJ. Suprascapular entrapment neuropathy. *J Neurosurg.* 1975;43:337–342.
4. Cohn L, Lowry RM, Hart S. Overuse syndromes of the upper extremity in interpreters for the deaf. *Orthopedics.* 1990;13:207–209.
5. Dumitru D, Walsh N, Visser B. Congenital hemihypertrophy associated with posterior interosseous nerve entrapment. *Arch Phys Med Rehabil.* 1988;69:696–698.
6. Gergoudis R, Barnes RW. Thoracic outlet arterial compression: prevalence in normal persons. *Angiology.* 1980;31:538–541.
7. Goldner JL. In discussion: Rengachary SS, Burr D, Lucas S, et al. Suprascapular entrapment neuropathy: a clinical, anatomical, and comparative study. II: anatomical study. *Neurosurgery.* 1979;5:451.
8. Gumley GJ. In discussion: Mackinnon SE, O'Brien JP, Dellon AL, et al. An assessment of the effects of internal neurolysis on a chronically compressed rat sciatic nerve. *Plast Reconstr Surg.* 1988;81:257–258.
9. Harter BT Jr. Indications for surgery in work-related compression neuropathies of the upper extremity. *Occup Med.* 1989;4:485–495.
10. Kiloh LG, Nevin S. Isolated neuritis of anterior interosseous nerve. *Br Med J.* 1952;1:850–851.
11. Luoma A, Nelems B. Thoracic outlet syndrome: thoracic surgery perspective. *Neurosurg Clin North Am.* 1991;2:187–226.
12. Mackinnon SE, McCabe S, Murray JF, et al. Internal neurolysis fails to improve the results of primary carpal tunnel decompression. *J Hand Surg Am.* 1991;16A:211–218.
13. Mackinnon SE, O'Brien JP, Dellon AL, et al. An assessment of the effects of internal neurolysis on a chronically compressed rat sciatic nerve. *Plast Reconstr Surg.* 1988;81:251–256.
14. Morgan RF, Stuart JD, Persing JA, et al. Peripheral nerve compression in the upper extremity. *Compr Ther.* May 1989;15:23–33.
15. Osterman AL. The double crush syndrome. *Orthop Clin North Am.* 1988;19:147–155.
16. Peimer CA. Compression neuropathies in the upper extremity. *Orthop Rev.* 1987;16:379–385.

17. Phalen GS. The birth of a syndrome, *or* carpal tunnel revisited. *J Hand Surg.* 1981;6:109–110.

18. Rengachary SS, Burr D, Lucas S, et al. Suprascapular entrapment neuropathy: a clinical, anatomical, and comparative study. II: anatomical study. *Neurosurgery.* 1979;5:447–451.

19. Rengachary SS, Burr D, Lucas S, et al. Suprascapular entrapment neuropathy: a clinical, anatomical, and comparative study, III: comparative study. *Neurosurgery.* 1979;5:452–455.

20. Rengachary SS, Neff JP, Singer PA, et al. Suprascapular entrapment neuropathy: a clinical, anatomical, and comparative study, I: clinical study. *Neurosurgery.* 1979;5:441–446.

21. Roles NC, Maudsley RH. Radial tunnel syndrome: resistant tennis elbow as a nerve entrapment. *J Bone Joint Surg BR.* 1972;54B:499–508.

22. Shabas D, Scheiber M. Suprascapular neuropathy related to the use of crutches: case report. *Am J Phys Med.* 1986;65:298–300.

23. Spinner M. The arcade of Frohse and its relationship to posterior interosseous nerve paralysis. *J Bone Joint Surg BR.* 1968;50B:809–812.

24. Spinner M, Spencer PS. Nerve compression lesions of the upper extremity: a clinical and experimental review. *Clin Orthop.* 1974;104:46–67.

25. Stern MB. The anterior interosseous nerve syndrome (the Kiloh-Nevin syndrome): report and follow-up study of three cases. *Clin Orthop.* 1984;187:223–227.

26. Wilbourn AJ. Thoracic outlet syndromes: a plea for conservatism. *Neurosurg Clin North Am.* 1991;2:235–245.

CHAPTER 5

Carpal Tunnel Syndrome

Brian K. Willis, MD

The carpal tunnel syndrome is the most common entrapment neuropathy. With the report by Cannon and Love[8] in 1946 of the favorable outcome in nine patients with median nerve entrapment at the wrist who underwent carpal tunnel release and neurolysis, the syndrome became increasingly recognized. During the next two decades, Phalen[30] championed and immensely popularized the relatively simple operation. Carpal tunnel release is now the most common hand operation performed.[24] Though the procedure is generally associated with low morbidity and relatively high success rates, failure of the surgeon to fully understand the anatomy, pathophysiology, and typical features of carpal tunnel syndrome, as well as the many pitfalls associated with its diagnosis and treatment, may lead to an unacceptable incidence of suboptimal results.

Anatomy

The median nerve originates from the lateral and medial cords of the brachial plexus and carries in it axons entering or leaving the spinal cord through the C6,7,8 and T1 nerve roots. It passes down the arm in the neurovascular compartment adjacent to the brachial artery but gives off no branches until the forearm and hand. In the forearm, the median nerve innervates numerous wrist and digital flexors of the preaxial muscular compartment. Though the sensory distribution of the median nerve in the hand closely approximates the C6 and 7 dermatomes, its motor fibers innervate intrinsic muscles of the hand within the C8 and T1 myotomes.

The abductor pollicis brevis, which abducts the thumb at a right angle to the palm, and the opponens pollicis, which flexes and opposes the thumb, are the most important of the median-innervated muscles of the hand. These two muscles of the thenar eminence are innervated by the recurrent motor branch that typically arises from the median nerve just distal to the flexor retinaculum. Damage to this nerve produces loss of thumb opposition and hence significant difficulties with grasp. Other muscles innervated include the superficial (flexor) pollicis brevis and the first and second lumbricals. The median nerve supplies sensory fibers to the radial three and one-half digits via the common palmar digital branches. The area over the thenar eminence, however, is supplied by the palmar cutaneous branch, which leaves the median nerve just proximal to and runs superficial to the transverse carpal ligament (Figure 1). Numerous variations in the origin and course of this surgically important cutaneous branch may be encountered. The branch may have origin on the ulnar side of the nerve, or it may course under or through the transverse carpal ligament.[10]

The transverse carpal ligament, or flexor retinaculum, is a dense ligament measuring approximately 4 cm in width, 5–6 cm in length, and 2.5–3.6 mm in thickness. It stretches transversely across the concavity of the carpal bones and converts their arch into a fibrous tunnel.[31] Referred to as the *carpal tunnel,* here the median nerve travels in its most superficial

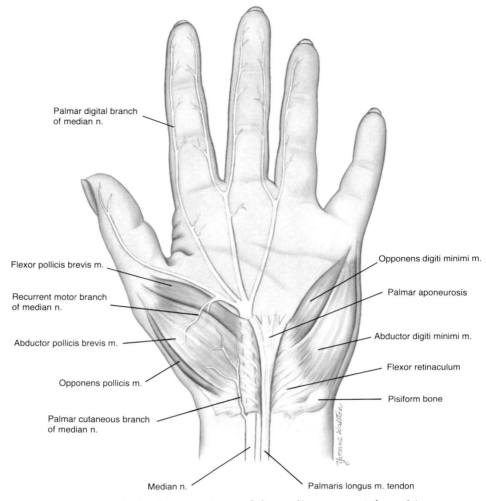

Figure 1. Pertinent anatomy of the median nerve at the wrist.

course as it and a number of synovium-invested tendons pass into the hand. In 10% of individuals, a small persistent median artery also will be found coursing through this tunnel. The tendon of the palmaris longus muscle passes superficial to the transverse carpal ligament and inserts into the palmar aponeurosis, a tough stratum of connective tissue that blends into the deep palmar aspect of the transverse carpal ligament. This tendon acts as a useful landmark as the median nerve lies just radial to it. The transverse carpal ligament acts in part as a point of origin for the muscles of the thenar and hypothenar eminences.

Like the palmar cutaneous branch, there are numerous variations in the course of the recur-

rent motor branch of the median nerve; however, in 95% of cases, the motor branch will take one of three courses. The most common point of origin is the radial side of the median nerve just distal to the transverse carpal ligament, frequently arising in common with the first common palmar digital nerve. The motor branch then courses directly to the thenar muscles (Figure 1). The second most common site is an origination from the median nerve as it travels beneath the transverse carpal ligament. The branch then passes around and over the distal edge of the ligament to the thenar muscles. An origin of the motor branch from beneath the transverse ligament with a transligamentous course is the third most common.[21] In rare cases, the motor nerve may arise from the ulnar aspect of the median nerve or may even travel for a short course on top of the distal edge of the transverse ligament. In cases of persistent median artery, the median nerve may have a high division; that is, the motor branch make take origin many centimeters proximal to the wrist.[10,18,21,32]

Epidemiology and Etiology

The carpal tunnel syndrome affects women somewhat more often than men, though the actual incidence in each sex is not entirely clear. Fifty percent of cases occur in the fifth and sixth decades.[14,15] Frequently, the patient's occupation will require repetitive wrist motion or prolonged pressure to the "heel" of the hand. Recreational-related trauma to the hand or wrist is increasingly becoming a factor in development of this entrapment syndrome. Five to ten percent of all patients will relate a history of recent or remote injury to the wrist.[30,31]

Numerous systemic diseases have been associated with an increased predisposition to development of carpal tunnel syndrome. Rheumatoid arthritis, amyloidosis, acromegaly, and hypothyroidism predispose the median nerve to compression within the carpal tunnel due to thickening and hypertrophy of the ligaments and other connective tissues. The carpal tunnel syndrome is also more likely to occur in association with diseases that produce demyelinating or ischemic neuropathies, such as diabetes mellitus, renal failure, or alcoholism. Pyridoxine (vitamin B6) deficiency has likewise been suggested to be an etiologic factor.[1,13] Transient symptoms of median nerve compression are very common during pregnancy and usually resolve spontaneously after delivery.[17,35] Any mass lesion within the carpal tunnel may produce median nerve impingement, such as neurofibromas, ganglion cysts, and other benign tumors. Anomalous muscles and tendons, as well as a persistent median artery or other vascular anomalies, have been reported to produce the carpal tunnel syndrome.[4,6,26] Other local conditions, such as synovial inflam-

mation and fibrosis (as is observed in tenosynovitis), fracture of the carpal bones, and thermal injuries to the hand or forearm may be associated with the carpal tunnel syndrome.[32]

Phalen argues for a common etiology for many of the idiopathic cases. During the course of decompressing the carpal tunnel, Phalen biopsied the synovium of the flexor tendon lying beneath the median nerve. Chronic inflammation and fibrosis of the flexor synovialis, consistent with tenosynovitis, were found in 126 of 148 biopsy specimens. Phalen also believes a vasomotor imbalance from sympathetic dysfunction may play a role in the disease process, though there is no scientific evidence to substantiate this.[30]

In essence, any disease process that reduces the cross-sectional area of the carpal tunnel or increases the volume of its contents may produce median nerve compression and entrapment, especially if a concurrent neuropathy predisposes the nerve to injury from compressive lesions.

Clinical Diagnosis

Symptoms

Carpal tunnel syndrome is characterized by a typical discomfort and numbness of the lateral three digits (radial half of the hand). The pain is often described by the patient as bothersome "pins and needles" paresthesias, though occasionally the pain will have more of a deep, aching quality. The pain may affect the entire hand or, in atypical cases, radiate proximally into the forearm, upper arm, or even the shoulder, producing symptoms that can be confused easily with a C6 nerve root compression syndrome.[14,20,32] The syndrome is frequently bilateral, though the symptoms are usually worse in the dominant hand.[15]

A feature quite distinctive of carpal tunnel syndrome is *nocturnal exacerbation* of the symptoms. The patient frequently complains of being awakened by pain during the early morning hours. Shaking and massaging the affected hand often relieve the discomfort. It has been suggested that akinesia during sleep leads to venous stasis in the extremities, which exacerbates compression of the median nerve within the already restrictive carpal tunnel. By shaking and moving the hands, venous return is improved, causing a reduction in the pressure within the tunnel, thus relieving the uncomfortable paresthesias.[33] Strenuous use of the hands, especially with repetitive or forceful flexion movements of the wrist, may also aggravate the symptoms.

In contrast to ulnar neuropathy at the elbow, it is unusual for weakness and atrophy to be present in the early stages of carpal tunnel syndrome. Thenar atrophy and weakness of thumb opposition are hallmarks of advanced disease. Interestingly, the rare patient who initially presents with weakness and atrophy frequently has little pain.[32]

Findings

The history alone usually establishes the diagnosis of carpal tunnel syndrome. Abnormal findings on neurologic examination may support the diagnosis in patients with less typical symptoms, though objective abnormalities are generally sparse except in more advanced cases. Hypesthesia in the median nerve distribution may be found, except over the thenar eminence and base of the palm. This is due to the palmar cutaneous branch of the median nerve arising proximal to and passing superficial to the transverse carpal ligament. This sensory branch is frequently spared the effects of entrapment within the carpal tunnel. Motor deficits are seen less frequently. The two most important muscles innervated by the distal median nerve are the opponens pollicis and the abductor pollicis brevis. The first is tested by having the patient oppose the thumb to the palm and draw it medially toward the base of the fifth digit against resistance. The latter is tested by resisting active abduction of the thumb away from the plane of the palm. Significant and long-standing denervation to these muscles leads to atrophy of the thenar eminence.

Two-thirds of patients will experience electrical sensations radiating into the palm and first three digits when the median nerve at the wrist crease is percussed.[15,30] This is known as *Tinel's sign,* which classically has been associated with median nerve entrapment at the wrist; however, recent reports suggest this test to be of dubious value in establishing the diagnosis of carpal tunnel syndrome due to a high incidence of false-positive results in otherwise asymptomatic individuals.[5,32] A more accurate predictor of carpal tunnel syndrome is *Phalen's wrist-flexion test.* The patient is asked to hold the forearms up in a vertical orientation with the wrists flexed for 60 seconds. Reproduction of the patient's painful dysesthesias provides a high degree of certainty of the diagnosis.[14,30] Likewise, inflating a blood pressure cuff placed around the arm may reproduce the symptoms. Again, symptom exacerbation in this test is likely due to venous distention within the rigid confines of the carpal tunnel.[33]

Electrodiagnostics

Electromyography and nerve conduction velocities should be obtained to confirm, not to establish, the diagnosis of carpal tunnel syndrome. Indications for surgery should not rest solely on the results of this test, but rather should be based on clinical judgment. Electrodiagnostic studies are helpful in differentiating the carpal tunnel syndrome from other disorders, such as cervical nerve root impingement or syndromes of the thoracic outlet.

The most sensitive and the earliest abnormality found is a prolonged sensory conduction latency across the wrist. Normally, the distal latency through the carpal tunnel to the abductor pollicis brevis is less than 4.5 milliseconds. A prolonged motor latency generally occurs later in the entrapment process. The amplitude of the action potential is frequently diminished. Denervation potentials in the opponens pollicis and abductor pollicis brevis indicate advanced and probably irreversible damage to the median nerve.

Nerve conduction velocities and latencies are subject to a number of physiologic variables, such as the age and metabolic status of the patient, as well as the temperature, vascular supply, and extent of edema in the arm. Numerous technical problems are associated with the determination itself. The treating physician or surgeon is responsible for being aware of the variability of the test and for assessing the results in light of the patient's clinical evaluation. Should the electrodiagnostic studies be equivocal, it might be prudent to wait up to 4–6 weeks to repeat the study before embarking on a course of surgical management.[14] Though electrical abnormalities may not be evident in up to 10% of clinical cases of carpal tunnel syndrome,[7,19] many surgeons will not consider decompression of the carpal tunnel without electrodiagnostic confirmation.[34]

Differential Diagnosis

The surgeon should be aware of the similarity between carpal tunnel syndrome and other pathologic processes that cause pain and neurologic dysfunction of the radial aspect of the forearm and hand. These include brachial plexopathy from tumor, trauma, or inflammation, and, less often, thoracic outlet syndrome. The most common of these, however, is C6 and C7 radiculopathy caused by cervical disk herniation or spondylosis. Typically, this pain seems to originate in the neck and shoulder and radiates down the arm in a lancinating fashion into the radial aspect of the hand. Exacerbation of the pain with movement of the cervical spine is a significant diagnostic factor in this pain syndrome. In general, C6 and C7 nerve root compression produces motor deficits in the upper arm, such as biceps or triceps weakness, and diminished deep tendon reflexes. The intrinsic hand muscles are relatively unaffected.

The median nerve may become entrapped at locations other than the carpal tunnel. The pronator syndrome is produced by median nerve compression at one of a number of locations around the distal humerus, elbow, and proximal forearm. Entrapment at these sites produces pain on the volar surface of the forearm and hypesthesia of the radial half of the hand. Weakness of the thenar muscles is observed less often. Symptoms are usually aggravated by exertion, especially with forceful flexion of the elbow or pronation of the forearm. Phalen's wrist-flexion test is typically negative. Likewise, the anterior interosseous syndrome causes pain in the proximal forearm. This pain is exacerbated by exercise and relieved by rest. Because it affects the anterior interosseous branch distal to where it leaves the median nerve in the cubital fossa, the motor and sensory innervation of the hand is not directly affected, though pain may be referred into the hand.

Carpal tunnel syndrome may coexist with other lesions of the nerve roots, brachial plexus, or median nerve. Concurrent cervical radiculopathy has been found in over 10% of electrically proven carpal tunnel syndrome. This is referred to as the *double-crush syndrome.*[25,27,36] This putative syndrome is based on the concept that proximal compression of a nerve may weaken the nerve's ability to withstand a more distal compression.

Management

Nonoperative Therapy

Many cases of carpal tunnel syndrome, especially mild cases or those that present early in the evolution of the disease process, are self-limiting and resolve spontaneously without need for surgical intervention. In cases related to systemic illnesses, such as hypothyroidism or acromegaly, treatment of the underlying illness may result in improvement or even resolution of entrapment symptoms.

The occurrence of the carpal tunnel syndrome in pregnancy is thought to be related to fluid retention in connective tissues about the wrist.[30,32] Nocturnal and exertional dysesthesias in the radial half of the palm occur in 10% to 25% of pregnant women. When the carpal tunnel syndrome occurs, the symptoms are more often bilateral. Onset of symptoms is typically during the third trimester. Relief occurs spontaneously, within a few weeks of delivery, in the majority of cases. Because of its transient nature, carpal tunnel syndrome during pregnancy is best treated by using conservative measures, such as splinting and analgesics.[17,35]

In the rare case of severe pain refractory to nonoperative therapy, it is reasonable to proceed with carpal tunnel decompression using a local anesthetic. That subsequent pregnancies are frequently associated with repeated episodes of carpal tunnel syndrome confirms the association of carpal tunnel syndrome and pregnancy.[14]

Short-term immobilization of the wrist by splinting is among the most commonly used of nonoperative therapies. In general, the splint is worn only at night, though patients with diurnal dysesthetic pain should wear the splint at all times. It is important that the splint be constructed such that no pressure overlies the median nerve at the wrist. In the author's experience, if symptoms are not alleviated or improved after 6-8 weeks of splinting, further conservative management is unproductive. The patient is then offered the option of surgical decompression.

Diuretics may prove helpful in patients with carpal tunnel syndrome related to excessive fluid retention, such as is observed in congestive heart failure.[3] Control of hyperglycemia in diabetics and weight loss in obese patients also may be of benefit in alleviating symptoms. Adequate analgesia may be obtained from nonsteroidal anti-inflammatory drugs, though their long-term efficacy in the treatment of carpal tunnel syndrome has not been determined. Pyridoxine administration has not gained widespread acceptance as a useful therapy. If development of the syndrome is occupation related, an alteration of work activities or even a change of occupation may be necessary.

Much has been written about the use of corticosteroid injections into the carpal tunnel, but few objective reports of positive results are available. Gelberman et al reported their results of a prospective trial of steroid injection and splinting. Patients with mild and early symptoms noted a beneficial effect after 3 weeks; however, those patients with more profound symptoms failed to respond to this therapy.[16] Others feel steroid injections may alleviate symptoms though only temporarily.[14,34] In the last decade, enthusiasm for this treatment modality has waned. Its primary indication, however, may remain as a means of controlling symptoms during temporary or reversible causes of carpal tunnel syndrome, such as is observed during pregnancy, or following failed carpal tunnel syndrome surgery.

Administration of corticosteroids into the carpal tunnel must be precise in order to avoid injury to the median nerve. A 25-gauge needle is inserted into the wrist at a point 1 cm proximal to the flexion crease between the tendons of the palmaris longus and the flexor carpi radialis and at an angle of 45 degrees to the long axis of the forearm. The needle is advanced approximately 1 cm until the flexor retinaculum is pierced. If painful dysesthesias in the distribution of the median nerve are produced, the needle is withdrawn and reinserted at a slightly different location. One to two milliliters of a mixture of triamcinolone or a similar corticosteroid and 1% lidocaine are slowly injected. If the patient does not obtain relief following the first injection, further injections, in general, should not be pursued.[16,30]

Surgical Therapy

The indications for carpal tunnel release are **(1)** rapidly progressive thenar wasting and hand dysfunction, or **(2)** substantial symptoms that are unrelieved by conservative measures. The surgeon should be confident of the diagnosis and have thoroughly excluded other causes of hand dysfunction and pain.

In cases of bilateral carpal tunnel syndrome, it is rarely necessary to operate on both hands simultaneously. The more severely affected hand (or in the case of symmetric disease, the nondominant hand) should be decompressed first. Surgery on the contralateral hand may be performed 6 weeks later, after the first hand has recovered and has regained full function. Most would agree that the patient undergoing simultaneous bilateral procedures would be rendered functionally impaired and quite dependent, albeit for a short period of time. Often the symptoms in the less severely affected hand will spontaneously resolve in the interim and will not require operative intervention. In Gainer and Nugent's series of 430 cases, only one-third of patients with bilateral carpal tunnel syndrome required bilateral operations. When bilateral surgery was needed, an interval between operations of at least 3 weeks was allowed.[15] Conversely, Cseuz et al[9] reported 313 cases of carpal tunnel syndrome; one-half of their patients presented with bilateral symptoms and underwent simultaneous bilateral decompressions.

Rarely does a patient require general anesthesia to undergo carpal tunnel release. The author prefers a regional block or, if the anesthesiologist is not well versed in this technique, a locally administered anesthetic agent. The use of a tourniquet is unnecessary.

There are as many methods of incision as there are surgeons performing carpal tunnel releases (Figure 2). The type of incision is of little importance as long as it follows three basic guidelines: **(1)** The incision should be designed to avoid potential division of the palmar cutaneous branch of the median nerve; **(2)** It should be carried far enough into the palm to confidently divide the most distal aspect of the ligament in its entirety; and **(3)** If it is to cross the flexion crease of the wrist, it should not do so in a perpendicular fashion.

A simple transverse wrist incision, though widely used in the past, is discouraged. This incision does not offer adequate exposure of the deep palm in order to ensure that the thickest and most distal portion of the transverse carpal ligament has been completely divided. In addition, the palmar cutaneous branch of the median nerve may be inadvertently divided, producing numbness over the thenar eminence or pain related to neuroma formation. As has been previously and eloquently stated, ''There is no doubt that unless the transverse carpal ligament is seen throughout its course, the completeness of division will remain a matter of hope, faith, and speculation.''[22]

Once the incision is made, sharp dissection is carried through the subcutaneous fatty tissue to the underlying anterior antebrachial fascia in the distal forearm and wrist and the palmar aponeurosis in the hand. Loupe magnification and headlamp illumination improve the visualization of anatomic structures. Hemostasis is maintained throughout the procedure by coagulating and dividing the small subcutaneous vessels using bipolar electrocautery. The author prefers to approach the transverse carpal ligament at its proximal extent, where tissue plains are thinner and more easily dissected. Beneath the superficial fascia, the tendon of the palmaris longus is encountered. The division of the transverse carpal ligament begins just radial to this easily identifiable tendon. Rarely, the palmaris longus tendon may overlie and appear to compress the median nerve when the wrist is extended. The author has on one occasion divided this tendon in order to complete the decompression with good results. Others have likewise described this phenomenon.[4,6,12]

The transverse carpal ligament is sharply divided using a No. 15 blade or fine Metzenbaum scissors. The division is performed under direct vision. The incision is made on the ulnar side of the median nerve where the palmar cutaneous and the recurrent motor branches are less likely to be encountered. As the dissection crosses the wrist into the palm, the transverse carpal ligament becomes noticeably tougher and thicker. The muscles of the thenar and hypothenar eminences originate from the transverse ligament at this site.

Deeper in the palm, the fibers of the palmar aponeurosis begin to blend with those of the transverse ligament, thus increasing its thickness and tenacity. Here it is of utmost importance to proceed cautiously and with vigilance for an aberrant course of the recurrent motor branch. A grooved dissector may be placed beneath the ligament in order to guide the knife blade through the tissues. The ligament may be incised likewise with a scissors throughout its entire length. The decompression is incomplete until the transverse ligament is divided in its entirety. The median nerve itself is then examined for pseudoneuroma formation or compression from adjacent masses, such as neurofibromas or ganglion cysts. The underlying flexor synovialis is also examined; presence of severe tenosynovitis is of prognostic importance. Internal neurolysis or epineurolysis is not routinely performed unless the procedure is a re-exploration with the only significant

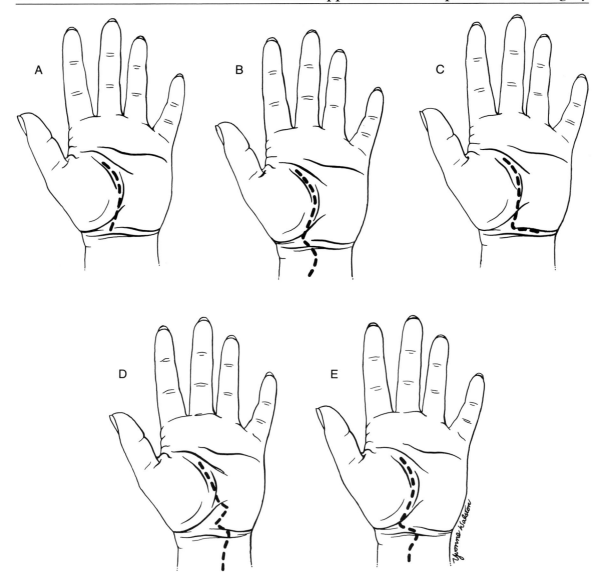

Figure 2. *Variations in incision for carpal tunnel release. A. Incision as described by Ariyan and Watson[2] and Ebob.[12] B. As described by Posch and Nugent.[29] C. By Das and Brown.[10] D. By Eversmann.[14] E. Author's preferred incision. Note that all incisions are carried deep into the palm and do not perpendicularly cross the wrist crease.*

finding being scarring in and about the nerve. The wound is then closed with a subcutaneous or subcuticular absorbable suture, taking care not to reapproximate the transverse carpal ligament over the median nerve. Nylon suture is used to reapproximate the thick palmar skin. Steristrips™ are placed over the incision at the wrist and distal forearm. A bulky dressing is placed and the hand wrapped lightly with an elastic bandage. It is important that the patient be reminded to keep the hand elevated above the level of the heart for at least 24 hours to limit postoperative edema and venous congestion.

Postoperative Management

The patient's hand should be bandaged with bulky dressing material in the palm for 1 week after surgery. Active flexion and extension of the digits as well as thumb abduction and opposition are encouraged to prevent the effects of prolonged immobilization. Bulky dressings are discontinued and the sutures are removed 1–2 weeks after surgery. The hand is placed back into night splints for the next few weeks. The patient is allowed to gradually increase the use of the hand but is discouraged from strong gripping or other exertional uses until 6 weeks postoperatively, at which time the patient is allowed to resume full activities. In patients with significant motor deficits, physiotherapy or hand rehabilitation is instituted at 4–6 weeks following surgery.

Generally, relief of painful dysesthesias occurs almost immediately following carpal tunnel release. Should the pain and tingling persist, the possibility of incomplete division of the transverse carpal ligament or of erroneous diagnosis should be entertained. A deep, aching sensation exacerbated by activity may develop in the thenar and hypothenar eminences and distal forearm related to swelling at the base of the palm. Referred to as "pillar pain," the condition is self-limiting and generally resolves within a few months.[14] Sensory deficits should show definite improvement by 6–12 weeks, though motor deficits are much slower to resolve. In cases of severe denervation and atrophy, complete recovery of motor function should not be expected.

Outcome

Results of Nonoperative Therapy

In Posch and Marcotte's[31] large review of over 1,200 patients with carpal tunnel syndrome, one-half obtained relief of their symptoms with nonoperative therapy. In those patients unrelieved by splinting and nonsteroidal analgesics, additional benefit may be obtained from steroidal injections into the carpal ligament; however, the effect is generally only temporary and 65% to 90% of patients undergoing this treatment modality will experience recurrence of symptoms.[14]

Results of Surgery

Relief of pain and improvement in motor and sensory deficits occur in 90% of patients undergoing carpal tunnel release. Gainer and Nugent[15] and Cseuz et al[9] reported their experience with 430 cases and 313 cases, respectively. Their surgical techniques were similar as were their results. Complete or near complete resolution of signs and symptoms was achieved in 82% of cases with an additional 10% obtaining moderate relief. The remaining 8% achieved little or no relief or were worse. Similarly, Posch and Marcotte[31] reported only a 10% failure to provide significant symptomatic relief in over 600 cases. Poor surgical outcomes fall into two main categories: **(1)** failure to relieve symptoms and **(2)** adverse effects and complications. The former is more common, probably related to failure to completely divide the transverse carpal ligament or to adequately manage other compressive lesions within the carpal tunnel. A significant number of surgical failures, however, may be due to misdiagnosis, such as mistaking cervical radiculopathy, brachial plexopathy, or diabetic neuropathy for carpal tunnel compression. This may be especially true if surgical indications are based on electrodiagnostic tests alone without appropriate regard for the clinical presentation and physical findings.

Mackinnon classified postoperative failures into four groups: **(1)** neurologic complications, such as injury to the palmar cutaneous branch and other neural elements, **(2)** vascular injury, including palmar hematomas, **(3)** tendon problems, such as bowstringing, tendon adhesions, and trigger finger, and **(4)** wound complications, including infection, wound dehiscence, and hypertrophic or painful scarring across the wrist crease.[24]

Except in cases of incomplete sectioning of the ligament and wound problems, reexploration following failed carpal tunnel release may prove disappointing and of limited benefit.[11]

Avoidance of Complications

Adverse effects and complications of carpal tunnel release are under-reported. Only those authors who deal with a large volume of patients referred for failure of prior decompressions have adequate data for evaluation.[24] Louis et al reported on such a group of patients, 26 of whom had undergone prior carpal tunnel release that resulted in postoperative complications. Fourteen patients had painful neuromas related to division of the palmar cutaneous branch, making this the most common complication. In two patients, failure to relieve symptoms was related to the use of transverse wrist incisions. Painful and hypertrophic scarring from perpendicular wrist incisions was observed in three patients. Two patients experienced stiffness of the interphalangeal joints following prolonged immobilization, two had neuromas of the superficial branch of the radial nerve, and three experienced dysesthesia, possibly secondary to reflex sympathetic dystrophy.[22] In a series of 186 patients reported by MacDonald et al[23], there were 34 complications in 22 patients. The complications included 12 cases of incomplete division of the transverse carpal ligament (in 8 of these cases, a transverse incision was used), 11 injuries to the palmar cutaneous branch of the median nerve, 4 cases of reflex sympathetic dystrophy, 2 each of hypertrophic scarring (from perpendicular incisions), palmar hematoma, and "bowstringing" of the flexor tendons, and 1 case of adherence of flexor tendons.[23] Superficial wound infections have been reported to occur in 0.5% to 6% of cases.[2,15] Fortunately, injury to the recurrent motor branch is a rarely reported complication.

In recent series by Eason et al analyzing suboptimal results of carpal tunnel release, over one-half of the patients evaluated were involved in litigation concerning Worker's Compensation or automobile, machinery, or medical malpractice liability.[11]

Retinaculotomy

This unique technique, about which little is written, deserves additional comment. In 1983, Paine and Polyzoidis described an innovative method of carpal tunnel release using a retinaculotome.[29] In their technique, a small transverse wrist incision is made centered over the palmaris longus tendon. The flexor retinaculum is opened medial to the median nerve and the retinaculotome is inserted. This instrument has a blunt foot plate beneath a sharp vertically oriented blade and is designed to acutely incise the ligament while deflecting the underlying median nerve. The instrument is passed beneath the transverse carpal ligament, dividing the ligament as it is advanced more distally into the palm. The procedure is repeated in a proximal direction to divide the remaining ligament. Adequacy of ligament division is determined by feel and sound, which the authors describe as being quite characteristic. In their review of 516 "closed" procedures using the retinaculotome, 89% of their patients reported satisfactory results. Their few failures were thought to be due to incomplete division of the ligament. Wound hematomas occurred in less than 1% of the cases. They reported no injuries to the recurrent motor branch.

Pagnanelli and Barrer reported a series of 577 hands decompressed using a slight modification of the Paine and Polyzoidis "closed" retinacultotomy.[28] Satisfactory results were obtained in 93% of cases. Complications were minor and few; no injuries to the median nerve or its branches occurred. Length of postoperative recovery appeared to be shorter with this technique as compared to the more traditional "open" procedure, and incisional discomfort was perhaps lessened.

Despite the comparable results achieved by closed retinaculotomy, it has not gained widespread acceptance among surgeons performing carpal tunnel release. However, the limited experience with this innovative technique challenges surgical dogma that the transverse carpal ligament must be divided its entire length under direct visualization. Further experience is needed to evaluate the role of this procedure in the surgical treatment of carpal tunnel syndrome.

Summary

Carpal tunnel syndrome is a common affliction, especially among persons whose occupations require repetitive wrist motion. Numerous systemic disease processes can predispose to the development of this disorder. Symptoms are quite characteristic as are physical findings; however, because of occasional similarity between other nerve compression syndromes, electrodiagnostic tests may be necessary to confirm the diagnosis of carpal tunnel syndrome. Early and mild cases are frequently self-limiting and resolve with time or conservative measures. This is especially true with regard to pregnancy-induced carpal tunnel syndrome. Symptoms are adequately managed in one-half of the cases by using wrist splinting, analgesics, physiotherapy, and occasionally steroid injections into the carpal tunnel. In those cases unrelieved by nonoperative means, surgical decompression of the carpal tunnel can be undertaken with an 80% to 90% success rate. Surgical failures can be minimized if care is taken to avoid injury to the palmar cutaneous and recurrent motor branches of the median nerve, and if an incision is made that avoids hypertrophic scarring in the wrist yet allows adequate visualization for division of the distal extent of the transverse carpal ligament.

With a proper understanding of the anatomy, pathophysiology, clinical presentation, and available treatment modalities for median nerve entrapment at the wrist, the surgeon can expect to offer substantial relief to the majority of his or her patients afflicted with carpal tunnel syndrome.

References

1. Amadio PC. Pyridoxine as an adjunct in the treatment of carpal tunnel syndrome. *J Hand Surg Am.* 1985;10A:237–241.

2. Ariyan S, Watson HK. The palmar approach for the visualization and release of the carpal tunnel: an analysis of 429 cases. *Plast Reconstr Surg.* 1977; 60:539–547.

3. Arnold AG. The carpal tunnel syndrome in congestive cardiac failure. *Postgrad Med J* 1977;53:623–624.

4. Backhouse KM, Churchill-Davidson D. Anomalous palmaris longus muscle producing carpal tunnel-like compression. *Hand.* 1975;7:22–24.

5. Bowles AP Jr, Asher SW, Pickett JB. Use of Tinel's sign in carpal tunnel syndrome. *Ann Neurol.* 1983;13:689–690.

6. Brones MF, Wilgis EFS. Anatomical variations of the *palmaris longus,* causing carpal tunnel syndrome: case reports. *Plast Reconstr Surg.* 1978;62:798–800.

7. Buchthal F, Rosenfalck A, Trojaborg W. Electrophysiological findings in entrapment of the median nerve at wrist and elbow. *J Neurol Neurosurg Psychiatry.* 1974;37:340–360.

8. Cannon BW, Love JG: Tardy median palsy, median neuritis; median thenar neuritis amenable to surgery. *Surgery.* 1946;20:210–216.

9. Csuez KA, Thomas JE, Lambert EH, et al. Long-term results of operation for carpal tunnel syndrome. *Mayo Clin Proc.* 1966;41:232–241.

10. Das SK, Brown HG. In search of complications in carpal tunnel decompression. *Hand.* 1976;8:243–249.

11. Eason SY, Belsole RJ, Greene TL. Carpal tunnel release: analysis of suboptimal results. *J Hand Surg Br.* 1985;10B:365–369.

12. Eboh N, Wilson DH. Surgery of the carpal tunnel: technical note. *J Neurosurg.* 1978;49:316–318.

13. Ellis JM, Folkers K, Levy M, et al. Response of vitamin B–6 deficiency and the carpal tunnel syndrome to pyridoxine. *Proc Natl Acad Sci USA.* 1982;79:7494–7498.

14. Eversmann WW Jr. Entrapment and compression neuropathies. In: *Operative Hand Surgery.* 2nd ed. Green DP, ed. New York, NY: Churchill Livingstone;1988;2:1423–1478.

15. Gainer JV Jr, Nugent GR. Carpal tunnel syndrome: report of 430 operations. *South Med J.* 1977;70:325–328.

16. Gelberman RH, Aronson D, Weisman MH. Carpal-tunnel syndrome: results of a prospective trial of steroid injection and splinting. *J Bone Joint Surg Am.* 1980;62A:1181–1184.

17. Gould JS, Wissinger HA. Carpal tunnel syndrome in pregnancy. *South Med J.* 1978;71:144–145,154.

18. Graham WP III. Variations of the motor branch of the median nerve at the wrist. *Plast Reconstr Surg.* 1973;51:90–92.

19. Grundberg AB. Carpal tunnel decompression in spite of normal electromyography. *J Hand Surg.* 1983; 8:348–349.

20. Kummel BM, Zazanis GA. Shoulder pain as the presenting complaint in carpal tunnel syndrome. *Clin Orthop.* 1973;92:227–230.

21. Lanz U. Anatomical variations of the median nerve in the carpal tunnel. *J Hand Surg.* 1977;2:44–53.

22. Louis DS, Greene TL, Noellert RC. Complications of carpal tunnel surgery. *J Neurosurg.* 1985;62:352–356.

23. MacDonald RI, Lichtman DM, Hanlon JJ, et al. Complications of surgical release for carpal tunnel syndrome. *J Hand Surg.* 1978;3:70–76.

24. Mackinnon SE. Secondary carpal tunnel surgery. *Neurosurg Clin North Am.* 1991; 2:75–91.

25. Massey EW, Riley TL, Pleet AB. Coexistent carpal tunnel syndrome and cervical radiculopathy (double crush syndrome). *South Med J.* 1981;74:957–959.

26. Maxwell JA, Kepes JJ, Ketchum LD. Acute carpal tunnel syndrome secondary to thrombosis of a persistent median artery. *J Neurosurg.* 1973;38:774–777.

27. Osterman AL. The double crush syndrome. *Orthop Clin North Am.* 1988;19:147–155.

28. Pagnanelli DM, Barrer SJ: Carpal tunnel syndrome: surgical treatment using the Paine retinaculotome. *J Neurosurg.* 1991; 75:77–81.

29. Paine KWE, Polyzoidis KS. Carpal tunnel syndrome: decompression using the Paine retinaculotome. *J Neurosurg.* 1983; 59:1031–1036.

30. Phalen GS. Reflections on 21 years' experience with the carpal-tunnel syndrome. *JAMA.* 1970;212:1365–1367.

31. Posch JL, Marcotte DR. Carpal tunnel syndrome: an analysis of 1,201 cases. *Orthop Rev.* 1976;5:25–35.

32. Rengachary SS. Entrapment neuropathies. In: Wilkins RH, Rengachary SS, eds. *Neurosurgery.* New York, NY: McGraw-Hill, 1985:1771–1795.

33. Sunderland S. The nerve lesion in the carpal tunnel syndrome. *J Neurol Neurosurg Psychiatry.* 1976;39:615–626.

34. Tindall SC. Chronic injuries of peripheral nerves by entrapment. In: Youmans JR, ed. *Neurological surgery.* Philadelphia, Pa: WB Saunders; 1990:2511–2542.

35. Voitk AJ, Mueller JC, Farlinger DE, et al. Carpal tunnel syndrome in pregnancy. *Can Med Assoc J.* 1983;128:277–281.

36. Yu J, Bendler EM, Mentari A. Neurological disorders associated with carpal tunnel syndrome. *Electromyogr Clin Neurophysiol.* 1979;19:27–32.

CHAPTER 6

Cubital Tunnel Syndrome

Brian K. Willis, MD

Because of the importance of hand function in most activities of daily living, the ulnar nerve, which provides the predominant motor innervation to the hand, is perhaps the single most important somatic peripheral nerve in the body. Neuropathy of the ulnar nerve may result in significant disability due to loss of hand function from pain, numbness, and weakness. The most common causes of ulnar nerve neuropathy are entrapment, impingement, stretching, and friction at or around the vicinity of the elbow.

Because of the multiplicity of pathological processes that can lead to ulnar neuropathy at the elbow, reviewing its causes and treatment as reported in the medical literature can be confusing and misleading. An example of the diversity of perspectives is the variety of names given throughout the last several decades to describe the phenomenon of ulnar neuropathy at the elbow. This disease process has been referred to as tardy ulnar palsy, traumatic ulnar neuritis, compression neuritis of the ulnar nerve, Feindel-Osborne syndrome, and the cubital tunnel syndrome.[8,18,25,28,29,30,32,34]

Some of these names, such as tardy ulnar palsy, are inappropriate when describing most ulnar neuropathies. Tardy ulnar palsy refers only to patients who develop a slow, chronic deterioration of ulnar nerve function months to years after trauma to the elbow, especially if associated with a supracondylar fracture or a fracture of the medial epicondyle. The preferred term in the current literature is cubital tunnel syndrome. This term is somewhat of an oversimplification: ulnar neuropathy at the elbow may be due to a number of factors other than compression within the cubital tunnel, such as recurrent subluxation of the ulnar nerve out of its groove, or entrapment proximal or distal to the cubital tunnel. The term *cubital tunnel syndrome*—in its broadest sense i.e. a focal neuropathy involving the ulnar nerve in the vicinity of the cubital tunnel—is used in this chapter.

Surgical Anatomy

Anatomic Course of the Ulnar Nerve

The ulnar nerve is the largest nerve derived from the medial cord of the brachial plexus. It carries nerve fibers from the eighth cervical and first thoracic nerves. In the upper arm, it courses medial to the brachial artery until the midarm, where it pierces the intermuscular septum and travels towards the dorsal and medial aspect of the elbow along with the medial head of the triceps. After passing behind the medial epicondyle of the humerus in a groove between it and the olecranon (referred to as the cubital tunnel), the ulnar nerve enters the forearm between the two heads of the flexor carpi ulnaris muscle.

Across this groove, the nerve passes from the extensor compartment in the arm into the flexor compartment of the forearm (Figure 1A). More distally in the forearm, the ulnar nerve joins the ulnar artery and emerges into a superficial location just lateral to the flexor carpi ulnaris before passing across the medial wrist

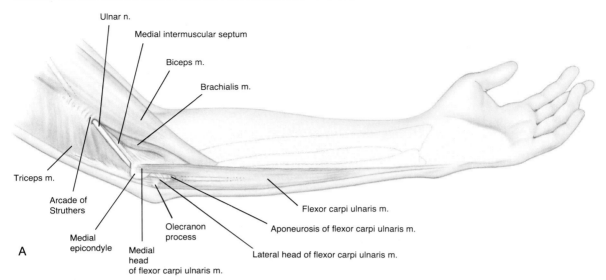

Figure 1A. *Anatomic relations of the ulnar nerve in the region of the elbow. After piercing the medial inter-muscular septum and passing under the inconstant arcade of Struthers in the extensor compartment of the arm, the nerve enters the cubital tunnel behind the medial epicondyle to pass into the flexor compartment of the forearm beneath the flexor carpi ulnaris.*

superficial to the transverse carpal ligament (flexor retinaculum) into the hand.

Innervation by the Ulnar Nerve

Like the median nerve, the ulnar nerve has no branches in the arm, but provides innervation to the forearm and hand. Unlike the median nerve, the motor fibers of the ulnar nerve predominately innervate the hand rather than the forearm.

Although the ulnar nerve gives rise to a number of small articular branches to the elbow joint, it is not until the nerve passes between the two heads of the flexor carpi ulnaris that it begins supplying motor and sensory innervation. As the nerve acquires a superficial location after passing beneath the belly of the flexor carpi ulnaris, where it supplies motor innervation to this and the flexor digitorum profundus muscles, it gives off the palmar cutaneous branch which pierces the fascia just proximal to the wrist and supplies the skin of the hypothenar eminence and medial aspect of the palm. The dorsal cutaneous branch of the ulnar nerve arises 5 cm proximal to the wrist

and turns dorsally, where it distributes sensory fibers to the medial one-half of the dorsum of the hand and the fourth and fifth digits.

Another surgically important cutaneous branch of the ulnar nerve is the medial antebrachial cutaneous nerve. Although not anatomically a branch of the ulnar nerve, it branches from the medial cord of the brachial plexus at the site of the origin of ulnar nerve. It pierces the brachial fascia at the lower part of the arm at its medial aspect. The larger anterior branch of this cutaneous nerve distributes sensory fibers to the ventral and medial aspect of the distal arm and proximal forearm, as well as to the cubital fossa. Its smaller ulnar branch passes ventral to the medial epicondyle of the humerus and supplies the skin on the dorsomedial aspect of the forearm. Division of one or both of these branches of the medial antebrachial cutaneous nerve during ulnar nerve decompression or transposition at the elbow can lead to postoperative numbness of the medial forearm or to painful neuroma formation.

After passing into the palm, the ulnar nerve divides into a superficial and a deep branch. The superficial branch carries sensory fibers to the palmar aspect of the fifth and medial one-half of the fourth digits. The deep (motor) branch passes deep into the palm through the muscles of the hypothenar eminence which it innervates. The hypothenar compartment contains three muscles: the abductor digiti minimi, flexor digiti minimi brevis, and opponens digiti minimi. Continuing its arch across the palm, it supplies innervation to the third and fourth lumbricales, all the interosseous muscles, and more laterally, the adductor pollicis.

Anatomy of the Cubital Tunnel

As the ulnar nerve passes through the groove behind the medial epicondyle of the humerus and past the articulation of the elbow, it lies beneath a fibrous arcade formed by dense fascial strands. This aponeurosis transversely bridges the groove from the attachment of one head of the carpi flexor ulnaris arising on the medial epicondyle of the humerus to the attachment of the other head arising from the medial aspect of the olecranon. This tunnel is referred to as the "cubital tunnel".

The most proximal edge of this fibrous arcade, known as Osborne's band, is frequently thickened and often is a site of compression of the underlying nerve.[11,30] Besides the ulnar nerve, the only contents of the cubital tunnel are the ulnohumeral ligaments encompassing the elbow joint (in particular the ulnar [or medial] collateral ligament) and a small amount of fibrofatty tissue.

The cubital tunnel can be anatomically divided into three parts: **(1)** the entrance of the tunnel just behind the medial epicondyle, **(2)** the area beneath the fascial aponeurosis joining the two heads of the flexor carpi ulnaris, and **(3)** and the muscle bellies of the flexor carpi ulnaris themselves.[14]

Anatomic and Physiologic Factors Related to Ulnar Neuropathy at the Elbow

Cubital tunnel syndrome may be caused by a number of pathologic processes. Not all of the pathologic processes are compressive lesions or entrapment-type processes. Neuritis related to friction may often play a significant role in the development of cubital tunnel syndrome. This may be especially true of those individuals with chronic and recurrent dislocation of the nerve from the ulnar groove.

Compression of the ulnar nerve within the cubital tunnel is most often due to constriction of the nerve by the overlying aponeurosis.[30,32] Less common compressive agents include inflammation, rheumatoid synovitis, lipomas and other tumors, bone fragments, osteophytes from the ulnohumeral articulation, and a rare anomaly known as the persistent epitrochleoanconeus muscle.[14,18,20,29] Entrapment outside the confines of the cubital tunnel is not unknown. Such areas as the medial intermuscular septum, arcade of Struthers, medial head of the triceps, and the groove between the two muscle bellies of the flexor carpi ulnaris have been implicated as sites of compression.

Another common etiology is repetitive trauma to or pressure on the nerve, such as habitual leaning on a desk with the elbows while working. Activities such as shoveling, swinging an axe or pick, and sleeping with the arms flexed at the elbows, lend themselves to the development of ulnar neuropathy.

The neuropathy is likely due to alterations in the volume of the cubital tunnel with flexion and extension. In extension, the tunnel is at its greatest volume, due to laxity in the overlying aponeurosis and the underlying ulnar collateral ligament. With flexion, the two points of attachment of the aponeurosis on the epicondyle and olecranon diverge, causing the fascial roof to become taut. Likewise, the ulnar collateral ligament along the floor of the tunnel comes under tension. Reduction in volume of the cubital tunnel results in compression and focal ischemia of the nerve.[8,32] Elbow flexion and repetitive stretching of the ulnar nerve around the medial epicondyle may also play a role in nerve damage in some patients.[2]

Chronic compressive processes such as those observed with malunited elbow fractures and cubitus valgus are the likely agents in tardy ulnar palsy. In contrast, single acute events have resulted in ulnar neuropathy at the elbow: a sharp blow to the elbow, injection of steroids into the elbow for bursitis or medial epicondylitis, and lying supine for a period of time on a hard surface with the elbows unprotected (as may occur in operating room settings or in a drunken stupor). Ten to 30% of cases are idiopathic and the etiology of the neuropathy cannot be explained.[2,18]

Like the median nerve in carpal tunnel syndrome, the ulnar nerve is made more susceptible to compressive lesions by metabolic processes that lead to demyelination, endoneurial/perineurial edema, and nerve ischemia such as occurs in diabetes mellitus, alcoholism and malnutrition, vitamin deficiency, or paraneoplastic syndromes.

Clinical Diagnosis

Symptoms and Findings

Numbness and tingling of the ulnar aspect of the hand, weakness and clumsiness, and noticeable thenar and first dorsal interossei atrophy are the most common complaints of patients with cubital tunnel syndrome. Unlike carpal tunnel syndrome, pain is less often a major component of the symptom complex. When pain does occur, it is described as an aching sensation in the medial elbow and forearm associated with dysesthetic tingling in the hand. Lancinating pain is less common and should alert the physician to other possible diagnoses, such as cervical radiculopathy. The patient may describe an abrupt worsening of the condition after a period of exertion or forceful and repetitive flexion-extension actions of the elbow. Patients who sleep with their hands beneath their head, causing prolonged "hyperflexion" at the elbow, may notice their symptoms are more pronounced upon awakening.

In a study of 100 patients with "tardy ulnar-nerve paralysis", Gay and Love[18] documented intrinsic hand muscle atrophy and weakness in 96%. In fact, onset of visually apparent atrophy frequently predated subjective weakness and sensory changes. Hypoesthesia in the sensory distribution of the ulnar nerve in the hand

was observed in 75% of patients. One-half were noted to have palpable enlargement or swelling of the ulnar nerve behind the elbow. Few had nerve tenderness.

Atrophic changes in the hand may be quite pronounced. The hypothenar eminence is often flattened, especially along the medial border of the hand. More impressive, however, is the depression between the thumb and index finger on the dorsal aspect of the hand, indicative of atrophy of the first dorsal interosseous muscle.

The three muscles of the hypothenar eminence abduct, adduct, flex, and rotate the fifth digit. The most easily tested is the abductor digiti minimi. Weakness of this muscle will manifest itself by difficulty with fanning (*abduction*) of the fingers. This is easier to detect when the weakness is unilateral, which allows comparison to the other hand. Weakness of *adduction* of the little finger is referred to as Wartenberg's sign, perhaps the most subtle and sensitive motor finding in cubital tunnel syndrome.[8]

Because most of the muscles innervated by the ulnar nerve are involved in flexion of the digits, grip strength can be an important indicator of ulnar nerve function. The ulnar-innervated adductor pollicis adducts the thumb. This muscle is tested by having the patient grip a piece of paper between his or her thumb and forefinger. Weakness of the adductor pollicis muscle will allow the paper to be easily pulled from the patient's grasp. Some patients will compensate for this weakness by flexing the interphalangeal joint of the thumb using the flexor pollicis longus, a muscle innervated by the anterior interosseous branch of the median nerve. This is referred to as Froment's sign, a finding typically associated with ulnar neuropathy.

Weakness of the flexor carpi ulnaris and flexor digitorum profundus muscles (innervated by the ulnar nerve just distal to the elbow) is rarely reported as a clinical finding in cubital tunnel syndrome. Many erroneously attribute this to the belief that the nerves innervating these muscles originate proximal to the elbow. Campbell et al dissected these nerves in 30 cadaveric arms and found only 3 arising at or proximal to the cubital tunnel. They concluded that sparing of the flexor carpi ulnaris is unrelated to the level of origin of its innervating branch, but rather is related to the internal neural topography and to the severity and level of the compression.[7] Others have confirmed why these muscles are spared loss of innervation: the fibers that innervate them lie in the deep aspect of the nerve and are spared the compressive effects of the more superficially-lying fibers to the hand.[2,16]

Weakness, however, is likely more common than reported. Due to the difficulty of detecting subtle motor changes in these muscles, weakness is often not tested for or is overlooked. Although they were unable to accurately assess function of the flexor carpi ulnaris muscle, Craven and Green detected weakness in the flexor digitorum profundus in 66% of their patients undergoing treatment for ulnar neuropathy.[8] In addition, Campbell et al found severe electromyographic abnormalities in the flexor carpi ulnaris in almost half of their cases of ulnar neuropathy.[7]

Percussing the area over the ulnar groove may produce tingling and numbness in the medial forearm and hand. This phenomenon is equivalent to the Tinel's sign found in patients with carpal tunnel syndrome. In the author's experience, a positive "Tinel's" of the ulnar nerve is a nonspecific finding of dubious pathologic significance and is frequently observed in individuals without any other evidence of ulnar neuropathy. Occasionally, maximal flexion of the elbow for 1–2 minutes may produce symptom exacerbation. The elbow flexion test, the usefulness of which has not been proven, is perhaps analogous to Phalen's wrist flexion test for median nerve entrapment.

The importance of careful examination of the elbow cannot be overstated. Cubitus valgus, medial epicondylitis, rheumatoid synovitis, and masses such as tumors or bone fragments may be discovered. Many of these findings may necessitate a course of treatment different than that indicated for idiopathic cu-

bital tunnel syndrome. This is especially true if ulnar nerve subluxation out of its groove and over the medial epicondyle is palpated.

Ancillary Diagnostic Tests

All patients with suspected cubital tunnel syndrome should have as part of their evaluation an electromyogram (EMG) with nerve conduction velocities (NCV), and x-rays of the elbows and cervical spine.

The EMG should be used to confirm the diagnosis and to assess the severity of cubital tunnel syndrome. It is also useful to evaluate for (1) a concomitant neuropathy of metabolic or nutritional origin, such as diabetic polyneuropathy and (2) secondary sites of entrapment, such as C8 nerve root impingement (the so-called "double-crush syndrome"). Results of electrodiagnostic tests should never be used as a primary diagnostic tool to indicate need for surgery.

Perhaps the most specific and reliable electrodiagnostic indicator of ulnar neuropathy at the elbow is slowed conduction velocity across the elbow.[8,24,32] Although normal values have not been firmly established, the conduction velocity (NCV) of the ulnar nerve generally ranges from 47–65 m/sec with an average velocity of 55 m/sec. A reduction in velocity of less than 25% is probably insignificant. Greater than a 33% reduction in velocity certainly indicates a neuropathic process at the elbow.[14]

Other EMG findings indicative of cubital tunnel syndrome include diminished numbers of motor units action potentials, fibrillations and positive waves, and, in more advanced cases, polyphasic reinnervation potentials. Another sensitive indicator of altered conduction is loss of evoked sensory potentials.[1,32,35] The position of the elbow must be standardized during the performance of electrodiagnostic studies. Variations in NCV readings may occur from flexion to extension, even in normal individuals.[4,24]

X-ray of the elbow provides useful information regarding etiology that assists in management decisions. Arthritic spurs, bony tumors, fractures, or cubitus valgus may be detected. A slightly oblique anteroposterior view, referred to as the cubital tunnel view, is most helpful.[16,32]

Differential Diagnosis

Many pathologic processes of the spinal cord can resemble cubital tunnel syndrome, all of which may present with a predominance of motor signs and symptoms. When patients complain of "numb and clumsy hands," consideration must be given to intrinsic cord lesions such as intramedullary tumors, syringomyelia, amyotrophic lateral sclerosis, and extrinsic cord lesions such as cervical spondylitic myelopathy. Other causes of hand dysfunction and pain include **(1)** cervical radiculopathy from osteophytes or herniated disc, **(2)** Pancoast tumors and other lesions of the lower and medial brachial plexus, and **(3)** other sites of ulnar nerve compression, such as at Guyon's canal. In addition, various systemic polyneuropathies, such as those observed in nutritional deficiencies or diabetes mellitus, may alone or in combination with cubital tunnel syndrome produce weakness, atrophy, pain, and numbness in the distal upper extremity. Occasionally, the effects of age will produce intrinsic hand atrophy and dysfunction.

Grading

A major difficulty in evaluating and comparing results of therapy for cubital tunnel syndrome is the lack of a widely accepted and uniform grading system for preoperatively categorizing patients by severity of symptoms and postoperatively grading their outcome. Perhaps the most often-used scheme is that proposed by McGowan in 1950.[28] This grading system categorizes ulnar neuropathy based on degrees of muscle weakness. Grade I patients have "minimal lesions, with no detectable motor weakness of the hand." *Intermediate lesions* are designated Grade II. Grade III includes patients with "severe lesions, with paralysis of

one or more of the ulnar intrinsic muscles." Unfortunately, the grades are poorly defined and neglect important features of the syndrome such as pain and numbness.

Dellon devised a detailed and well-defined staging system based on sensory and motor changes as well as other physical findings, such as Tinel's sign and the elbow flexion test.[10] His three-tiered system grades severity of preoperative symptoms into mild, moderate, and severe. Although an excellent system for categorizing and comparing patients according to degree of preoperative deficits, its use for postoperative classification of outcome is complex and unwieldy.

Another method of comparison is using a system of scoring by points, described by Gabel and Amadio.[17] Points are given based on the severity of three factors: motor function, sensation, and pain (Table 1). No points are given for the most severe symptoms; an increasing number of points are given for less severe symptoms. Postoperative outcome can also be graded into excellent, good, fair, and poor based on this scoring system (Table 2). Regardless of what grading scheme is eventually used, a standard and uniform system should be adopted for the assessment of treatment results.

Nonoperative Management

Historically, cubital tunnel syndrome was thought to be a malady remediable only by surgical treatment. Gay and Love stated "the course of tardy paralysis of the ulnar nerve is characterized by unrelenting progression, and no known conservative form of treatment has been found to be of any permanent benefit."[18] Reports are now emerging that suggest nonoperative means of treatment in selected cases may provide symptomatic relief.[10,13,31,35] Having the patient avoid activities and positions which produce **(1)** friction from repetitive elbow movements or **(2)** stretching and compression of the nerve from excessive elbow flexion may be all that is required in many pa-

TABLE 1
Gabel and Amadio's Preoperative and Postoperative Rating Scale for Ulnar Nerve Entrapment*

Score (points)	Motor	Sensory	Pain
3	Normal (McGowan Grade I)	No numbness	No pain
2	Weaker than opposite side	2-point discrimination normal; intermittent paresthesias	Intermittent pain
1	Obvious atrophy (McGowan Grade II)	2-point discrimination >6 mm; constant numbness	Constant pain, intermittent meds
0	Intrinsic paralysis with claw deformity (McGowan Grade III)	2-point discrimination >10 mm; anesthesia	Needs narcotics regularly

*Reference 17

TABLE 2
Classification of Outcome Based on Gabel and Amadio Scores*

Excellent — score of 9

Good — score of 2 or more points in each category with an increase in score in each category of 1 or more points, or an increase in total score of 4 or more points

Fair — score less than 2 points in any category, but with an increase in total score of 1–3 points

Poor — no change or decline in total score

*Reference 17

tients with early symptoms. A loose-fitting towel may be wrapped around the affected elbow at night to prevent folding of the arms under the body or head during sleep.[11] In some cases, an elbow splint placed in slight flexion (approximately 30° of flexion) worn only at night may prove to be of benefit. Dimond and Lister suggested in a nonrandomized retrospective study that long-arm splinting of the elbow compares favorably to surgical intervention.[12] Unfortunately, data regarding the results of conservative therapy remain too limited to be meaningful.

Surgical Options and Results

Unlike the limited amount of data on nonoperative therapy, a voluminous amount of information exists regarding surgical options, techniques, and results. Dellon reviewed the literature from 1898–1988 and found more than 50 reports of series totalling more than 2,000 patients treated for cubital tunnel syndrome.[10] Unfortunately, due to the lack of controlled, randomized, or otherwise adequately constructed scientific studies, the data are inconclusive.

Statistically significant comparison of surgical techniques and their results remains virtually impossible. The surgeon has available a number of operations devised to relieve the ulnar nerve of the effects of compression or friction in and around the vicinity of the cubital tunnel. Each procedure has proponents heralding the superiority of their preferred technique. To decide on the appropriateness of each procedure, the surgeon must rely only on speculation and his or her personal bias, which is usually a manifestation of the surgeon's training colored by recent experiences, especially those that involve complications or failures.

At least five distinct surgical procedures are advocated for the relief of symptomatic cubital tunnel syndrome. They can be grouped into the categories of: **(1)** decompressive procedures and **(2)** transposition procedures. Decompressive procedures address the compressive process without surgically mobilizing the nerve from its location in the ulnar groove. The principal decompressive procedures are simple decompression and medial epicondylectomy. The transposition procedures mobilize the nerve and move it anteriorly into a purportedly more protected location. They can be further divided by the position in which the ulnar nerve is placed— subcutaneous, intramuscular, or submuscular. The advantages and disadvantages of each procedure are summarized in Table 3.

Operative Techniques

Surgical decompression or transposition of the ulnar nerve rarely requires general anesthesia. The exception is an extensive procedure such as a submuscular transposition with Z-plasty muscle lengthening.

The author prefers a regional block (axillary or supraclavicular) placed by the anesthesiologist immediately prior to the procedure. The affected arm is placed outstretched, with the humerus abducted and externally rotated and the elbow slightly flexed. Several folded surgical towels beneath the elbow help maintain this position. A tourniquet is not necessary and, in fact, may be harmful.

The author prefers a regional block (axillary or supraclavicular) placed by the anesthesiologist immediately prior to the procedure. The affected arm is placed outstretched, with the humerus abducted and externally rotated and the elbow slightly flexed. Several folded surgical towels beneath the elbow help maintain this position. A tourniquet is not necessary and, in fact, may be harmful.

The argument against the use of a tourniquet during any type of peripheral nerve surgery is convincing. With increasing extraneural pres-sure, segmental intraneural blood flow is diminished. At 80 mm Hg, complete intraneural ischemia occurs.[19,33] Soon, epineural and endoneural edema develops, which further aggravates the compression and ischemia of the nerve. Distal to the tourniquet, the already chronically ischemic nerve at the entrapment site is further deprived of blood flow due to regional loss of blood flow. Venous congestion within the nerve can further complicate endoneural edema and ischemia.[9] Furthermore, hemostasis is best acquired if the small arterioles and veins are electrocoagulated and divided as they are encountered.

Simply closing the wound, wrapping the extremity tightly, then releasing the tourniquet places the wound at risk for hematoma formation. Ultimately, the entire procedure is placed at risk for failure. Near bloodless surgery can be easily accomplished without use of a tourniquet if adequate attention to detailed hemostasis is given. Visualization is improved by using headlamp illumination and loupe magnification.

The most common operative techniques are described in the next section and their advantages and disadvantages are discussed.

Simple Decompression

Simple decompression, also known as cubital tunnel release, is the simplest of the five procedures. Other techniques are more extensive variations of this basic operation. Osborne was among the first to advocate the procedure more than three decades ago.[30] In recent years, an increasing number of surgeons appear to be turning from the use of the transposition procedures for "typical" cubital tunnel syndrome to this simpler, safer, and perhaps equally efficacious mode of therapy.

The patient is positioned in the standard fashion described above. A 6–7 cm linear incision is made parallel to the ulnar nerve and centered between the medial epicondyle and the prominence of the olecranon.[14,36] Dissection is carried down to the underlying fascia. The ulnar nerve is approached as it courses under the

TABLE 3
**Advantages and Disadvantages of the Surgical Procedures
for the Cubital Tunnel Syndrome**

I. Decompressive Procedures

    A. Simple decompression

        Advantages—**(1)** simpler and quicker to perform with low risk of complications, **(2)** small linear incision avoids injury to medial antebrachial cutaneous nerve, **(3)** no need to mobilize nerve from its bed and risk disrupting vascular supply (vasa nervorum) or injuring articular or muscular branches, **(4)** shorter postoperative recovery.

        Disadvantages—**(1)** exposure not adequate to explore the proximal and distal extent of nerve for additional sites of entrapment, **(2)** does not address (and may predispose to) neuropathy from recurrent subluxation, **(3)** potential for entrapment in scar tissue from overlying incision, **(4)** possibly less efficacious in advanced stages of disease.

    B. Medial epicondylectomy

        Advantages—**(1)** easy to perform, **(2)** does not require mobilization of the nerve, **(3)** relieves compressive effects of medial epicondyle in elbow flexion, **(4)** addresses recurrent subluxation over the medial epicondyle.

        Disadvantages—**(1)** nerve is more vulnerable to external trauma both within the ulnar groove and in its anterior position over the flexor-pronator origin, **(2)** potential for friction neuritis, elbow instability from injury to the ulnar collateral ligament, or flexor-pronator weakness related to detachment of its origin, **(3)** bone tenderness at site of epicondylectomy, **(4)** length of nerve visualized and explored may be inadequate.

II. Transposition Procedures

    A. Subcutaneous transposition

        Advantages—**(1)** removes the ulnar nerve away from the compressive agent at the elbow, even if the pathology is unidentified, **(2)** reduces tension on the nerve with elbow flexion, **(3)** allows complete visualization of the nerve from its proximal to distal extent.

        Disadvantages—**(1)** may devascularize the nerve, **(2)** may constrict or kink the nerve proximally at the intermuscular septum, "arcade of Struthers", or medial head of the triceps or distally at or between the two heads of the flexor carpi ulnaris, **(3)** stretching/angulation of nerve over epicondyle and flexor-pronator mass when elbow is fully extended, **(4)** fascial sling created to hold nerve into anterior position may entrap nerve, **(5)** nerve prone to injury due to its unprotected and superficial location, **(6)** longer and complex postoperative recuperation and rehabilitation, **(7)** longer incision and undermining of skin increases risk of bleeding and hematoma formation.

    B. Intramuscular transposition

        Advantages—same as for subcutaneous transposition.

        Disadvantages—same as for subcutaneous transposition, but for significantly increased risk of scarring/fibrosis around transposed nerve (cicatrix formation).

    C. Submuscular transposition

        Advantages—same as for subcutaneous transposition but for **(1)** ulnar nerve is better protected from external trauma, **(2)** deeper position of nerve causes less anterior angulation, **(3)** less risk for stretching, kinking, or constriction, **(4)** less risk for entrapment of nerve in scar tissue.

        Disadvantages—**(1)** procedure is complex and relatively lengthy, **(2)** mobilization may devascularize nerve or injure distal muscular branches, **(3)** may produce weakness of flexor-pronator muscle group, **(4)** longer recovery period required, **(5)** extensive procedure possibly of greater risk but no greater efficacy than simple decompression for most patients.

medial epicondyle just proximal to the point where it passes under Osborne's band, the thickened aponeurotic edge of the roof of the cubital tunnel. The rare, anomalous epitrochleoanconeus muscle may be observed in the place of the aponeurotic roof stretching over the cubital tunnel.[20]

Tracing the nerve distally, the aponeurosis is sharply divided, thereby "releasing" the nerve from the confines of the cubital tunnel. Division of the tissues over the nerve is continued distally as the nerve passes into the muscular cleft between the two heads of the flexor carpi ulnaris. If a point of constriction along the nerve is observed after decompression, the epineurium at the constricted site may be longitudinally incised and opened for 1–2 cm—i.e. an epineurotomy. Internal neurolysis plays little role in the initial surgical procedure.

The nerve itself is not removed from its bed; hence, the "extrinsic circulation" of the nerve is not adversely altered and division of the small articular branches of the ulnar nerve is not necessary. The wound is then closed and the elbow placed in a soft, bulky dressing. The patient is instructed to gently flex and extend the elbow for its full range of motion for the first 2 weeks but not to use it for strenuous or exertional activities. Use of a nocturnal splint is recommended for patients who tend to flex their elbows at night.

Medial Epicondylectomy

This procedure, first described by King and Morgan in 1950,[25] has not gained wide acceptance despite several favorable reports.[8,16,23,29] Based on the premise that the offending agent in ulnar neuropathy at the elbow is the median epicondyle, proponents advocate the logic of removing the epicondyle as one would remove any offending mass to relieve tension on the nerve and allow it to find its own optimal position.[25,29] In this sense, the operation can also be considered a transposition procedure.

The technique for medial epicondylectomy approximates the technique for simple decompression, with the exception of the centering of the short linear incision over the medial epi-

condyle and the removal of the medial epicondyle. The periosteum over the epicondyle is incised in a longitudinal or curvilinear fashion and retracted off the bone along with the origin of the flexor-pronator muscle group. The flexor-pronator muscle group includes the pronator teres, flexor carpi radialis, medial head of the flexor carpi ulnaris, flexor digitorum superficialis, and the palmaris longus, all of which share a common tendinous origin on the anterior aspect of the medial epicondyle.

Using rongeurs or an osteotome, the epicondyle is then completely removed. Incomplete amputation of the tip of the epicondyle may leave a sharp edge at the condylar base which may abrade and damage the ulnar nerve. Care should also be taken not to disrupt the ulnar collateral ligament at the base of the epicondyle; injury to this ligament may lead to elbow instability. The periosteum and tendinous origin of the flexor-pronator muscle group are repaired over the waxed bony defect as the elbow is held in extension. Before closure, the elbow is placed through a full range of motion. The nerve should slide freely to and fro over the resected condylar mass and the reattached muscle mass. The wound is then closed in a routine manner. Postoperative care is provided in the same manner as in the simple decompression.

Subcutaneous Transposition

Subcutaneous transposition is the oldest and most commonly performed of the anterior transposition procedures. It has been widely applied since the turn of the century. A 12–15 cm curvilinear incision arching anteriorly over the medial epicondyle is utilized (Figure 1B). As compared to the smaller linear incision, the curvilinear incision lessens the possibility of adhesions and scarring of the incision to the underlying nerve and provides better exposure with which to deal with proximal and distal compressive areas.

As in the simple decompression, the aponeurotic roof of the cubital tunnel is sharply divided and the ulnar nerve is "released". Division of the tissues over the nerve is continued distally as the nerve passes into the muscular cleft between the two heads of the flexor carpi ulnaris. Taking care not to injure the motor branches to the flexor carpi ulnaris, the dissection is continued into the proximal forearm until it is certain no further sites of distal compression exist. Similarly, the ulnar nerve is followed proximally along the medial head of the triceps for 7–8 cm to the often sharp edge of the intermuscular septum, which is also divided. The arcade of Struthers, an inconstant fascial band extending from the medial head of the triceps to the intermuscular septum, is likewise divided.

Once the ulnar nerve is adequately decompressed from beneath the flexor carpi ulnaris to the medial intermuscular septum, the nerve is elevated, encircled with a vessel loop, and dissected from its bed within the ulnar groove. The small articular branches from the nerve are divided, as are any small vessels passing into the epineurium from the surrounding soft tissues. As much epineurium and perineural fatty tissue as possible should be left around the nerve to limit post-operative adhesions and to preserve perineural vasculature.

Mobilization of the ulnar nerve continues proximally and distally for at least 12 cm. The nerve is moved anterior to the epicondyle and the flexor-pronator muscle group arising from it. Occasionally, the length of immobilization necessary to prevent stretching or acute angulation of the nerve over the anterior aspect of the extended elbow is 16 cm, a length which precariously places the ulnar nerve at risk for ischemia. Adequate decompression of overlying fascial bands or planes must be carried out at the proximal and distal extents of the nerve exposure prior to transposition. Sacrifice of the muscular branch to the flexor carpi ulnaris should be avoided. Should the muscular branch cause distal tethering during anterior transposition, intrafascicular dissection for 2–3 cm may be necessary to free it from the nerve proper.

A fascial sling is created over the ulnar nerve to prevent it from slipping back into the ulnar groove; care must be taken not to recreate a new site of ulnar nerve compression or entrap-

ment. The nerve is carefully examined along its entire exposure with the elbow both in flexion and extension to be sure the nerve does not slip back into the ulnar groove and that there are no additional sites of entrapment or kinking. The wound is then closed in a routine fashion. The elbow is usually placed in a plaster long-arm splint postoperatively.

Intramuscular Transposition

This procedure protects the ulnar nerve in a vascularized muscle bed. However, it is looked upon less favorably because of the development of circumferential scarring and adhesions, or cicatrix, making the nerve more vulnerable to traction forces. The operation is carried out in the manner of the subcutaneous transposition. Instead of creating a fascial sling over the nerve, however, an intramuscular trough is created by incising the flexor-pronator muscle mass. The ulnar nerve is placed into the muscular bed and oversewn.

Submuscular Transposition

Also known as the Learmonth procedure, submuscular transposition was developed to overcome some of the deficiencies of the subcutaneous and intramuscular techniques. The literature is replete with descriptions of this technique and its numerous modifications.[11,26,27] As with the intramuscular transposition, the transposed nerve is more protected and is less angulated over the flexor-pronator mass as compared to the subcutaneous technique. Unlike the intramuscular transposition, the ulnar nerve is free to slide to and fro with elbow movement and is less prone to scarring and adhesions with the submuscular technique.

Once the ulnar nerve has been adequately mobilized from the medial intermuscular septum to its course deep to the flexor carpi ulnaris, but prior to its transposition anterior to the epicondyle, the origin of flexor-pronator muscle mass is detached from the medial epicondyle. Levy and Apfelberg described detaching the tip of the epicondyle along with the tendinous origin and reattaching it with wire suture after transposing the ulnar nerve beneath the muscle mass.[27] The flexor-pronator muscle mass is elevated using a periosteal elevator; caution must be exercised to avoid injury to the nearby median nerve and brachial artery bifurcation.

The ulnar nerve is transposed anteriorly and placed beneath the muscle mass to lie upon the brachialis fascia a centimeter or so medial to the median nerve. A gentle anterior curve of the nerve should occur with this technique, a decided advantage over the subcutaneous transposition. The elbow is flexed and the forearm pronated to assist in reattaching the flexor-pronator mass. Dellon describes elongation of the muscle mass through a Z-plasty and muscle slide technique so that no additional tension is placed on the ulnar nerve.[11] 2-0 gauge nonabsorbable suture is used, being careful not to catch the transposed nerve in the suture line. The wound is closed and the elbow is placed in a long-arm splint in a flexed and pronated position.

Additional Techniques

Most other techniques are, in one form or another, modifications of the five listed above. One particularly novel technique deserves further comment. Some surgeons have long used Silastic as an adjunct to peripheral nerve repair. Campbell et al reported the use of a Silastic envelope placed around the ulnar nerve in patients undergoing reoperation for painful dysesthesia and progressive neurologic deficit following failed subcutaneous transposition procedures.[6]

Their rationale is that the Silastic will prevent rescarring and entrapment of the nerve and preserve its free, unrestricted movement across the elbow. Once the nerve is separated and elevated from its scarred postoperative bed, a piece of Silastic measuring 15 cm long and 3 cm wide is folded around the nerve and sutured. Campbell does not advocate the use of this technique as a primary procedure as he be-

lieves the presumed risks of rejection due to infection associated with the implantation of a foreign body outweigh the relatively low risk of entrapment in scar tissue. Benoit et al described the use of a 6 cm long Silastic sheath sutured around the ulnar nerve after simple decompression as a primary procedure.[3]

Author's Preferred Technique

The author's technique uses the many advantages of simple decompression, yet addresses its shortcomings by more extensively exploring and decompressing the nerve. Though perhaps an overly long title, the author refers to this technique as "extended cubital tunnel release with partial osteotomy of the medial epicondyle". This hybrid of the simple decompression and medial epicondylectomy uses the excellent exposure of the transposition procedures without accruing their disadvantages.

As in the transposition techniques, the classic 12–15 cm curvilinear incision arches anteriorly over the medial epicondyle (Figure 1B). Care is taken not to inadvertently divide branches of the medial antebrachial cutaneous nerve. The roof of the cubital tunnel is incised and the section of the ulnar nerve from just proximal to the medial intermuscular septum to its location deep to the flexor carpi ulnaris is explored and decompressed. An epineurotomy is performed at any observed site of nerve constriction if needed.

At this point, any similarity to the transposition procedures is abandoned. Because the nerve is not dissected free from its relatively vascular and fatty-cushioned bed, risks for nerve ischemia and injury to the distal muscular branches are avoided and the potential for cicatrix formation is diminished. The periosteum over the tip of the medial epicondyle is incised parallel to the ulnar nerve for 2–3 cm. There is no risk for postoperative flexor weakness as the flexor-pronator origin is not detached.

Using a small periosteal elevator, the periosteum is removed off the posterior aspect of the

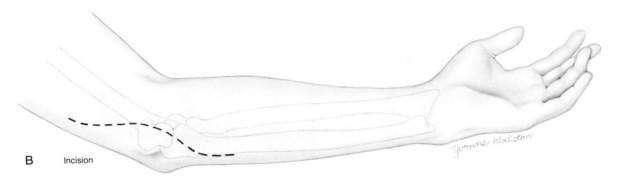

Figure 1B. *Topographic depiction of the "classic" incision for surgical relief of ulnar neuropathy at the elbow.*

epicondyle down to the floor of the ulnar groove and reflected over the nerve. The ulnar collateral ligament is not disturbed. A malleable ribbon retractor and the periosteum is used to cover and protect the nerve as the posterior aspect of the epicondyle is drilled down. This partial osteotomy of the medial epicondyle is performed with an air-powered microdrill with a burr bit. High-speed drills are not advised due to the risk of severe injury to the nerve if the drill bit deflects off the bone. The periosteum is reapproximated over the bony defect which is waxed only if significant bone bleeding occurs (Figure 2).

Before skin closure the elbow is passively flexed and extended, closely observing the anatomic relations and movements of the ulnar nerve and the medial epicondyle. If flexion causes the nerve to easily slip anteriorly over the medial epicondyle, consideration is given to extending the surgery to include a transposition procedure. Only after hemostasis is assured is the wound closed using absorbable sutures in the subcutaneous and subcuticular layers and adhesive strips on the skin. The patient is discharged from the hospital on the first postoperative day.

Postoperatively, the elbow is immobilized for 1 week in a well-padded long-arm splint long enough to also support the wrist. The patient is encouraged to use and exercise the hand as often as possible. After 1 week, the splint is removed during the day but replaced at night for an additional 2–3 weeks. Gentle range-of-motion exercises of the shoulder, elbow, and hand are prescribed. The patient is allowed to resume full activities 3–6 weeks after surgery.

Advantages of the extended decompression with partial osteotomy are similar to those of the simple decompression. It is simple to perform, entails little manipulation of the nerve, and patients have shorter postoperative recovery periods. Unlike the simple decompression, the nerve is more fully explored and compression at other sites are more likely to be discovered and appropriately treated. Like the medial epicondylectomy, this technique relieves to some degree the tension on the ulnar nerve in elbow flexion by enlarging the ulnar groove.

Unlike the medial epicondylectomy, the ulnar nerve retains the protective effect of the epicondyle and the ulnar groove. The attachment of the flexor-pronator group to the epicondyle does not require division. Friction neuritis from recurrent dislocation of the nerve is not a potential cause of postoperative failure as it is with the medial epicondylectomy technique. Advantages over the transposition procedures are the relative simplicity of the procedure, minimal manipulation of the ulnar nerve itself, and shorter recovery time. Disadvantages are **(1)** the potential for callus formation and subsequent nerve entrapment at the site of the partial osteotomy, and **(2)** risk to the ulnar nerve and ulnar collateral ligament from the proximate use of an air-powered drill.

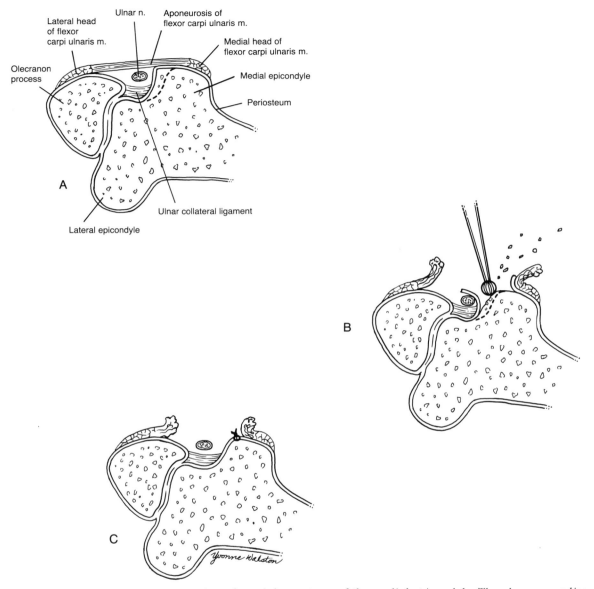

Figure 2 *(A) Schematic representation of partial osteotomy of the medial epicondyle. The ulnar nerve lies adjacent to the posterior aspect of the medial epicondyle and beneath the aponeurosis traversing between the heads of the flexor carpi ulnaris muscle. (B) The aponeurosis is divided and the nerve is released along its length from the medial intermuscular septum to the deep aspect of the flexor carpi ulnaris. The periosteum over the tip of the epicondyle is incised and reflected over the nerve. The cubital tunnel is widened by drilling down the posterior aspect of the epicondyle. (C) The periosteum is repaired over the bony defect.*

Results of Surgery

Numerous and obvious difficulties are encountered when evaluating and comparing the results of different authors. A major difficulty is the lack of well-designed, controlled or randomized studies. The few studies which attempt to compare results are neither truly randomized nor prospective, do not have comparable control groups, and rarely use statistical analyses. None has been able to clearly demonstrate, in terms of outcome, an advantage of one surgical technique over another.

Retrospectively comparing results of patients undergoing a particular operation is also difficult. Some series report a mixture of procedures.[1,18] For example, in McGowan's report of 42 cases of anterior transposition, 25 underwent placement subcutaneously, 17 intramuscularly, and 4 submuscularly.[28] This makes the interpretation of the outcome data tenuous. Other series may report results of one particular technique, but include in their patient population patients undergoing "re-do" operations.[26] Lack of a widely accepted classification system for grading preoperative severity of symptoms and postoperative outcome also hampers attempts at retrospective review of large numbers of series. These series differ significantly with regard to the severity of symptoms of their respective patient populations, and with regard to the duration of symptoms.

Definitions of excellent, good, fair, and poor results also vary widely. In one study, only 22% of patients undergoing surgery by a variety of techniques had good results, while 54% had fair results (defined as "little to no improvement, but not worsened").[1] Most surgeons would not consider "no improvement" as a fair result, but rather would classify it as a poor result or failure. Another study defined satisfactory outcome as "normal use of the hand and the patient's satisfaction with the results."[18] Future studies would do well to use a well-defined standardized grading system such as that suggested by Dellon or by Gabel and Amadio.[10,17]

Personal biases are overtly present in a number of reports. Advocates of the lesser procedures profusely extol a number of disadvantages of transposition procedures, but fail to substantiate with clinical data an increased morbidity with these procedures. Conversely, the proponents of anterior transposition champion their procedures as having better results, although this contention has little scientific validity.

Although simple decompression is one of the more widely used techniques in recent years, very little data regarding the outcome can be found in the literature. Advocates of the procedure claim equal efficacy to the transposition procedures, with much less risk and morbidity. Wilson and Krout reported good or excellent outcomes in 13 of 16 patients (81%) undergoing simple decompression.[36] Thomsen reported 32 decompressive procedures followed from 7 months to 5 years postoperatively; 16 resulted in complete alleviation of symptoms, while 12 resulted in improvement and 4 in no improvement. None experienced complications or deterioration.[34]

Results of medial epicondylectomy are more variable. Some surgeons reported good to excellent results in 45% to 85% of their patients. Complete resolution of symptoms and neurologic deficits occurred less frequently than in many series reporting outcome of transposition procedures. The best results were obtained in patients with early or mild symptoms. Poor outcomes, defined as those with no improvement or worsening, occurred in 0% to 32% of cases.[8,16,22,23,25,29] Eversmann suggests the best indications for medial epicondylectomy may be recurrent subluxation of the nerve, cubitus valgus deformity, or an irritating nonunited medial epicondyle fracture with callus formation.[14]

Advocates of the anterior transposition, particularly those who use the subcutaneous technique, argue that this operation has been shown to most consistently relieve symptoms and has withstood the test of time. Transposition procedures clearly have certain advantages over the lesser procedures, but they also entail certain risks and disadvantages (Table 3). Most reports, unfortunately, combine the results of the different techniques of transposition. Perhaps the best results have been achieved by Leffert using the Learmonth (submuscular transposition) technique.[26] More than half of his patients, including those undergoing "re-do" procedures, experienced complete resolution of all pain and neurologic deficits. Complications were "minimal" and no patients were worsened as a result of the operation. Likewise, Levy and Apfelberg performed three subcutaneous transpositions and seven submuscular transpositions to achieve a 60% rate of excellent results, defined as complete resolution of symptoms.[27] In most series, the results of the anterior transposition are similar to those obtained by simple decompression and medial epicondylectomy.[15,18,21]

The incidence of post-transposition failure or complications is not clear. Surgeons having poor results with this technique generally do not report their experiences. Some authors imply a high failure rate in their prior experiences with transpositions, leading them to adopt lesser procedures as the initial treatment of choice.[14,16] In fact, the series reporting reoperation for failure of surgical therapy predominately consist of failed transposition operations.[5,6,17,26] Although the literature suggests a slightly greater chance of symptom resolution after transposition procedures, especially in patients with more advanced disease, it also suggests a greater likelihood of postoperative worsening as compared to the lesser procedures.

Perhaps the best indications for anterior transposition are failure of simple decompression to alleviate symptoms, recurrent subluxation of the ulnar nerve, persistent or progressive valgus deformity, and persistently positive elbow flexion test with severe neuritic signs with prolonged flexion of the elbow.[14]

The data regarding results of decompression or transposition followed by the ensheathing of the ulnar nerve in Silastic are sparse. There appears to be no added advantage to this procedure.[3,6]

The author, until recently, used the subcutaneous transposition technique for initial surgical treatment of cubital tunnel syndrome. However, six of the last seven patients treated by the author underwent extended cubital tunnel release with partial osteotomy of the medial epicondyle. The seventh had a chronically-subluxating ulnar nerve and underwent transposition. Based on the grading scale of Gabel and Amadio, all had at least a good outcome and two had excellent results defined as alleviation of all symptoms and deficits. No complications have occurred.

Summary

The course of the ulnar nerve from the extensor compartment of the arm across the elbow joint into the flexor compartment of the forearm lends itself to injury from a wide range of compressive, tractional, and frictional forces in the vicinity of the elbow. Subsequent damage to the nerve produces a neuropathic process known as the cubital tunnel syndrome. Characteristic symptoms are weakness and atrophy of the intrinsic muscles of the hand, and numbness and painful dysesthesias of the medial aspect of the hand. A number of surgical techniques have been designed to relieve entrapment of the ulnar nerve as it passes around the medial epicondyle of the elbow. They either remove the compressing agent or remove the nerve from its bed. Each procedure has its proponents. The efficacy and morbidity of any of the five basic techniques have not been shown to be significantly better or worse than any other.

References

1. Adelaar RS, Foster WC, McDowell C. The treatment of the cubital tunnel syndrome. *J Hand Surg Am.* 1984;9A:90–95.
2. Apfelberg DB, Larson SJ. Dynamic anatomy of the ulnar nerve at the elbow. *Plast Reconstr Surg.* 1973; 51:76–81.
3. Benoit BG, Preston DN, Atack DM, et al. Neurolysis combined with the application of a silastic envelope for ulnar nerve entrapment at the elbow. *Neurosurgery.* 1987;20:594–598.
4. Bielawski M, Hallett M. Position of the elbow in determination of abnormal motor conduction of the ulnar nerve across the elbow. *Muscle Nerve.* 1989;12:803–809.
5. Broudy AS, Leffert RD, Smith RJ. Technical problems with ulnar nerve transposition at the elbow: findings and results of reoperation. *J Hand Surg Am.* 1978;3:85–89.
6. Campbell JB, Post KD, Morantz RA. A technique for relief of motor and sensory deficits occurring after anterior ulnar transposition. *J Neurosurg.* 1974; 40:405-409.
7. Campbell WW, Pridgeon RM, Riaz G, et al. Sparing of the flexor carpi ulnaris in ulnar neuropathy at the elbow. *Muscle Nerve.* 1989;12:965–967.
8. Craven PR Jr, Green DP. Cubital tunnel syndrome: Treatment by medial epicondylectomy. *J Bone Joint Surg Am.* 1980;62A:986–989.
9. Dahlin LB. Aspects on pathophysiology of nerve entrapments and nerve compression injuries. *Neurosurg Clin North Am.*1991;2:21–29.

10. Dellon AL. Techniques for successful management of ulnar nerve entrapment at the elbow. *Neurosurg Clin North Am*. 1991;2:57–73.

11. Dellon AL. Review of treatment results for ulnar nerve entrapment at the elbow. *J Hand Surg Am*. 1989;14A:688–700.

12. Dimond ML, Lister GD. Cubital tunnel syndrome treated by long-arm splintage (abstract). *J Hand Surg Am*. 1985;10A:430. Abstract.

13. Eisen A, Danon J. The mild cubital tunnel syndrome: its natural history and indications for surgical intervention. *Neurology*. 1974;24:608–613.

14. Eversmann WW Jr. Entrapment and compression neuropathies. In: Green DP, ed. *Operative Hand Surgery*, 2nd ed. New York, NY: Churchill Livingstone; 1988:2:1423–1478.

15. Freidman RJ, Cochran TP. Anterior transposition for advanced ulnar neuropathy at the elbow. *Surg Neurol*. 1986;25:446–448.

16. Froimson AI, Zahrawi F. Treatment of compression neuropathy of the ulnar nerve at the elbow by epicondylectomy and neurolysis. *J Hand Surg Am*. 1980;5:391–395.

17. Gabel GT, Amadio PC. Reoperation for failed decompression of the ulnar nerve in the region of the elbow. *J Bone Joint Surg Am*. 1990;72A:213–219.

18. Gay JR, Love JG. Diagnosis and treatment of tardy paralysis of the ulnar nerve: Based on a study of 100 cases. *J Bone Joint Surg Am*. 1947;29:1087–1097.

19. Gelberman RH, Szabo RM, Williamson RV. Tissue pressure threshold for peripheral nerve viability. *Clin Orthop*. 1983;178:285–289.

20. Gessini L, Jandolo B, Pietrangeli A, et al. Ulnar nerve entrapment at the elbow by persistent epitrochleoanconeus muscle. *J Neurosurg*. 1981;55:830–831.

21. Hagstrom P. Ulnar nerve compression at the elbow: results of surgery in 85 cases. *Scand J Plast Reconstr Surg*. 1977;11:59–62.

22. Heithoff SJ, Millender LH, Nalebuff EA, et al. Medial epicondylectomy for the treatment of ulnar nerve compression at the elbow. *J Hand Surg Am*. 1990; 15A:22–29.

23. Jones RE, Gauntt C. Medial epicondylectomy for ulnar nerve compression syndrome at the elbow. *Clin Orthop*. 1979;139:174–178.

24. Kincaid JC, Phillips LH, II, Daube JR. The evaluation of suspected ulnar neuropathy at the elbow: Normal conduction study values. *Arch Neurol*. 1986;43: 44–47.

25. King T, Morgan FP. Late results of removing the medial humeral epicondyle for traumatic ulnar neuritis. *J Bone Joint Surg Br*. 1959;41B:51–55.

26. Leffert RD. Anterior submuscular transposition of the ulnar nerves by the Learmonth technique. *J Hand Surg*. 1982;7:147–155.

27. Levy DM, Apfelberg DB. Results of anterior transposition for ulnar neuropathy at the elbow. *Am J Surg*. 1972;123:304–308.

28. McGowan AJ. The results of transposition of the ulnar nerve for traumatic ulnar neuritis. *J Bone Joint Surg Br*. 1950;32B:293–300.

29. Neblett C, Ehni G. Medial epicondylectomy for ulnar palsy. *J Neurosurg*. 1970;32:55–62.

30. Osborne G. Compression neuritis of the ulnar nerve at the elbow. *Hand*. 1970;2:10–16.

31. Payan J. Anterior transposition of the ulnar nerve: an electrophysiological study. *J Neurol Neurosurg Psychiatry*. 1970;33:157–165.

32. Rengachary SS. Entrapment neuropathies. In: Wilkins RH, Rengachary SS, eds. *Neurosurgery*. New York, NY: McGraw Hill; 1985:2:1771–1795.

33. Rydevik B, Lundborg G, Bagge U. Effects of graded compression on intraneural blood flow: an in vivo study on rabbit tibial nerve. *J Hand Surg Am*. 1981;6:3–12.

34. Thomsen PB. Compression neuritis of the ulnar nerve treated with simple decompression. *Acta Orthop Scand*. 1977;48:164–167.

35. Wadsworth TG. The external compression syndrome of the ulnar nerve at the cubital tunnel. *Clin Orthop*. 1977;124:189–204.

36. Wilson DH, Krout R. Surgery of ulnar neuropathy at the elbow: 16 cases treated by decompression without transposition. *J Neurosurg*. 1973;38:780–785.

CHAPTER 7

Entrapment Neuropathies of the Lower Extremity

Lee Kesterson, MD

Entrapment neuropathies of the lower extremities are less common than those of the upper extremities. The mere existence of several of them, much less their surgical management, is controversial. In this chapter, the more common syndromes as well as their pathophysiology, electrodiagnostic and clinical features, differential diagnoses, and treatment are addressed.

Lateral Femoral Cutaneous Nerve Entrapment

Clinical Features

Lesions of the lateral femoral cutaneous nerve were first described by Bernhardt and Roth in 1895.[3,20] The term meralgia paresthetica, previously used to define any pain in the thigh, was applied.[6] This term now refers to a condition that manifests itself as discomfort in the distribution of the lateral femoral cutaneous nerve. This discomfort may be in the form of formication, coldness, burning, or lightning pains, which may progress to hypesthesia or frank anesthesia.[8] Relief is usually realized by assuming the supine position or by flexing the thigh while in the erect position. The symptoms are usually unilateral.[6,8]

Physical examination reveals only sensory loss over the affected area. The sensory loss occupies a region much less than that usually described for the lateral cutaneous nerve distribution. The area of sensory loss for pinprick is usually less than that observed with light touch. Importantly, the response to sensory testing may be one of hyperesthesia rather than hypesthesia in some cases.

Etiology

Ghent described four variations of the course of the lateral femoral cutaneous nerve, each of which may produce the classical picture of this disorder: **(1)** the nerve passes through the inguinal ligament; **(2)** nerve deformation by a sharp edge of iliacus fascia lying posterior to a normally placed nerve (compression occurs when the patient is in the supine position); **(3)** the nerve enters the sartorius muscle near its origin at the anterior superior iliac spine and passes distally in the muscle before emerging beneath the fascia lata; and, **(4)** the lateral cutaneous nerve enters the thigh, crossing the iliac crest lateral and posterior to the anterior superior iliac spine.[8]

Factors that precipitate symptoms include obesity, adoption of the recumbent position in debilitating disease or following anesthesia, increased intra-abdominal pressure (usually associated with pregnancy, ascites, or tumor), and altered mechanics of the hip joint secondary to intraspinal disease such as a herniated disc).[6,8,14]

Differential Diagnosis

Proximal lesions should be ruled out before surgical therapy is considered. The differential diagnosis includes femoral neuropathy and radiculopathy involving the second or third lumbar nerve roots. In these conditions, whether caused by intraspinal or extraspinal disease, motor disability consisting of weakness of the hip flexors or the quadriceps muscle is generally present. A herniated disc at L1–2 or L2–3 may also mimic meralgia paresthetica. In addition, lesions in the ilium, cecum, sigmoid colon, or any lesion in the upper retroperitoneal space may compress the nerve at the level of the psoas muscle.[6,11]

Electrodiagnostic evaluation

Electromyographic (EMG) studies of the quadriceps muscle are useful because the diagnosis of meralgia paresthetica is unlikely if abnormalities are found. Sensory action potentials may be abnormal in meralgia paresthetica. It is important to test the asymptomatic thigh to assure the validity of the technique, especially in obesity.[6]

Treatment

A conservative approach to this mild condition is usually indicated. Initial attempts should include altering physical activity or removing constricting belts, corsets, or binders. If weight gain or pregnancy is a provocative factor, weight reduction or passage of time will often improve matters. If these measures do not relieve the symptoms, local nerve blocks or steroid injections may be helpful.[6,25]

On rare occasions, severe symptoms persist despite attempts at conservative measures. In these cases, surgical decompression may be entertained. The lateral femoral cutaneous nerve is exposed, either through a vertical (Figure 1A) or horizontal incision.[1,11]

Kempe describes a vertical incision that begins approximately 2.5 cm above and medial to the anterior superior iliac spine and extends caudally. This exposes the interval between the tensor fascia lata and the sartorius muscle. The fascia lata is then incised and retracted, permitting the nerve to be identified (Figure 1B). The

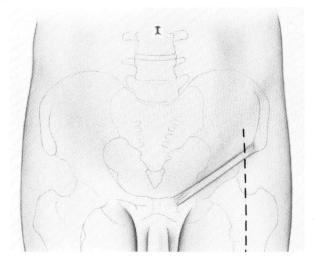

Figure 1A. Surgical exposure for management of meralgia paresthetica. A vertical incision located just medial to the anterior superior iliac spine exposes the lateral femoral cutaneous nerve. This incision will more readily allow medial retraction of an abdominal panniculus in an obese patient.[19]

nerve then can be dissected proximally to the inguinal ligament, where it is released into the subcutaneous tissue. Failures of surgical management are not uncommon, and are sometimes blamed on the difficulties associated with nerve identification and/or the performance of an inadequate decompression.[1,6,11] Sectioning of the nerve should be avoided because the symptoms may worsen postoperatively.[1]

Proximal Sciatic Nerve Entrapment

The piriformis syndrome represents a clinical entity characterized by neurologic symptoms referable to the distribution of the sciatic nerve. It is one of many pathological processes that may cause symptoms in a sciatic nerve distribution of nonspinal origin. Patients with these symptoms may have associated lumbosacral spine disease.[6] The legitimacy of the piriformis syndrome is often questioned. The

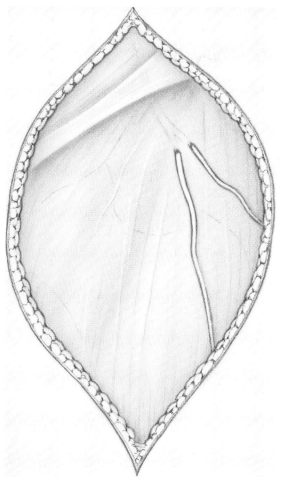

Figure 1B. *Occasionally, the nerve is difficult to differentiate from surrounding adipose tissue. It is best identified at the medial border of the sartorius muscle where it penetrates the fascia lata. Once identified, it can be traced to the inguinal ligament, which is then incised. Release of the nerve into the subcutaneous tissue then occurs.*

diagnosis of a proximal sciatic nerve lesion is difficult to establish with certainty.

Clinical Features

Symptoms are not unlike those associated with a herniated lumbar disc. Sensory and motor deficits are more extensive than those associated with a single nerve root, however. Complete palsy of the sciatic nerve is unusual.

Partial involvement with weakness of any or all of the knee flexors, ankle flexors or extensors, and foot intrinsics may occur. Sensory loss may involve all of the foot except for the small region supplied by the saphenous nerve over the medial malleolus.

Pathophysiology and Differential Diagnosis

Yeoman first stressed the clinical significance of the anatomical relationships of the sciatic nerve and the piriformis muscle.[30] The pathophysiologic mechanisms of nerve irritation or injury by this muscle are still unclear. It is thought that the variable anatomical relationship of the nerve or its branches to the muscle are the principal factors.

Pecina examined 130 cadavers and discovered that in 6% the sciatic nerve passed between the two tendinous parts of the piriformis muscle (Fig. 2A).[17] A high bifurcation of the nerve, with the peroneal portion of the nerve passing through the muscle, was not uncommon. Inward rotation rather than outward rotation of the hip was noted to cause nerve compression by the two tendinous portions of the muscle. However, this anatomical variation is much more common than the existence of the syndrome.[17]

Other causes of sciatic nerve entrapment are also rare. A case in which a myofascial band in the distal portion of the thigh trapped the sciatic nerve was reported by Banerjee and Hall.[2] Entrapment has been reported to occur secondary to fibrosis induced by pentazocine injection.[20] Symptomatic compression of the sciatic nerve may be caused by a retroperitoneal hematoma due to a complication of anticoagulant therapy or hip surgery.[6,7,22,28] Sciatic nerve compromise may be caused by the leakage of acrylic into the region posterior to the hip joint during total hip replacement.[7] Abnormal subclinical EMG findings have been observed in the majority of patients undergoing hip replacement. An aneurysm of the iliac artery may also involve the sciatic nerve.[6] Finally, nonstructural etiologies should be considered: diabetic and vascular neuropathies may cause symptoms similar to those mentioned earlier.[6]

Electrodiagnostic and Radiographic Evaluation

The most important role of electrodiagnostic studies is to separate proximal sciatic nerve entrapment from the more common root compression syndromes. EMG studies are invaluable: the proximal paraspinous muscles, as well as the muscles supplied by the inferior and superior gluteal nerves (tensor fascia lata, and the gluteus minimus and medius muscles) are usually abnormal with a root lesion, but normal with a sciatic nerve entrapment. If the superior gluteal nerve is involved, the gluteus minimus and medius muscles and the tensor fascia lata often demonstrate abnormal EMG readings.

Somatosensory evoked potentials may be assessed over the gluteal fold, over the spine at L5 region, and over the T12–L1 region. These potentials are thought to respectively originate from the sciatic nerve, the roots of the cauda equina, and the dorsal root entry zone of the spinal cord. Cutaneous sensory action potentials recorded from the sural, peroneal, or plantar nerves may be abnormal with sciatic lesions and normal with root lesions. The H-reflex and F-responses are not useful regarding the differential diagnosis.

Abdominal and pelvic computed tomography (CT) may demonstrate structural lesions impinging upon the sciatic nerve. Magnetic resonance imaging (MRI), however, is increasingly being used for this purpose.[6,27]

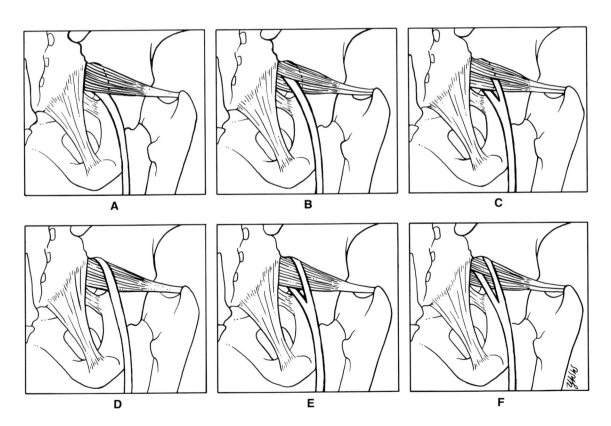

Figure 2A. *As described by Pecína, there are a number of anatomical variations of the relationship between the sciatic nerve and the piriformis muscle. A and B are the most commonly encountered variations while E and F are the least common. C and D are of intermediate frequency.*

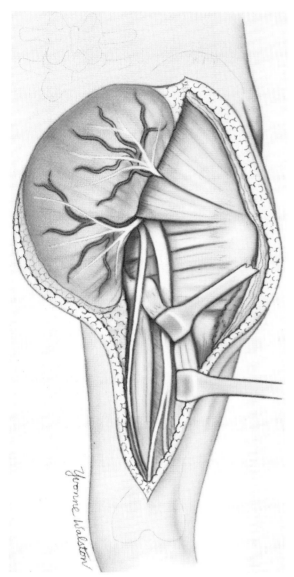

Figure 2B. *Surgical exposure of the proximal sciatic nerve. The "gluteal lid" is lifted to expose the sciatic nerve as it exits the pelvis. Note its anatomical relationship to the surrounding musculature and neural structures.*

Treatment

Since the true etiology of proximal sciatic nerve dysfunction is often in question, a reasonable course of conservative treatment should nearly always precede surgical management. Although this management scheme is nonspecific, a trial with a nonsteroidal anti-inflammatory agent and rest should be the initial therapy in most cases.

The surgical approach for the management of the piriformis syndrome is discussed in Chapters 11 and 12, and is illustrated in Figure 2B. It consists of the sectioning of the piriformis muscle at its tendinous insertion on the greater trochanter.

When sciatic neuropathy is due to hematoma as a complication of anticoagulant therapy, operative exploration may occasionally be appropriate, following correction of the coagulation abnormalities.[7,15] Fleming demonstrated that, in the setting of postoperative hematomas following hip surgery, neural recovery appears to occur sooner and more completely in those patients who undergo early decompression compared to those who do not.[7]

Posterior Tarsal Tunnel Syndrome

Two forms of the tarsal tunnel syndrome exist, but the posterior form is usually called the tarsal tunnel syndrome and is much more common. The less common anterior tarsal tunnel syndrome involves the deep peroneal nerve.[6] In this chapter, each is referred to separately as the posterior and the anterior tarsal tunnel syndromes.

Clinical and Electrodiagnostic Features

Patients with posterior tarsal tunnel syndrome present with a slow and insidiously progressive course of burning pain and paresthesias involving the plantar surface of the foot and toes.[16] The distribution of involvement depends on which branch of the posterior tibial nerve is involved. Occasionally, the pain radiates proximally into the leg. The pain is usually exacerbated by standing and/or activity and is relieved by rest and/or by rubbing the foot. Symptoms are often worse at night. The heel is frequently spared because the calcaneal branch more often arises proximal to the flexor retinaculum and, hence, is less frequently involved.[13,18]

Clinical signs of the posterior tarsal tunnel

syndrome are frequently difficult to detect. The intrinsic foot musculature may be weak and atrophied; it is best evaluated by examining toe plantar flexion strength, especially in the lateral toes. Intrinsic muscle weakness leads to a change in conformation of the foot and to instability of the phalanges, which impairs the pushing-off phase of walking.[6] This motor disturbance may lead to a pes cavus deformity, with clawing of the toes.[14] A flat-foot gait with a short stride length may result. The sensory loss is dependent on which of the branches is involved. The sensory examination is also difficult because of the thickness of the skin on the plantar surface of the foot. Hypesthesia along the medial surface of the foot, if present, is easier to detect.

A positive Tinel's sign may be present with distal paresthesias and pain occurring following gentle percussion over the tarsal tunnel. This is located inferior and posterior to the medial malleolus. A Tinel's sign may also be present over the course of each of the plantar nerves.[6]

Electrodiagnostic studies are often useful. Baylen found an abnormal EMG in 11 of 48 patients with rheumatoid arthritis. Only 2 had symptoms of the posterior tarsal tunnel syndrome.[3] When conduction latencies are performed, they should be determined in both plantar nerves in order to increase the accuracy of pathology detection.

Sensory action potentials recorded proximal to the flexor retinaculum may be abnormal and are more sensitive than motor conduction velocities for detecting pathology. Motor conduction latencies, recorded distally following stimulation proximal to the flexor retinaculum, are considered abnormal when prolonged more than 1 millisecond (comparing the two feet). Prolonged distal motor latency to the abductor hallucis is indicative of involvement of the medial plantar branch, while prolonged latency to the abductor digiti quinti represents involvement of the lateral branch. Typically, the conduction velocities in the posterior tibial nerve in the leg are normal.[6,18] EMG has been infrequently reported because of difficulty in testing the intrinsic foot musculature.

Pathophysiology

The posterior tarsal tunnel syndrome is the counterpart of the carpal tunnel syndrome. The site of compression is located posterior and inferior to the medial malleolus. The roof of the tarsal tunnel is comprised of the flexor retinaculum and the floor comprised of the bones of the ankle. Numerous structures are present within this tunnel, including tendons, synovial sheaths, and neurovascular structures. Any or all of the three terminal branches of the posterior tibial nerve (the medial and lateral planter and the calcaneal nerve) may lie within the tunnel.[6] The tarsal tunnel also differs from the carpal tunnel in that numerous fibrous septa connect the roof of the tunnel and the floor.

Fifty percent of patients presenting with symptoms of the posterior tarsal tunnel syndrome have a history of trauma. However, the symptoms may develop some time after injury.[18] Symptoms may be due to intraneural scarring or to nonspecific scarring of the surrounding osseous and soft-tissue structures. Prolonged standing and venous stasis also have been reported to be associated with this syndrome.

The etiology may be a nonspecific tenosynovitis or venous congestion within the tunnel.[6] The tarsal syndrome has been reported in association with rheumatoid arthritis, and in hyperlipidemias, where the etiology is lipid deposition within the tunnel.[21]

Treatment

Conservative treatment should begin by minimizing local trauma and/or by bracing the foot with a medial arch support. An arch support immobilizes the affected region, similar to the use of a wrist splint in the carpal tunnel syndrome. Nonsteroidal anti-inflammatory agents may be beneficial in the presence of a local phlebitis or tenosynovitis. A block of the posterior tibial nerve with a local anesthetic agent just proximal to the flexor retinaculum may relieve symptoms and aid in predicting a favorable operative result.[18] Operative treatment should be performed only following failure of conservative management, and in patients in whom the clinical features are typical and the electrodiagnostic studies support the diagnosis. Wilemon reported that fewer than 200 patients with tarsal tunnel syndrome had been reported prior to 1979; only about 60% underwent surgery.[29]

The surgical approach is usually through a curvilinear incision 1.5 cm behind and below the medial malleolus (Figure 3A). The incision may be extended proximally to identify the posterior tibial nerve in the distal calf. Following incision of the flexor retinaculum, most authors recommend external neurolysis of both branches, which may be bound by the numerous fibrous bands and septations that exist in this region (Figure 3B).[14,18]

Anterior Tarsal Tunnel Syndrome

Clinical Features

The anterior tarsal tunnel syndrome refers to compression of the deep peroneal nerve at the ankle. The clinical features are mainly sensory, with numbness and paresthesias in the first dorsal web space. Occasionally, complaints relate to aching and tightness around the ankle and dorsum of the foot with centripetal radiation up the entire peroneal trunk. Pain in-

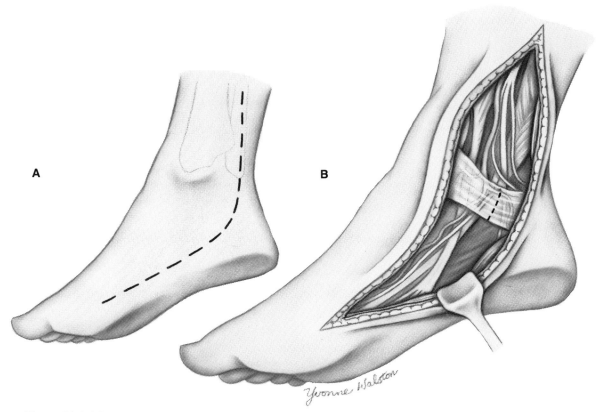

A

B

Figure 3(A) The incision for exposure of the posterior tibial nerve for tarsal tunnel release. Note the location of the incision posterior and inferior to the medial malleolus. (B) The flexor retinaculum is depicted with its underlying structures, including the medial and lateral plantar nerves and the medial calcaneal branch. The terminal branches of the posterior tibial nerve should be freed of the many fibrous attachments.

creases with certain positions and with inactivity, often awakening the patient from sleep.[5,6]

This syndrome has been reviewed extensively by Borges et al. There are, however, very few reports and little investigation regarding the syndrome's frequency, etiology, or electrophysiologic features. Borges et al, in an autopsy study, demonstrated that the deep peroneal nerve was flattened and widened by the overlying extensor retinaculum.[5] This study demonstrated that firm plantar flexion at the ankle with dorsiflexion of the toes stressed the nerve to the maximum degree. This is the same position that is induced by wearing high-heel shoes. The position of the nerve at the dorsum of the ankle also makes it susceptible to compression, for example by tight shoes.[6]

Treatment

If the patient does not experience relief with rest, removal of possible external aggravating pressure, or anti-inflammatory medication, operative intervention may be necessary. Decompression is undertaken in a similar manner to that performed for the posterior syndrome. During decompression of the nerve, a branch of the superficial peroneal nerve should not be mistaken for a parallel branch of the deep peroneal nerve. The nerve also should be traced proximally to exclude a lesion in the ankle region.[14]

Peroneal Nerve Entrapment

Clinical and Electrodiagnostic Features

Peroneal neuropathy is a common and well-known clinical entity. It is manifested as paralysis or weakness of the foot dorsiflexors and as weakness of foot eversion. A steppage gait may be present.[28] The peroneal nerve, as well as its superficial and deep branches, may be affected by compression. Superficial branch compression, however, is more common. The lateral surface of the leg, the lateral malleolus, the dorsum of the foot, and the web interspaces of the second and third toes are usually hypesthetic. The superficial branch also innervates the peroneus longus and brevis muscles. This leads to weakness of foot eversion.

If the deep branch is affected, motor involvement is more prominent because of the innervation of the anterior tibial muscles, as well as the extensors of all the toes. The deep branch provides sensation to a relatively small area between the first and second toes and the adjacent portion of the dorsum of the foot. The branch to the extensor digitorum brevis is observed to be weak early in the course when nerve damage occurs. It is consequently important to examine the activity of this muscle. Although the extensor digitorum brevis muscle may receive innervation from both branches, it is innervated by the deep peroneal nerve in 72% of cases.[6] When the common peroneal nerve is compressed, clinical features attributable to both the deep and superficial branches may be present.

The clinical features of peroneal entrapment vary, depending on the nature of the condition. Acute compressive lesions tend to be associated with more motor than sensory involvement. More chronic forms of compression, such as those caused by cysts or tumors, may be associated with radiating pain and subsequent progressive motor and sensory disturbances.[6] An electrodiagnostic evaluation is useful diagnostically, and for establishing a prognosis.[6] If the motor conduction velocity is normal or nearly normal, the prognosis for recovery is excellent. The prognosis is poor if the conduction velocity is slow.

Motor nerve conduction velocities are measured from the tibialis anterior muscle with stimulation at the ankle, lateral popliteal fossa, and below the fibular head. Recording from the tibialis anterior rather than the extensor digitorum brevis muscles may be more useful because of the frequent presence of complete denervation when the extensor digitorum is involved. The loss of amplitude of the compound motor action potential is also a useful observation regarding motor nerve conduction studies. Again, recording from the tibialis anterior muscle is more beneficial than from the extensor digitorum muscle for the same reason.

Distal stimulation at the ankle, with nerve action potential recording distal and proximal to the fibular head, is more accurate than motor conduction velocity regarding identification of focal slowing.[9] In fact, absolute focal slowing of sensory conduction is a more sensitive measurement with fewer false positives than relative focal sensory conduction slowing, decrease of sensory action potential, and dispersal of the sensory action potential.[3] Axonal features are more common than features associated with demyelination.

EMG readings are frequently abnormal, but may be confusing because of the tendency of proximal lesions to involve the peroneal innervated muscles. However, EMG of the peroneal innervated muscles is a good indicator of recovery because reinnervation occurs prior to clinical recovery.[6]

Pathophysiology

Peroneal palsies are relatively common, but true entrapment neuropathies are uncommon. The fibular tunnel syndrome is an entrapment phenomenon in which the peroneal nerve is compressed against the fibula by the tendinous edge of the peroneus longus muscle, which originates at the neck of the fibula. External compression of the peroneal nerve at the fibular head can occur secondary to a number of processes, however: plaster casts, tight stockings, bandages, and garters may cause compression. External compression may also occur in a patient who is stuporous or in a coma secondary to drug ingestion, with the leg laying against a protruding object. It also may occur when a patient is under general anesthesia or in the lithotomy position.

A number of masses, including ganglia, nerve tumors, or tumors of neighboring structures have been noted to lead to compression neuropathy.[6] Peroneal nerve compression has also been associated with increased intra-articular pressure within the knee, which leads to herniation of synovial tissue posteriorly. This may manifest as fullness or swelling and pain in the posterior aspect of the knee. In some instances, surgical exploration may be required to differentiate entrapment from external nerve compression from a variety of masses, including ganglia or tumors.

Occupational practices such as prolonged kneeling or squatting may also predispose to a peroneal compression neuropathy.[7,13,24] Compression is thought to occur at the tendon of the posterior border of the peroneus longus muscle at the level of the head of the fibula.[15] Peroneal palsy may develop following loss of a large amount of weight.[6] This most probably is related to an increased susceptibility of the nerve to trauma at the fibular head.

Differential Diagnosis

A complete palsy of the foot dorsiflexors is strongly suggestive of a peroneal nerve palsy. Most radiculopathies partially spare these muscles due to overlap of nerve root innervation. An L5 radiculopathy resembles a peroneal palsy, but is differentiated from it by: **(1)** weakness of foot inversion, **(2)** sensory loss occurring well above the midpoint of the calf, **(3)** more weakness of the extensor hallucis than of the anterior tibialis muscle (which receives more L4 innervation than does the extensor hallucis muscle and is, thus, less involved), and **(4)** back pain.[6]

The peroneal nerve may be damaged at different levels below the knee. The deep peroneal nerve may be injured by an anterior compartment syndrome with resultant footdrop, but with sparing of the foot evertors. The distal deep peroneal nerve may be involved in an anterior tarsal tunnel syndrome. This may produce asymptomatic atrophy of the extensor digitorum brevis as well as a sensory loss in the web space between the first and second toes.

A sciatic nerve lesion may present with predominantly peroneal signs because of the more frequent and severe involvement of the peroneal nerve compared to the tibial nerve. The additional absence of the ankle reflex, atrophy or weakness of the hamstring or calf muscles, or sensory loss on the sole of the foot may indicate that the sciatic nerve is affected.[6]

Peripheral neuropathies may also cause peroneal nerve dysfunction. The common peroneal nerve is also a frequent site of involvement of diabetic peripheral neuropathy.[6]

Treatment

Patients who experience a chronic progressive course of pain and sensory and/or motor loss should be considered to have an entrapment neuropathy (Figure 4A,B), tumor, or ganglion cyst. Early exploration is indicated, since little will be gained from waiting. Those patients with an acute compressive lesion due to the more common etiologies should be treated expectantly with alteration of behavioral patterns that predispose to the neuropathy. A brace should be used to provide stability to the ankle during ambulation.

Saphenous Nerve Entrapment Syndrome

The saphenous nerve is the largest cutaneous sensory branch of the femoral nerve. It is a

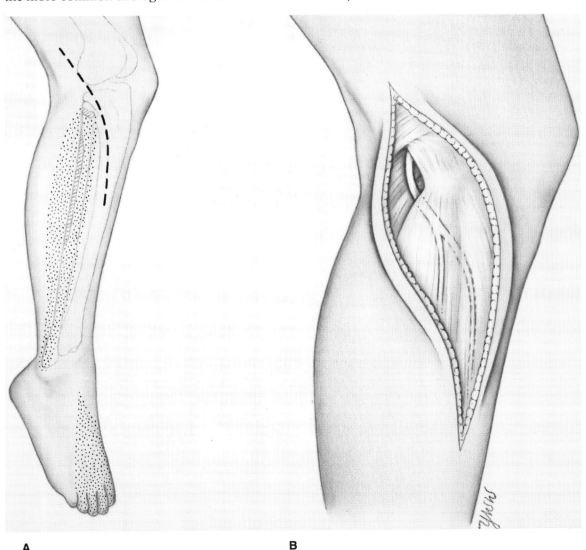

A   **B**

Figure 4 (A) Surgical exposure for the management of peroneal nerve comparison at the lateral aspect of the knee. (B) Note the course of the peroneal nerve underneath the peroneus longus muscle as it passes through the fibular tunnel.

pure sensory nerve with two terminal branches. The infrapatellar branch supplies the anteromedial aspect of the knee, while the descending branch supplies the anteromedial aspect of the leg and ankle.

Clinical Features and Anatomy

The saphenous nerve originates just below the inguinal ligament. It then enters the adductor canal (Hunter's canal), crosses the femoral artery from lateral to medial and leaves the canal by piercing its roof together with the descending genicular artery. The nerve penetrates the subsartorial fascia, the roof of the canal. It is here that the site of entrapment is thought to occur, approximately 10 cm above the medial condyle of the femur. After piercing the deep fascia, the nerve branches into its two terminal branches.

Physical examination reveals tenderness over the point of emergence of the nerve from the subsartorial canal. A Tinel's sign may be noted at this point, as well as along the course of the nerve. Sensory loss usually occurs along the medial aspect of the knee and/or leg.[6,19]

The saphenous nerve may be injured during vascular surgical procedures (arterial and venous) or by lacerations. The infrapatellar branch may be injured during knee surgery, with numbness occurring over the region of the patellar tendon.[6]

Treatment

If the syndrome remains refractory to conservative measures, neurolysis should be performed at the point of penetrance through the roof of Hunter's canal. This is carried out via an incision centered at the nerve's point of emergence from the canal. The deep fascia along the anterior border of the sartorius muscle is then incised. The sartorius muscle is retracted medially to identify the roof of Hunter's canal. The point of emergence is then identified, as well as its association with the descending genicular artery. Finally, the fascia should be widely opened.[6]

References

1. Aldrich EF, Van den Heever CM. Suprainguinal ligament approach for surgical treatment of meralgia paresthetica. *J Neurosurg.* 1989;70:492–494.
2. Banerjee T, Hall CD. Sciatic entrapment neuropathy. *J Neurosurg.* 1976;45:216–217.
3. Baylan SP, Paik SW, Barnert AL, et al. Prevalence of the tarsal tunnel syndrome in rheumatoid arthritis. *Rheumatol Rehabil.* 1981;20:148–150.
4. Bernhardt M. Ueber isolirt in gebiete des nervus cutaneus femoris externus vorkommende parästhesien. *Neurol Centralbl.* 1895;14:242–244.
5. Borges LF, Hallet M, Selkoe DJ, et al. The anterior tarsal tunnel syndrome: report of two cases. *J Neurosurg.* 1981;54:89–92.
6. Dawson DM, Hallet M, Millender LH. *Entrapment Neuropathies.* 2nd ed. Boston, Mass: Little Brown and Company;1990.
7. Fleming RE Jr, Michelsen CB, Stinchfield FE. Sciatic paralysis. *J Bone Joint Surg Am.* 1979;61A:37–39.
8. Ghent WR. Further studies on meralgia paresthetica. *Can Med Assoc J.* 1961;85:871–875.
9. Gilliatt RW, Goodman HV, Willison RG. The recording of lateral popliteal nerve actions potentials in man. *J Neurol Neurosurg Psychiatry.* 1961;24:305–318.
10. Kaplan PE, Kernahan WT. Tarsal tunnel syndrome. *J Bone Joint Surg Am.* 1981;63A:96–99.
11. Kempe LG. *Operative Neurosurgery.* New York, NY:Springer-Verlag; 1970;2:203–232.
12. Kernohan J, Levack B, Wilson JN. Entrapment of the superficial peroneal nerve: three case reports. *J Bone Joint Surg Br.* 1985;67B:60–61.
13. Koller RL, Blank NK. Strawberry picker's palsy. *Arch Neurol.* 1980;37:320.
14. Kopell HP, Thompson WAL. *Peripheral Entrapment Neuropathies,* 2nd ed. Huntington, NY: Robert E Krieger Publishing Company; 1976.
15. Leonard MA. Sciatic nerve paralysis following anticoagulation therapy. *J Bone Joint Surg Br.* 1972;54B:152–153.
16. Mann RA. Tarsal tunnel syndrome. *Orthop Clin North Am.* 1974;5:109–115.
17. Pećina M. Contribution to the etiological explanation of the piriformis syndrome. *Acta Anat (Basel).* 1979;105:181–187.
18. Rengachary SS. Entrapment neuropathies. In: Wilkins RH,Rengachary SS, eds. *Neurosurgery.* New York, NY: McGraw Hill Book Company; 1985:1771–1795.
19. Roth WK. *Meralgia Paresthetica.* Berlin, Germany: S Karque; 1985.
20. Rousseau J-J, Reznik M, LeJeaune GM, et al. Sciatic nerve entrapment by pentazocine induced muscle fibrosis. *Arch Neurol.* 1979;36:723.
21. Ruderman MI, Palmer RH, Olarte MR, et al. Tarsal tunnel syndrome caused by hyperlipidemia: reversal after plasmapheresis. *Arch Neurol.* 1983;40:124–125.
22. Sandhu HS, Sandhey BS. Occupational compression of the common peroneal nerve at the neck of the fibula. *Aust NZ J Surg.* 1976; 46:160–163.
23. Seletz E. *Surgery of Peripheral Nerves.* Springfield, IL: Charles C Thomas; 1951.
24. Sherman DG, Easton JD. Dieting and peroneal nerve palsy. *JAMA.* 1977:238:230–231.
25. Sotaniemi KA. Slimmer's paralysis: peroneal neuropa-

thy during weight reductions. *J Neurol Neurosurg Psychiatry*. 1984;47:564–566.

26. Teng P. Meralgia paresthetica. *Bull L Neurol Soc.* 1972;37:75–83.

27. Wallach HW, Oren ME. Sciatic nerve compression during anticoagulation therapy: computerized tomography aids in diagnosis. *Arch Neurol*. 1979;36:448.

28. Weber ER, Daube JR, Coventry MB. Peripheral neuro-

pathies associated with total hip arthroplasty. *J Bone Joint Surg*. 1976;58A:66–69.

29. Wilemon WK. Tarsal tunnel syndrome: a 50-year survey of the world literature and a report of two new cases. *Orthop Rev*. November 1979;8:111–117.

30. Yeoman W. The relation of arthritis of the sacro-iliac joint to sciatica with an analysis of 100 cases. *Lancet*. 1928;2:1119–1122.

PART III

TRAUMA

CHAPTER 8

Traumatic Peripheral Nerve Injuries

George E. Omer, Jr., MD, MS, FACS

A peripheral nerve lesion is a severe complication of a traumatic extremity injury, since recovery of muscle and tendon activity and restoration of sensibility are essential for a functional extremity. Principles for the initial management of the traumatized extremity have been well established. A clean wound, structural alignment, and prevention of deformity are important goals[3,16]; however, the more extensive and severe the injury to the involved extremity, the longer the time required for the attainment of homeostasis in the tissues. Vascular insufficiency, chronic osteomyelitis, and articular incongruity all contribute to fibrotic infiltration and decreased activity. Clinical studies of traumatic peripheral nerve injuries in humans show considerable variation because return of useful function depends as much on the total response of the extremity to the injury as on the regeneration of the injured nerve. Furthermore, peripheral nerves are only as functional as the pertinent sensory receptors and motor end plates. An overview of the traumatically injured nerve is thus presented within the context of neurologic evaluation, outcome, and global extremity injury.

Initial Evaluation

The initial clinical examination is a broad assessment of functional loss designed to determine the level of peripheral nerve injury. In the conscious patient, this may be done with voluntary muscle testing and the testing of the threshold for sensibility. The voluntary muscle

test, with manual grading as introduced by Robert W. Lovett's text on infantile paralysis, published in 1917, will determine the level of the nerve lesion on the basis of active and inactive muscles, as reported by Omer.[22,23]. Common gestures are easier to elicit in a distracted patient than sequential muscle contractions; for example, "cross your fingers" is an adequate test for intact motor function of the ulnar nerve.[29] Passive muscle stretching will alert the examiner to a potential compartment syndrome with associated loss of peripheral nerve function. Sensibility threshold also is related to the responsiveness of the conscious patient. A tuning fork can be used to determine threshold recognition of sensibility, which then can be quantitated with either static or moving two-point discrimination distance.[25] In the unconscious patient with fractures or dislocations, the examiner should maintain a high index of suspicion for a compartment syndrome[12] and consider electrodiagnostic studies to establish the integrity of any potentially involved peripheral nerves.[31,43]

The severity of the overall injury alone may dictate exploration of the extremity. This decision is usually based on the involvement of other anatomic structures in addition to the peripheral nerves, such as an abnormal angiogram or an open fracture. Magnetic resonance imaging is useful when there is a two-level extremity injury and the extent of peripheral nerve involvement is unknown. This point will be addressed later in this chapter. If an emergency operation is indicated, the nonfunctional peripheral nerve should be assessed by direct observation. A disrupted nerve should be repaired as soon as clinically practical. If debridement exposes the nerve and judgment indicates delayed repair, the nerve stumps can be tagged with fine monofilament wire sutures to prevent retraction and enhance roentgenographic identification.[17]

Nerve Injury Classification Scheme

During World War II, Seddon[36] introduced a simple classification of traumatic nerve injuries with specific terminology: neurapraxia, axonotmesis, and neurotmesis. Sunderland identified five degrees of injury, of increasing severity, that produce loss of function.[40] It seems logical to use three degrees of injury, however, in the clinical situation. These are: **(1)** a peripheral nerve so severely disorganized that spontaneous regeneration cannot occur. This could result from nerve division, traction, impalement, or injection with subsequent scarring. The involved segment requires excision as part of the surgical repair. This condition is termed *neurotmesis* by Seddon and *fourth-* or *fifth-degree injury* by Sunderland; **(2)** a peripheral nerve with interruption of axons and their myelin sheaths, but connective tissue planes, such as the perineurium, are maintained. There is a reduction in the number of axons available for regeneration and there may be intrafascicular bundle fibrosis. This commonly results from penetrating missiles or impalement, traction, or compression with related ischemia. This condition is termed *axonotmesis* by Seddon and *second-* or *third-degree injury* by Sunderland; and **(3)** a peripheral nerve with a segmental interruption of the myelin sheaths, but intact axons and connective tissue planes. No Wallerian degeneration occurs, and the disturbance that is responsible for blocking conduction is fully reversible. This commonly results from contusion, such as a fracture, or compression, such as "Saturday night palsy." Functional recovery occurs in weeks to months. This condition is termed *neurapraxia* by Seddon or a *first-degree injury* by Sunderland.

Factors Affecting the Decision-Making Process

Age

Age is the most significant single factor in recovery following nerve injury and suture.[30] Almost all patients up to the age of puberty have good clinical results following nerve suture. The young patient has a greater intrinsic capacity for sensibility re-education and motor adaptability than does the older patient.[1]

Distance from End Organ

The proximal (high) nerve injury presents a difficult dilemma with regard to both prognosis for recovery and indications for surgery.[21] There may be considerable distance from the site of injury to the first motor point to be reinnervated. From the moment of injury, there is progressive distortion and degeneration of the distal motor and sensory end organs. Over time, distortion of the nerve distal to the site of injury occurs, with associated slowing of the regenerative process for axon regrowth. The more proximal the injury, the longer the denervation of the distal tissues and the slower the recovery of function. One should expect axon regeneration to be vigorous for the first year after injury in an adult,[41] but if the interval between injury and end organ reinnervation is longer than 4–5 years, functional recovery will be quite limited. A proximal injury of the ulnar or sciatic nerves may be more than 20–30 cm from the most proximal end organ.

Associated Injury

The more extensive the injury to the involved extremity, the longer the time required for the establishment of tissue homeostasis. Peripheral nerves are only as functional as their sensory receptors and muscle-tendon motor plates. A nerve gap often reflects the severity of the traumatic insult. Multiple nerve involvement is a more serious problem for functional recovery of the entire extremity than is an isolated nerve injury. Severe vascular deficiency or chronic osteomyelitis involving the soft tissue around the nerve both contribute to fibrotic infiltration and delayed healing.

The incidence of nerve injuries associated with fractures is unknown. A fracture of the humerus is the fracture most likely to be associated with a nerve injury.[25] Most injuries associated with diaphyseal (shaft) fractures leave the peripheral nerve in continuity. The radial nerve is involved in 60%, the ulnar nerve in 18%, the common peroneal nerve in 15%, and the median nerve in 6% of all neuropathies resulting from fractures.[30] Epiphyseal-level fractures or dislocations can result in vascular disruption and nerve injury. Tight fascial constraints about joints enhance the potential for ischemic damage and traction. Nerve dysfunction occurs in 18% of knee dislocations. These are usually traction injuries that vary from neurapraxia to neurotmesis. The sciatic nerve is injured in approximately 13% of posterior dislocations of the hip or posterior acetabular fractures. Shoulder dislocations are associated with axillary nerve stretch injuries in 5% of cases. Infraclavicular brachial plexus injuries often accompany shoulder subluxation, whereas supraclavicular injuries are often signaled by fractures of the first rib, transverse process of the cervical spine, or the clavicle.[9] The prognosis for spontaneous recovery is poorer for dislocations or epiphyseal-level fractures than for diaphyseal-level fractures. The prognosis is different for closed and open fracture injuries and is related to the severity of damage to the extremity. Seddon[37] reported an 83.5% spontaneous recovery rate in 109 cases of closed fractures of the upper extremity with associated nerve injury, but only 65% in 37 cases of open fractures with neuropathy. Omer[18] found 83% spontaneous recovery for all neuropathies associated with fractures.

Mechanism of Injury

Nerve injury associated with traction or stretch has a poorer prognosis than does neuropathy related to fracture. Traction usually involves a long segment of the nerve trunk. A World War II experience demonstrated that only 58% of patients with traction injuries at the knee in the presence of continuity of the peroneal nerve had functional motor recovery. Furthermore, the prognosis of traction injuries was unaffected by surgical exploration.[6]

Gunshot wounds are a fact of life in our society. Their incidence is increasing worldwide.[35] Surgeons will therefore be dealing with these injuries more and more often. These injuries include those caused by sophisticated weapons that deliver substantial kinetic injury to tissue. High-velocity gunshot wounds can result in internal explosions and may be associated with fractured bones remote from the missile tract[32]; however, the pressure-related disturbances related to increased missile velocity are pertinent only with deep tissue penetration by the missile.[8] With gunshot wounds there is often a loss of function without disruption of the nerve. Foerster reported retrospectively on 2,915 cases of motor paralysis during World War I, of which 1,980 (67%) improved with conservative treatment. This was first reported in the American literature by Omer and Spinner.[32] Sunderland[41] studied a small series of military patients during World War II and documented spontaneous recovery in 68% of the cases. In a prospective study of 595 gunshot wounds during the Vietnam War, Omer[18] determined that spontaneous recovery occurred in 227 of 331 (69%) low-velocity gunshot wounds and 183 of 264 (69%) high-velocity gunshot wounds. Neurapraxia and axonotmesis injuries are approximately equal in gunshot wounds, with the clinical time scale for spontaneous recovery being 1–4 months for neurapraxia and 4–9 months for axonotmesis.[18] Rakolta and Omer[34] noted that spontaneous regeneration may be delayed up to 11 months without excluding the possibility of complete recovery in femoral nerve combat injuries.

Low-velocity gunshot wounds result in a higher percentage of peripheral nerve axon loss (neurotmesis) than do high-velocity missile wounds. Low-velocity wounds with a smaller shock wave tend to directly involve structures such as peripheral nerves, blood vessels, and bone. Shotgun wounds have a higher percentage of associated peripheral nerve injuries than low-velocity handgun wounds. In addition, shotgun wounds require thorough debridement with early exploration of neurovascular structures and, usually, a delayed primary closure. Spontaneous recovery of peripheral nerve injuries resulting from shotgun wounds has been reported as only 45%.[33]

Lacerations, injections, and penetrating impalement are low-velocity injuries that often do not demonstrate significant spontaneous recovery from the initial injury.[21] Lacerations with associated loss of peripheral nerve function, therefore, should be diagnosed clinically as severed-nerve lesions (neurotmesis) until proven otherwise through intraoperative examination.

Surgical Technique

A disrupted peripheral nerve (neurotmesis) should be repaired as soon as clinically practical.[13] Anastomosis should be done with adequate magnification and appropriate instruments and suture. There should be minimal circumferential and longitudinal tension at the suture line in order to avoid internal disorganization of the fascicular bundles.[7] Epineurial suture technique may be used in all peripheral nerve injuries with single (monofascicular) or less than four (oligofascicular) bundle patterns.[5] Fascicular bundle suture techniques may be preferred in peripheral nerves with many (polyfascicular) bundles in segment avulsion, or in chronic lesions with either a nerve gap or a neuroma-in-continuity.

Current reports indicate the superiority of primary repair over delayed repair of peripheral nerves. Kline and Nulsen[11] recorded a 72% good or better motor recovery after primary repair of the median nerve at the wrist. Moneim and Omer[15] reported an 83% good or better motor recovery of the ulnar nerve after primary group fascicular repair at wrist level, whereas Birch and Raji[2] obtained an 81% good or better motor recovery of the median and ulnar nerves after primary repair at wrist level.

Trophic Factors

A variety of trophic factors that influence nerve regeneration have been identified.[13] These include nerve growth factor and axon outgrowth factor. Brushart[4] has found random evidence that reinnervation of the distal nerve stump usually occurs, with subsequent survival of correct projections and loss of malaligned neùrons. Badalamente and Hurst[1] have attempted to inhibit calcium-activated neutral protease through intramuscular injections of tripeptide leupeptin. Inhibition of the calcium-activated neural protease facilitates morphologic recovery in peripheral nerve injuries.

Time Frame for Recovery

The time frame for recovery following neurapraxia is 1–4 months, and following axonotmesis is 4–9 months.[18,25] As previously addressed, proximal extremity injuries take longer to demonstrate clinical function than distal injuries, and extensive extremity injuries producing multiple nerve lesions require a longer period for return of clinical function than do injuries resulting in isolated nerve dysfunction.[29]

Assessment of Recovery Potential

Assessing the specific etiology of the nerve injury, the level of functional loss, and the overall severity of extremity involvement will provide a clinical classification of the nerve injury and indicate the potential for spontaneous recovery. Lacerations require exploration and suture of disrupted nerves at the time of injury. A disrupted nerve should be repaired as soon as clinically practical. It is appropriate at 4 months to electively explore the clinically complete nerve lesion in high-velocity, low-velocity, and shotgun wounds above the elbow or knee, severely comminuted fractures, and fractures adjacent to joints.[21] At this point, 100% of neurapraxia injuries and 50% of axonotmesis lesions should have recovered.[21] However, approximately 60% of these nerves will have a neuroma-in-continuity,[10] and a decision must be made concerning resection of the neuroma (strategies for intraoperative decision making have been discussed in Chapter 3). Because the degree of functional loss is very influential in brachial plexus injuries, these should be explored somewhat earlier (perhaps at 3 months) if there has been no recovery from a clinically complete nerve lesion.[9,28]

The progress of regeneration cannot be assessed without evaluating functional loss and recovery. Assessment of the established peripheral neuropathy requires a series of quantitative tests that are repeated at regular intervals of approximately 12 weeks.[27] The sensibility level related to the individual peripheral nerve and the motor strength of individual reinnervated muscles are the most important studies in the series of quantitative tests.

Sensibility testing evaluates the patient's capacity for precise interpretation of sensation.[19] All current tests that assess sensibility are related to cutaneous touch pressure; for example, the Weber two-point discrimination test is a judgment more than the recognition of sensation. The Weber-Moberg static two-point discrimination test determines if the patient can discriminate between being touched with one or two points and the minimal distance at which two points are recognized.[14] The testing instrument can be an ordinary paper clip, a blunted eye caliper, or a Boley gauge. The normal threshold for the volar surface of the hand varies from 2–5 mm at the fingertip to 7–10 mm at the base of the palm.[14,23,24] The Dellon moving two-point discrimination test is normal between 2–3 mm at the volar fingertip.[24] Other sensibility techniques in current use include Von Frey monofilaments[44] and the ridge sensitometer test.[23,24] Functional results should be measured against the contralateral extremity. Functional sensation may be tested with the stem of a tuning fork (30 cycles per second) over the anatomical trunk of the involved peripheral nerve (Tinel's sign). This percussion stimulation begins at the distal portion of the extremity to delay the patient's potential discomfort until the positive point of the test.

The voluntary muscle test used to determine muscle strength is based on the use of gravity and resistance, first devised by Lovett in 1912 as reported by Omer.[22] The examiner grades muscle strength by palpation of the involved muscle-tendon unit and by resistance to movement of a bone-joint lever arm motored by the involved muscle. The active range of motion can be quantitated with a goniometer across an appropriate joint. Trick movements must be detected. Strength can be quantitated with the aid of resistance instruments, such as grip and pinch meters. The contralateral (if normal) extremity should be used for comparison.

Electrodiagnostic studies are more objective than clinical tests. Determination of the conduction velocity of sensory nerves is the only objective study to measure sensation. Electromyography cannot be used to predict the quantity or quality of reinnervation.

These studies may become redundant if early research in nuclear magnetic resonance (NMR) spectroscopy is fruitful. Despite the most refined histochemical techniques, the nature of the critical early stages of nerve degeneration remains unclear; however, using high-field NMR, reproducible patterns of biophysical changes occurring during wallerian degeneration and nerve regeneration have been recorded.[39] Although the NMR data may demonstrate that metabolic perturbations occur within hours after nerve injury, the corresponding histologic findings show virtually no edema and no remarkable changes in nerve morphology. The loss of spin-spin correlations in NMR studies is dramatic after 5 hours. As the nerves undergo repair and regeneration, the spin-spin correlations return, indicating that an ongoing evaluation of nerve degeneration and regeneration is feasible.

Rehabilitation Program

From the time of injury, the extremity is kept in a functional position and in a dynamic state. Fibrotic tissue is stretched and mobilized. The principle of active motion cannot be neglected and daily activities should be emphasized.[17] An important aspect of treatment is the use of dynamic splints, which should be fabricated for each patient and changed whenever indicated.

In the upper extremity, function will improve with a motor and sensibility re-education program. Motor re-education will prevent abnormal motor habits such as the extended and "divorced" insensible index finger following median nerve loss. Sensibility re-education should allow recovery of the full potential of the regenerating nerve.

Motor re-education consists of two phases: **(1)** visual monitoring of activity patterns and **(2)** early tendon transfers (which function as internal splints). The principles for early tendon transfers are: **(1)** use only one tendon and **(2)** use a transfer that will not result in deformity should spontaneous nerve recovery occur.[26] For example, transfer of the pronator teres tendon to the tendon of the extensor carpi radialis brevis muscle will result in active extension of the wrist and passive mobilization of the collateral ligaments of the metacarpophalangeal joints in a patient with radial palsy. Recovery of the radial nerve will not result in a deformity.

Sensibility re-education consists of conscious handling of objects with the eyes open and then closed. The purpose is to use items in the patient's occupation, such as nails for a carpenter. Sensibility re-education is not effective if the patient cannot recognize vibratory sensation (250 cycles per second tuning fork) over the autonomous zone of the involved nerve. A timed picking-up test will quantitate improvement in a patient with median or ulnar palsy.[20]

Excellent re-education requires a team approach, including an occupational therapist, physical therapist, and brace maker (orthotist), as well as a cooperative patient and an interested surgeon.

Outcome Assessment

Evaluation can be done at several levels: individual nerve recovery, extremity coordination, medical impairment and disability. This is accessed through the motor strength of individual reinnervated muscles, and the sensibility level of the individual's nerve recovery.[27]

Voluntary muscle testing is based on the use of gravity and resistance. The examiner grades muscle strength by palpation of the involved muscle-tendon unit and by resisting movement of a bone-joint lever arm motored by the involved muscle: zero (no contractibility), trace (contractility), poor (complete range of motion with gravity eliminated), fair (motion against gravity), good (motion against gravity and some resistance), and normal (complete function). The range of motion can be quantitated with a goniometer across an appropriate joint.

Sensibility is the capacity for precise interpretation of sensation.[19] All current tests to assess sensibility are related to cutaneous touch/pressure. The static two-point discrimination test has the greater application. Normal levels are between 3–5 mm at the fingertips, and 7–10 mm at the base of the palm.[23] Moving two-point discrimination is normal between 2–3 mm at the fingertips.[24] Other techniques in current use include monofilaments[44] and the ridge sensitometer. Functional levels should be measured against the contralateral (if normal) extremity.

The British Medical Research Council report of 1954[38] and the United States Veterans Administration monograph of 1956[45] were the first studies to develop specific criteria for assessment of motor and sensibility recovery. The British scales (Tables 1, 2, and 3) are the most frequently used today. Motor recovery is based on combined motor activity. This is most useful in proximal (high) lesions (Table 2). The British sensibility grading scale is considered inadequate by Moberg[14,23,27] (Table 3).

Extremity coordination is the end product of motor and sensibility function.[28] Grasp and pinch can be measured with dynamometers, which should be adjusted to fit the finger span of the patient. Tactile gnosis can be tested by writing numbers on a digit, identifying a coin, or palpating type or arrows. In all tests the patient's eyes are closed. The best comparison is the contralateral (if normal) extremity.

The degree of medical impairment is affected by pain. A simple grading scheme has been presented: 100% = P4 (prevents all activity); 75% = P3 (prevents some activity); 50% = P2 (interferes with activity); 25% = P1 (annoying); and 0% = PO (normal).[42]

The best current reference for the evaluation of permanent impairment is the American Med-

TABLE 1
Motor Recovery

Grade	Description
M5	Complete recovery
M4	All synergic and independent movements are possible
M3	All important muscles act against resistance
M2	Return of perceptible contraction in both proximal and distal muscles
M1	Return of perceptible contraction in proximal muscles
M0	No contraction

Adapted from References 23, 24, 38, 45.

TABLE 2
Proximal and Distal Muscles Innervated by Peripheral Nerves

Proximal Muscle	Distal Muscle
Radial Nerve	
Brachioradialis	Abductor pollicus longus
Extensor carpi radialis longus	Extensor pollicis longus
	Extensor indicis
Extensor digitorum communis	
Extensor carpi ulnaris	
Median Nerve	
Pronator teres	Abductor pollicis brevis
Flexor carpi radialis	
Flexor digitorum superficialis	
Flexor pollicis longus	
Ulnar Nerve	
Flexor carpi ulnaris	Abductor digiti quinti
Flexor digitorum profundus (ring and little)	Interossei
Common Peroneal Nerve	
Tibialis anterior	Extensor digitorum brevis
Extensor digitorum longus	
Extensor hallucis longus	
Peronei	
Tibial Nerve	
Gastrocnemius and soleus	Abductor hallucis
Tibialis posterior	Intrinsic muscles of sole of foot
Flexor digitorum longus	
Flexor hallucis longus	

Adapted from References 23, 24, 38, 45.

TABLE 3
British and Moberg Sensibility Scale

British Code	Sensibility Description	Moberg Scale
S4	Normal sensibility	
	Two-point discrimination distance of 12 mm or less—tactile gnosis	Good
	Two-point discrimination distance of 12–15 mm	Fair
S3 +	Some recovery of two-point discrimination within the autonomous area of the nerve	Poor
S3	Return of superficial cutaneous pain and tactile sensibility throughout the autonomous area with disappearance of any previous over-reaction	Bad
S2	Return of some degree of superficial cutaneous pain and tactile sensibility within the autonomous area of the nerve	
S1	Recovery of deep cutaneous pain sensibility within the autonomous area of the nerve	
S0	Absence of sensibility in the autonomous area of the nerve	

Adapted from References 23, 24, 27.

ical Association's *Guides to the Evaluation of Permanent Impairment* (3rd ed. [revised], 1990). This is a comprehensive publication. One must remember, however, that disability determination is an administrative and non-medical decision that defines the patient's ability to engage in personal, social, and occupational activities related to earning capacity in a given social and economic situation.

References

1. Badalamente MA, Hurst LC, and Stracher A. Neuromuscular recovery using calcium protease inhibition after median nerve repair in primates. *Proc Nat Acad Sci USA*. 1989;86:5983–5987.
2. Birch R, Raji ARM. Repair of median and ulnar nerves: primary suture is best. *J Bone Joint Surg Br.* 1991;73B:154–157.
3. Brown PN. Open injuries of the hand. In: Green DP ed. *Operative Hand Surgery.* 2nd ed. New York, NY: Churchill Livingstone; 1988;2:1619–1653.
4. Brushart TME. Preferential motor reinnervation: a sequential double-labeling study. *Restorative Neurol Nuro Sci.* 1990;1:281–287.
5. Buck-Gramcko D. Evaluation of perineurial repair with nerve injuries. In: Jupiter JB, ed. *Flynn's Hand Surgery.* 4th ed. Baltimore, Md. Williams and Wilkins; 1991:472–480.
6. Clawson DK, Seddon HJ. The late consequences of sciatic nerve injury. *J. Bone Joint Surg. Br.* 1960;42B:213–225.
7. Edshage S. Peripheral nerve suture. *Acta Chir Scand Suppl.* 1964;331:1–104.
8. Fackler ML. Wound ballistics: a review of common misconceptions. *JAMA.* 1988;259:2730–2736.
9. Kanaya F, Gonzalez M, Park C-M, et al. Improvement in motor function after brachial plexus surgery. *J Hand Surg Am.* 1990;15A:30–36.
10. Kline DG. Evaluation of the neuroma in continuity. In: Omer GE Jr, Spinner M, eds. *Management of Peripheral Nerve Problems.* Philadelphia, Pa: WB Saunders Co; 1980:450–461.
11. Kline DG, Nulsen FE. Management of peripheral nerve injuries producing hand dysfunction. In: Jupiter JB, ed. *Flynn's Hand Surgery,* 4th ed. Baltimore, Md: Williams and Wilkins; 1991:481–489.
12. Lundborg G, Gelberman RH, Minteer-Convery M, et al. Median nerve compression in the carpal tunnel: functional response to experimentally induced controlled pressure. *J Hand Surg.* 1982;7:252–259.
13. Millesi, H. Peripheral nerve surgery today: turning point or continuous development? *J Hand Surg Br.* 1990;15B:281–287.
14. Moberg E. Relation of touch and deep sensation to hand reconstruction. *Am J Surg.* 1965;109:353–355.
15. Moneim MS, Omer GE, Jr. Results of nerve suture under ideal conditions. Presented at 104th Annual Meeting, American Orthopaedic Association; Orlando, Fla: June 9–13, 1991.
16. Omer GE Jr. The early management of gunshot wounds of the extremities. *S D J Med.* 1956;9:340–346.
17. Omer GE Jr. Evaluation and reconstruction of the forearm and hand after acute traumatic peripheral nerve injuries. *Amer Acad Orthop Surg.* 1962–1969;18(J1): 93–119.
18. Omer GE Jr. Injuries to nerves of the upper extremity. *J Bone Joint Surg Am.* 1974;56A:1615–1624.
19. Omer GE Jr. Sensation and sensibility in the upper extremity. *Clin Orthop.* 1974;104:30–36.

20. Omer GE Jr. Sensory evaluation by the pick up test. In: Jewett DL, McCarroll HR Jr, eds. *Nerve Repair and Regeneration: Its Clinical and Experimental Basis.* St. Louis, Mo: CV Mosby Co; 1980;250–251.

21. Omer GE Jr. The results of untreated traumatic injuries. In: Omer GE Jr, Spinner M, eds. *Management of Peripheral Nerve Problems.* Philadelphia, Pa: WB Saunders Co; 1980:502–506.

22. Omer GE Jr. The evaluation of clinical results following peripheral nerve suture. In: Omer GE Jr, Spinner M, eds.: *Management of Peripheral Nerve Problems.* Philadelphia, Pa: WB Saunders Co: 1980:431–442.

23. Omer GE Jr. Physical diagnosis of peripheral nerve injuries. *Orthop Clin North Am.* 1981;12:207–227.

24. Omer GE Jr. Methods of assessment of injury and recovery of peripheral nerves. *Surg Clin North Am.* 1981;61:303–319.

25. Omer GE Jr. Results of untreated nerve defects. *Clin Orthop.* 1982;163:15–19.

26. Omer GE Jr. Early tendon transfers in the rehabilitation of median, radial, and ulnar palsies. *Ann Chir Main.* 1982;1:187–190.

27. Omer GE Jr. Report of the committee for evaluation of the clinical result in peripheral nerve injury. *J Hand Surg.* 1983;8:754–759.

28. Omer GE Jr. Evaluation of the extremity with peripheral nerve injury and timing for nerve suture, part II. In: Murray JA, ed. *American Academy of Orthopedic Surgeons Instructional Course Lectures.* St. Louis, Mo: CV Mosby Co; 1984;33:463–486.

29. Omer GE Jr. Acute management of peripheral nerve injuries. *Hand Clin.* 1986;2:193–206.

30. Omer GE Jr. Complications of peripheral nerve injuries. In: Epps. CH Jr, ed. *Complications in Orthopaedic Surgery.* 2nd ed. Philadelphia, Pa: JB Lippincott; 1986:865–908.

31. Omer GE Jr. War injuries in the hand. In: Tubiana R, ed. *The Hand.* Philadelphia, Pa: WB Saunders Co; 1988;3:903–924.

32. Omer GE, Spinner M. Peripheral nerve testing and suture techniques. In: Evans EB, ed. *American Academy of Orthopaedic Surgeons Instructional Course Lectures.* St. Louis, CV Mosby Co; 1975;24:122–143.

33. Paradies LH, Gregory CF. The early treatment of close-range shotgun wounds to the extremities. *J Bone Joint Surg Am.* 1966; 48A:425–435.

34. Rakolta GG, Omer GE Jr. Combat-sustained femoral nerve injuries. *Surg Gynecol Obstet.* 1969;128:813–817.

35. Russotti GM, Sim FH. Missile wounds of the extremities: a current concepts review. *Orthopedics.* 1985; 8:1106–1116.

36. Seddon HJ. Three types of nerve injury. *Brain.* 1943; 66:237–288.

37. Seddon HJ. Nerve lesions complicating certain closed bone injuries. *JAMA.* 1947; 135:691–694.

38. Seddon HJ. Peripheral nerve injuries. *Medical Research Council Special Report Series.* London, England: Her Majesty's Stationery Office, 1954:282.

39. Sillerud, LO, Kirsch CF, Pennino RP, et al. Monitoring of early Wallerian degeneration in rat sciatic nerve using high-field proton NMR spectroscopy. *Surg Forum.* 1987;38:555–558.

40. Sunderland S. A classification of peripheral nerve injuries producing loss of function. *Brain.* 1951; 74:491–516.

41. Sunderland S. *Nerves and Nerve Injuries.* 2nd ed. New York, NY: Churchill Livingstone; 1978.

42. Swanson AB, Göran-Hagert C, Swanson GD. Evaluation of impairment of hand function. In: Hunter JM, Schneider LH, Mackin EJ, et al, eds. *Rehabilitation of the Hand.* St. Louis, Mo: CV Mosby Co; 1978:31–69.

43. Thompson LL. *The Electromyographer's Handbook.* Boston, Mass: Little Brown & Co Inc; 1981.

44. Werner JL, Omer GE Jr. Evaluating cutaneous pressure sensitivity of the hand. *Am J Occup Ther.* 1970; 24:347–356.

45. Woodhall B, Beebe GW, eds. *Peripheral Nerve Regeneration.* Washington, DC: US Government Printing Office; 1956.

PART IV

SURGICAL ANATOMY AND EXPOSURE

CHAPTER 9

Surgical Exposure of the Brachial Plexus*

Steven S. Weinshel, MD

The anatomy of the brachial plexus is accurately depicted in standard anatomy texts. Once the anatomy is mastered, the anatomic considerations often take a back seat to the more complicated issues such as timing of operation, intraoperative physiologic testing, and resecting and grafting neuromas.[8,9] This chapter focuses on brachial plexus anatomy and surgical approaches.

Anatomy

A review of the anatomy of the brachial plexus is necessary before a discussion of surgical approaches can be made. The brachial plexus is composed of ventral rami of C5, C6, C7, C8, and T1. The plexus lies in the posterior triangle of the neck between the scalenus anterior and scalenus medius muscles. It passes deep to the clavicle, a structure often conveniently used as a landmark in plexus surgery. The distal plexus surrounds the axillary artery, which is also an important operative landmark.

The structure of the plexus has many variations, but the basic outline is as follows[3,10.]

1. Ventral C5 and C6 roots become the upper trunk. The C7 ramus forms the middle trunk and C8 and T1 rami form the lower trunk.
2. The trunks divide into anterior and posterior divisions with all three posterior divisions becoming the posterior cord. The anterior divisions of the upper and middle trunks form the lateral cord. The remaining division—the anterior division of the lower trunk—forms the medial cord.
3. The cords terminate in the major branches. The lateral cord becomes the musculocutaneous nerve and contributes to the median nerve. The posterior cord divides into the radial and axillary nerves. The ulnar nerve and a portion of the median nerve are formed by the medial cord (Figure 1).

In addition to the main terminal branches, numerous branches exit the plexus at other levels. Often in traumatic injuries, many of the smaller branches were destroyed by the traumatic event or result from post-traumatic scarring.

Branches from Rami and Trunks

1. The phrenic nerve receives contributions from the C5 ramus. The phrenic nerve then travels along the anterior surface of the scalenus anterior muscle. This nerve is often visualized early in an anterior dissection of the brachial plexus.
2. The long thoracic nerve arises from the C5–7 anterior and rami to innervate the serratus anterior muscle.
3. The dorsal scapular nerve arises from the C5 ramus and innervates the rhomboid muscles as well as the levator scapulae muscle.
4. The nerve to the subclavius muscle is a branch of the upper trunk.
5. The suprascapular nerve is a relatively large nerve that exits the upper trunk and travels

*The views expressed in this material are those of the author, and do not reflect the official policy or position of the U.S. government, the Department of Defense, or the Department of the Air Force.

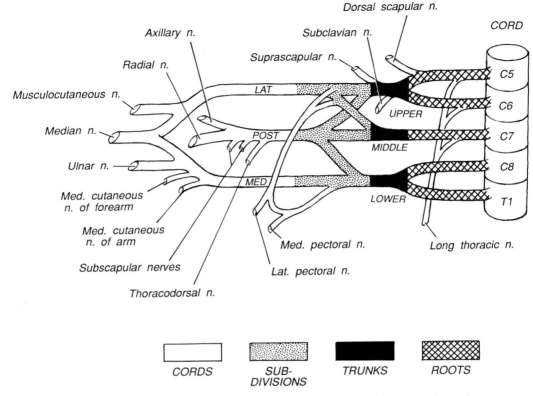

Figure 1. *Schematic diagram of the brachial plexus and its major branches.*

in a lateral direction to innervate the infraspinatus and supraspinatus muscles.

Branches from Cords

Lateral Cord

The lateral pectoral nerve innervates the pectoralis major muscle.

Medial Cord

1. The medial pectoral joins the lateral pectoral nerve to innervate the pectoral muscles.
2. The medial brachial and antebrachial cutaneous nerves supply cutaneous sensation to the arm and forearm. These nerves are important in that they can be sacrificed for nerve cable grafting if necessary with the only deficit being loss of sensation to the skin in a relatively insignificant distribution.

Posterior Cord

1. The subscapular nerve innervates the subscapulous muscle and the teres major muscle. This nerve often leaves the cord in two branches.
2. The thoracodorsal nerve innervates the latissimus dorsi muscle.

Operative Approaches

The two fundamental operative approaches to the brachial plexus are the *anterior* and *posterior* approaches. The anterior approach may be divided into a supraclavicular and an infraclavicular exposure, which often are combined to expose the entire plexus. The posterior approach is used infrequently because of fewer indications and greater operative complications; however, it may be helpful in isolated cases.

General Considerations

Since it is important to be able to observe the upper extremity during the entire procedure, either the entire arm should be included in the surgical field or draped so that the major muscle groups can be palpated during the operation. The position of the patient is important and is discussed along with each operative approach here.

The choice of anesthetic agents depends on the need for intraoperative electrodiagnostic studies. Since these studies are usually required in trauma, tumor, and the vast majority of brachial plexus stretch injury cases, the anesthetic technique should involve no agents that interfere with nerve action potentials. Pharmacologic muscle paralysis is contraindicated. Nitrous oxide, narcotics, and inhalation agents are the agents of choice.

If it is necessary to graft gaps in plexus elements, both legs should be prepared for sural nerve harvesting prior to the operation. Although the medial antebrachial cutaneous nerve to the forearm may be harvested, it is often not long enough. Magnification may be used for the surgical dissection and the suturing of grafts. Either surgical loupes or the operating microscope can be used, depending on the preference of the surgeon. Loupes with 3.5× magnification are often satisfactory for most purposes.[5]

Finally, the plexus surgeon must possess basic vascular surgical skills in his or her armamentarium. Post-traumatic brachial plexus explorations often involve dissecting through scar tissue around vascular structures such as the axillary artery and vein. Following months of healing, both vascular and neural structures may be embedded in thick scar. The vascular and plexus elements, therefore, need to be separated during the operative procedure. In this situation, it may be necessary to repair vascular injuries that may arise. If this skill is not possessed by the plexus surgeon, a vascular surgeon should be available to assist in the operation, if needed.

Once the plexus is exposed, meticulous dissection must be performed to expose all neural and vascular elements. Small branches of the plexus must be identified and reserved. Often in delayed traumatic explorations, all elements will be encased in scar tissue. Sharp dissection is the best way to dissect the elements from the scar tissue. When the elements are exposed, Penrose drains may be placed around the large neural elements in order to retract and isolate the elements. Smaller nervous structures may be retracted using smaller vessel loops. This will allow isolation of single elements to facilitate the electrophysiologic testing, which was described in Chapters 1 and 2.[4]

Anterior Approach

The anterior approach to the brachial plexus is the most common approach and can be used in most circumstances. The entire plexus, from nerve roots to terminal branches can be exposed using this technique. The patient is positioned supine on the operating table. A roll is placed under the ipsilateral shoulder and the head is slightly rotated toward the contralateral side. The ipsilateral arm is best placed on an arm board laterally. This will allow the arm to be either palpated under sterile drapes or visualized if included in the operative field.[5,7] Also, this arrangement will allow one surgeon to stand next to the neck above the arm board and the other surgeon to stand in the apex between the arm and the chest. The neck, shoulder, axilla, and chest wall should be prepared along with both legs if a grafting procedure is anticipated.

Supraclavicular Approach

An incision is made along the posterior border of the sternocleidomastoid muscle. This incision should be carried down across the clavicle and may be extended farther if an infraclavicular approach is required (Figure 2). The skin is opened and the platysma muscle, which is enveloped by the superficial fascia of the neck, is visualized. It is useful to split the muscle and later close the platysma muscle as a separate layer if possible, as this often will allow a good cosmetic closure of the neck. The external jugular vein is often found under the pla-

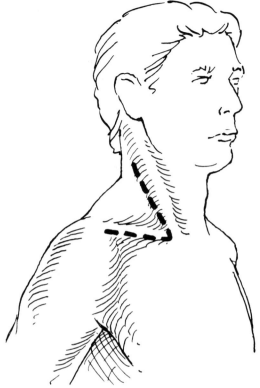

Figure 2. *Surgical incision for the supraclavicular approach to the brachial plexus.*

tysma muscle and can be ligated if needed. The sternocleidomastoid muscle may be detached from its lateral attachment to the clavicle. The spinal accessory nerve crosses the sternocleidomastoid muscle and must be preserved. This nerve is often located more cephalad than the operative exposure.

A deep fascial layer separates the superficial portion of the posterior triangle from its deep portion. This contains the brachial plexus. The first structure seen will be the omohyoid muscle, which may be divided between two sutures and retracted. This muscle can be reapproximated when closing. The transverse cervical artery and vein can be ligated or retracted as necessary. The brachial plexus is observed between the scalenus anterior and scalenus medius muscle. The phrenic nerve, which is usually found on the anterior surface of the scalenus anterior muscle, needs to be preserved. Dissection now may be carried in a medial direction by cutting fibers of both scalenus muscles to fully expose the plexus and the roots (Figure 3).

Care must be taken to avoid injury to vascular structures other than the transverse cervical

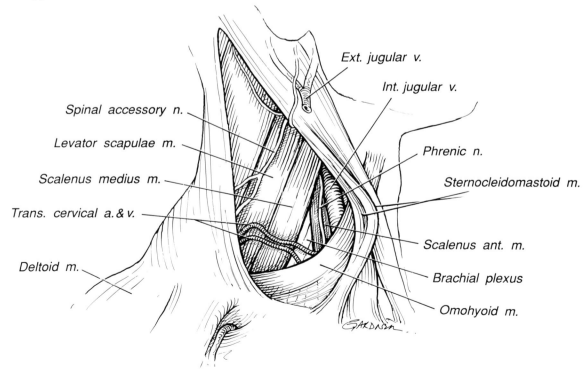

Figure 3. *Posterior triangle of the neck showing the brachial plexus and surrounding structures.*

vessels. Important vascular structures include the subclavian artery and vein inferior to the plexus and the vertebral artery located in front of the scalenus anterior muscle and medial to the phrenic nerve. The thoracic duct can be sealed off with cautery if a lymphatic leak is encountered. The supraclavicular approach will expose the nerve roots as they exit the neuroforamina, become trunks, and divide. If the cords need to be exposed, the skin incision can be extended into an infraclavicular approach.

Infraclavicular Approach

The supraclavicular incision may be continued over the clavicle or the incision started at the clavicle if a supraclavicular incision was not made. The incision should extend laterally in the deltopectoral groove, which usually can be palpated. After the skin and the subcutaneous tissue are incised, the incision of the fascial plane over the deltoid and pectoralis muscles exposes the cephalic vein (Figure 4A and B).

Blunt dissection between the deltoid and pectoralis major muscles is performed with gentle retraction of the cephalic vein. Self-

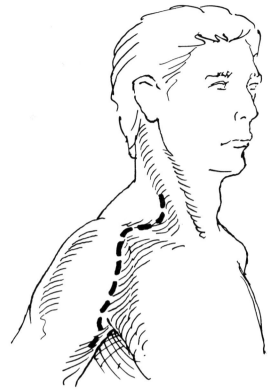

Figure 4A. Surgical incision for the infraclavicular approach to the brachial plexus.

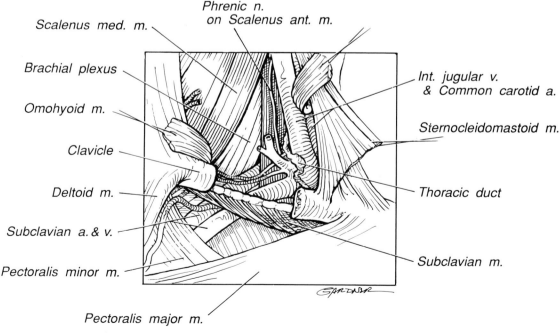

Figure 4B. The underlying plexus as exposed with the infraclavicular approach.

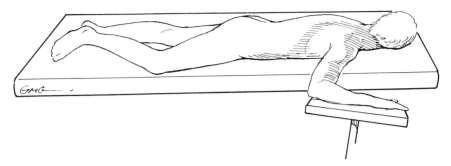

Figure 5. Patient position for the posterior subscapular approach.

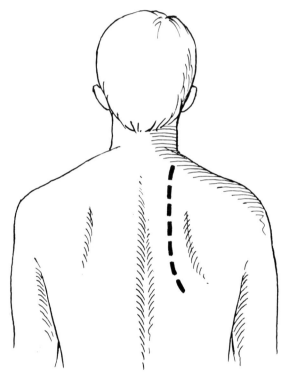

Figure 6. Surgical incision for the posterior sub-scapular approach.

retaining retractors are placed between the two muscles. The lateral and medial pectoral nerves are then visualized. The nerves can be sacrificed, if needed, to expose the plexus.[5] The pectoralis minor muscle is located below these muscles and the pectoral nerves. This muscle should be ligated between two sutures and cut. This muscle must not be reapproximated. Constriction of a repaired plexus may result.[5]

Dissection toward the clavicle will expose the subclavius muscle on the inferior surface of the clavicle. This muscle can be sacrificed if necessary, especially when dissection must be done under the clavicle. Often, numerous small vessels are in this area. They must be cauterized or profuse bleeding will occur. Under normal conditions, the first neural element visualized is the lateral cord. Deeper dissection will reveal the other cords and the axillary artery. The cords are named for their anatomic relationships to the artery, however, with post-traumatic scarring, these relationships often are obliterated. Distal dissection that identifies the major branches may be necessary to allow backtracking to the cords in order to label the cords.

Combined Approach

The supraclavicular and infraclavicular approaches can be combined or either approach extended if necessary. In the past, the clavicle was often resected followed by internal fixation during the closure of the procedure. Recently more and more plexus surgeons are not resecting the clavicle due to the higher-than-expected incidence of nonunion. The skeletonized clavicle has a poor vascular supply and often does not heal well.[7] If the clavicle has been fractured by previous trauma, it is easy to remove loose pieces to gain more exposure for the nerve dissection, but if the clavicle is intact, it should be retracted. By wrapping an unfolded surgical sponge around the clavicle,

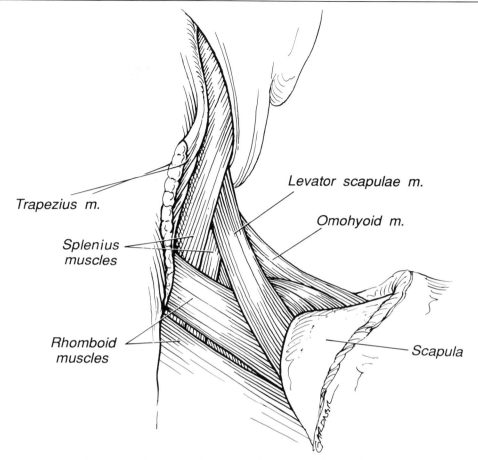

Figure 7A. Muscular dissection in the posterior subscapular approach.

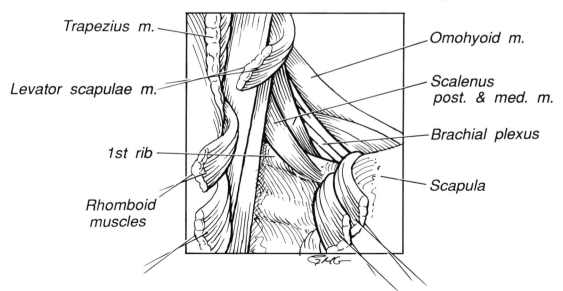

Figure 7B. Exposure of the brachial plexus with the subscapular approach.

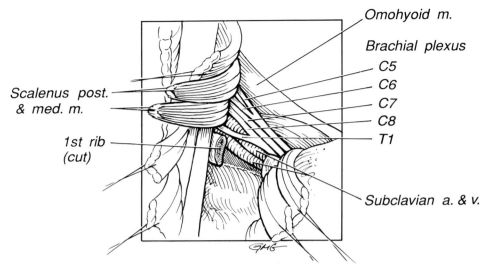

Omohyoid m.

Brachial plexus

C5

C6

C7

C8

T1

Scalenus post. & med. m.

1st rib (cut)

Subclavian a. & v.

Figure 8. Deep exposure showing the brachial plexus elements.

clamping the sponge, and pulling on the clamp, the clavicle can be retracted in both directions. This provides adequate exposure in nearly all cases.

Closure

Following a supraclavicular exposure, the omohyoid muscle can be reapproximated. The platysma is closed. This will pull most of the neck structures together.[8] This is followed by closing the subcutaneous tissue and the skin closure.

Following an infraclavicular approach, the pectoralis minor muscle should not be resutured; however, fascia over the deltoid and pectoral muscles is sutured, followed by closure of the subcutaneous tissue and skin.

Posterior Approach

The posterior approach was used originally in the treatment of empyema in the preantibiotic era.[1,2] Recently it has been used in selected cases of brachial plexus pathology. The approach is useful for proximal plexus lesions involving roots and trunks. It is also a useful approach in patients who have had a prior ante-

rior plexus operation or who have undergone radiation therapy of the anterior chest wall. Finally, it is useful for the treatment of thoracic outlet syndrome in patients who have had a previous operation, especially a transaxillary approach.[6]

The patient is positioned prone on the operating table with the head turned toward the contralateral side. The ipsilateral arm is abducted and flexed at the shoulder. The arm is then flexed at the elbow (Figure 5). The incision is made midpoint between the spinous processes and medial border of the scapula (Figure 6). The patient's position causes external rotation of the scapula and affords more space between the scapula and spine. The incision can be extended onto the neck if further exposure is needed.

The trapezius muscle is divided along the length of the incision. The muscle can be divided between clamps, and the fibers can be sutured prior to the clamps' removal. This will allow reapproximation of the muscle at the time of closure. Under the trapezius muscle in a cephalad to caudad direction, the levator scapulae, the rhomboid minor, and the rhomboid major muscles are observed. These muscles also can be divided by a clamp and tagged with a suture to facilitate closure. A self-retaining retractor is then placed between the ventral scapula and spinous processes (Figure 7A and B).

Ribs are easily palpated at this time. The second rib is identified and may need to be removed along its medial aspect to identify the first rib. The goal is resection of the first rib and its periosteum from the transverse process of T1 to the costoclavicular ligament. The first rib has been observed to regenerate if the periosteum has not been removed.[6] After the first rib has been removed, the scalenus posterior and medius muscles will be identified and can be removed. At this point, the brachial plexus trunks will be identified. The subclavian artery and vein will be inferior to the lower trunk and should be protected. The trunks can be followed laterally to the division level or medially to the root level (Figure 8).

Often, this approach can result in a small pleural leak, and a chest tube may need to be inserted.[6] Closure of this exposure involves reapproximating the cut muscle groups. This muscle cutting provides the major morbidity of this procedure. Complications include occasional winged scapula and decreased shoulder strength, especially if a prior shoulder injury has caused muscle weakness.

References

1. Brown HS, Smith RA. First rib resection for neurovascular syndromes of the thoracic outlet. *Surg Clin North Am.* 1974;54:1277–1289.
2. Clagett OT. Presidential address: research and prosearch. *J Thorac Cardiovasc Surg.* 1962;44:153–166.
3. Devinsky O, Feldman E. *Examination of the Cranial and Peripheral Nerves.* New York, NY: Churchill Livingstone; 1988;1–54.
4. Kline DG, Hackett ER, May PR. Evaluation of nerve injuries by evoked potentials and electromyography. *J Neurosurg.* 1969;31:128–136.
5. Kline DG, Judice DJ. Operative management of selected brachial plexus lesions. *J Neurosurg.* 1983;58:631–649.
6. Kline DG, Kott J, Barnes G, Bryant L. Exploration of selected brachial plexus lesions by the posterior subscapular approach. *J Neurosurg.* 1978;49:872–880.
7. Leffert RD. In: Green DP, ed. *Operative Hand Surgery.* New York, NY: Churchill Livingstone; 1988;1569–1591.
8. Leffert RD. The brachial plexus. In: Evarts CM, ed. *Surgery of the Musculoskeletal System.* New York, NY: Churchill Livingstone; 1983;1:2:387–406.
9. Seddon HJ. *Surgical Disorders of the Peripheral Nerves.* Baltimore, Md: Williams and Wilkins; 1972;250–287.
10. Wright PE. *Campbell's Operative Orthopedics.* St Louis, Mo.: CV Mosby Company; 1987;2783–2842.

CHAPTER 10

Surgical Exposure of the Peripheral Nerves of the Upper Extremity

Miguel A. Pirela-Cruz, MD, FAAOS, FACS; George E. Omer, Jr., MD; and Edward C. Benzel, MD, FACS

The nuances of the surgical exposure of the nerves of the upper extremity are, perhaps, better understood by most surgeons than those of any other region of the body. The more commonly surgically approached maladies, the carpal and cubital tunnel syndromes, are discussed in Chapters 5 and 6, respectively. The discussion of these entities therefore will be abbreviated in this chapter. Instead, this chapter focuses on the less frequently surgically encountered segments of nerves and on the surgical principles of upper extremity peripheral nerve surgery.

Although the nerves of the upper extremity can be studied in a variety of ways, the approach taken here focuses on regional anatomy. The nerves of the upper extremity have therefore been divided into three regions of surgical exposure:

1. the subaxilla and upper arm (which include the nerves of the distal brachial plexus and the musculocutaneous, median ulnar, radial, and axillary nerves)
2. the elbow and forearm (which include the median, ulnar, and radial nerves on the anterior and medial aspects of the elbow and forearm)
3. the palm and wrist (which include the median and ulnar nerves on the anterior aspect of the wrist and palm, as well as the digital nerves)

Variants of the nerves of the upper extremity also will be presented. The implications of these variants, both clinical and surgical, are addressed. Throughout this chapter, unless otherwise specified, the works of Grant,[6] Hollinshead,[7] Kempe,[13] Gray,[8] and Seletz[22] provide additional anatomic reference material.

Subaxilla and Upper Arm
Lower Brachial Plexus

The surgical exposure of the brachial plexus has been discussed in detail in the previous chapter. The lower brachial plexus is again briefly discussed here in order to focus on the exposure of the region of the distal cords.

The lower brachial plexus is approached through an infraclavicular brachial plexus incision (as described in Chapter 10) that extends over the pectoralis muscles' insertion on the humerus and drops down onto the intermuscular septum (between the biceps and the triceps muscles). The incision of the pectoralis major muscle should be made in close proximity to the humerus while leaving enough tendon for suturing at the time of closure. If the incision is made too far from the humerus, the tendon thins and is inadequate for a strong suture-fixation to the insertion site (see Chapter 9).

Following the reflection of the pectoralis major muscle medially (if indicated), the cords of

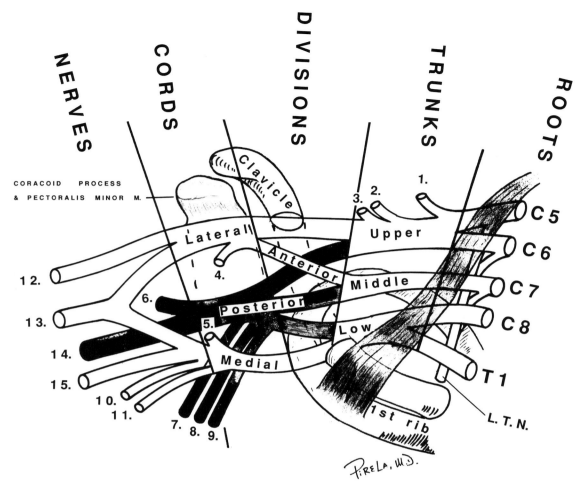

Figure 1. *The brachial plexus of the right upper extremity. L.T.N. is the long thoracic nerve. 1. Dorsal scapular nerve, 2. Suprascapular nerve, 3. Subclavian nerve, 4. Lateral Pectoral nerve, 5. Medial Pectoral nerve, 6. Axillary nerve, 7. Lower Subscapular nerve, 8. Thoracodorsal nerve, 9. Upper Subscapular nerve, 10. Medial Antebrachial nerve, 11. Medial Brachial nerve, 12. Musculocutaneous nerve, 13. Median nerve, 14. Radial nerve, 15. Ulnar nerve. As a review exercise, cover the legend and identify the nerves in the above drawing.*

the brachial plexus and the proximal nerves of the upper arm are easily observed and identified (Figure 1). In this region, the relationship of the axillary (brachial) artery to the radial, median, and ulnar nerves is consistent and aids the surgeon in nerve identification.

Proximal Brachial Nerves

The proximal axillary and musculocutaneous nerves are readily visualized with this approach. The brachial and antebrachial cutane-

ous nerves also may be identified in the intermuscular septum. It is important to recognize their proximal separation from their parent nerve (ulnar nerve). The antebrachial cutaneous nerve does not pass through the cubital fossa with the ulnar nerve despite its parallel relationship over a significant portion of its course. The thoracodorsal nerve is visualized along the chest wall. This nerve readily is observed following medial chest wall exposure. Finally, the radial nerve (a direct extension of the posterior cord) is visualized just before it passes behind the humerus as it begins its descent by spiraling around the humerus.

Medial Upper Arm

The musculocutaneous, median, and ulnar nerves are located in the medial aspect of the upper arm. Both the median and ulnar nerves descend in the intermuscular septum, along the brachial artery and vein. Their relationship to these vascular structures as well as their relationship to the medial brachial and antebrachial cutaneous nerves are illustrated in Figures 1 and 2. The medial arm incision described before gains access to the intermuscular septum as described. It is emphasized that this region is straightforward with respect to anatomic relationships; therefore, an exhaustive discussion of the anatomic details will not be undertaken.

The musculocutaneous nerve is readily visu-

alized by retracting the biceps muscle. Its branches, which innervate the biceps and brachialis muscles, can then be observed.

Lateral and Posterior Upper Arm

In contrast to the medial upper arm, the lateral and posterior upper arm is more complex regarding peripheral nerve exposure. As the radial nerve spirals around the humerus, it passes under and through several muscles enroute to the forearm. An incision, as illustrated in Figure 3A, gains access to the entire course of the radial nerve in the proximal upper extremity, in addition to the distal axillary nerve (the proximal axillary nerve may be approached best through the subaxillary approach). Following opening of the brachial fascia (which is a fairly significant fascial covering), the axillary nerve

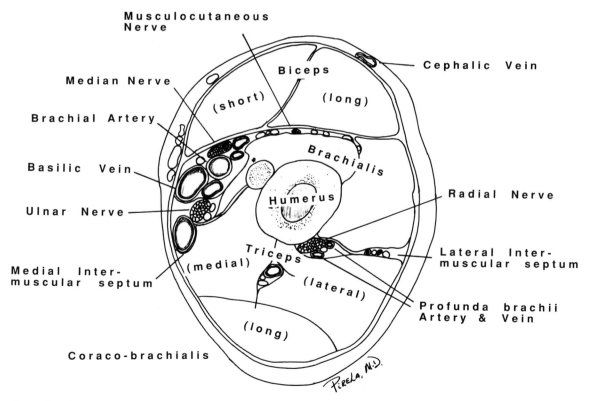

Figure 2. Cross-section through the midarm. Note the relationship of the median, ulnar, and radial nerves to the brachial artery and the compartments of the arm.

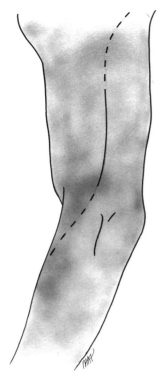

Figure 3A. Incision for the exposure of the proximal radial nerve.

must be taken to minimize lateral muscle dissection, which could injure the motor branches to the muscle. Multiple motor branches and the posterior antebrachial cutaneous nerve branch from the radial nerve and can be visualized through this exposure (see below).

Elbow and Forearm Region

Ulnar Nerve

The cubital tunnel begins at the condylar groove between the medial epicondyle of the humerus and the olecranon of the ulna. The floor of the cubital tunnel is the medial collateral ligament (ulnar lateral ligament) of the elbow joint, and the sides are formed by the two heads of the flexor carpi ulnaris muscle. The roof is formed by the triangular arcuate ligament (aponeurotic band) that bridges from the medial epicondyle of the humerus to the me-

as it approaches the deltoid muscle is observed. The separation of the triceps muscle bellies (long and lateral heads) along their fibers allows a view and exposure of the radial nerve throughout its course in the upper arm. This is achieved by simply mobilizing the muscle bellies from side to side. After mobilizing these muscles, the radial nerve can be observed underneath. The planes between the muscle bellies can be identified by palpation. Blunt dissection allows their separation and, thus, the desired deeper exposure (Figure 3B). A radial compressive neuropathy caused by the triceps muscle in this region may occur.[18,19]

The radial nerve spirals around the humerus, staying in relatively close proximity to the bone. Distally in the upper arm, however, it pierces an intermuscular septum between the brachioradialis and the brachialis muscles. Reflection of the brachioradialis muscle laterally allows the reidentification of the nerve medial to the muscle and underneath the septum. Care

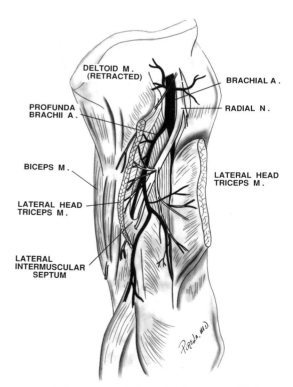

Figure 3B. Course of the radial nerve as it pierces the lateral intermuscular septum.

dial aspect of the olecranon.[20] The capacity of the cubital tunnel is greatest when the elbow is in extension. Measurements in cadaveric material demonstrate that the distance between the humeral and ulnar attachments of the triangular arcuate ligament lengthens 5 mm for each 45 degrees of flexion.[21] Refer to Chapter 6 for details regarding cubital anatomy and surgical approaches.

After penetrating the flexor carpi ulnaris muscle, the ulnar nerve continues throughout the entire forearm under the cover of the flexor carpi ulnaris muscle (Figure 4). Just above the middle of the forearm, the ulnar artery veers toward the nerve from the radial aspect and continues to lie close to the nerve until it reaches the wrist joint. The neurovascular bundle becomes more superficial in the distal third of the forearm, where it is barely under cover of the radial border of the flexor carpi ulnaris muscle.[2]

The surgical approach to the ulnar nerve at the elbow is through a posteromedial longitudinal curvilinear or zigzag incision (Figure 5A). The ulnar nerve should be freed for at least 8 cm proximal to the medial epicondyle to ensure release from the arcade of Struthers or entrapment on the medial intermuscular septum. Fixation of the nerve at the level of the medial epicondylar groove can result in traction neuritis.[10] The fibrous arcade over the flexor carpi ulnaris muscle must be excised, and the ulnar nerve should be explored to the midportion of the proximal third of the forearm. The superior ulnar collateral artery, which accompanies the ulnar nerve in the condylar groove, should not be injured (see Chapter 6 for further detail).

Exposure of the ulnar nerve in the forearm is best accomplished through a longitudinal "stepped" or 60-degree "turned" incision along the ulnar border of the forearm about 5 cm volar to the palpable portion of the ulnar bone (Figure 5B). After opening the antebrachial fascia, the nerve is approached by separating the flexor carpi ulnaris from the flexor digitorum superficialis muscle. After creating this division, the flexor carpi ulnaris is elevated from the flexor digitorum profundus to expose the ulnar nerve throughout the forearm.[10]

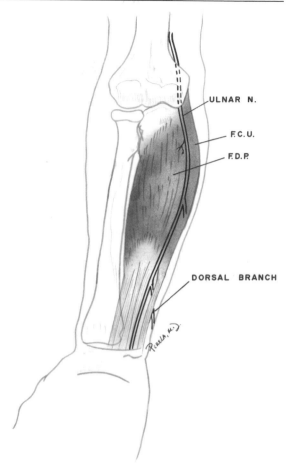

Figure 4. Ulnar nerve as it crosses the elbow and enters into the forearm. Note the relationship of the ulnar nerve to the flexor digitorum profundus (F.D.P.) and the flexor carpi ulnaris muscles (F.C.U.)

The cubital tunnel syndrome and, occasionally, median nerve entrapment can occur in the region of the elbow. Nerve injury from percutaneous or open attempts at vascular access or angiography may result in median nerve injury as well.

Median Nerve

The median nerve begins just below the pectoralis minor muscle as a union of branches from the lateral and medial cords of the brachial plexus. The median nerve continues on the

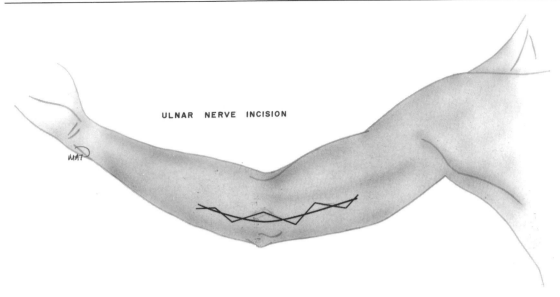

ULNAR NERVE INCISION

Figure 5A. *Incision to expose the ulnar nerve in the elbow region. This exposure can be performed through either a curvilinear incision or multiple zigzag incisions.*

medial side of the biceps brachii muscle and accompanies the brachial artery to the elbow. The median nerve is closely related to the vessels through most of the arm, and in those injuries that damage the vessel, the nerve is almost always involved. The nerve lies in the medial bicipital groove and anterior to the medial intermuscular septum.[2,23]

As it approaches the elbow joint, the median nerve is directly covered by the lacertus fibrosis (bicipital aponeurosis). The nerve passes out of the cubital fossa between the humeral and ulnar heads of the pronator teres muscle (Figure 6). Just beyond the exit of the median nerve from between the heads of the pronator teres, the anterior interosseous nerve branch passes forward to supply the deep muscles of the forearm. The median nerve passes behind the flexor superficialis arch and comes to lie deeply in the middle of the volar surface of the forearm, between the flexor digitorum superficialis and the flexor digitorum profundus muscles (Figure 6). The median nerve becomes superficial to the flexor digitorum superficialis muscle bellies about 5 cm proximal to the transverse carpal ligament.

The operative approach to the median nerve in the forearm is a longitudinal approach along the medial ulnar border of the biceps brachii muscle in the distal arm, curving transversely at the elbow flexion crease, then taking either a gentle S-curve or a zigzag course along the ulnar (medial) distal border of the pronator teres muscles, and continuing longitudinally to the wrist crease (Figure 7A). An incision into the palm should cross the wrist crease obliquely at a point in line with the long axis of the ring finger. The safe side of the median nerve in the proximal forearm is the radial side, since the branches are ulnarward. The best surgical approach is to identify the median nerve proximal to the lacertus fibrosis and to trace it distally through the region of the pronator teres and the flexor superficialis arch (Figure 7B).

Entrapment of the median nerve in the proximal forearm is termed the *pronator syndrome*. Most commonly the entrapment occurs by the deep head of the pronator muscle. At least two other areas of potential entrapment exist in close proximity: at the lacertus fibrosis and at the flexor superficialis arch.[26] When forearm pain is reproduced by resistance to pronation of the forearm, and is aggravated by extending the elbow, the localization is to the pronator teres. When the pain is reproduced by resistance to flexion of the elbow and supination of

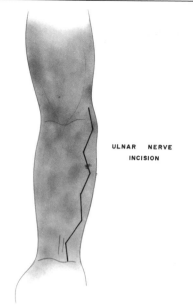

Figure 5B. Incision for exposing the ulnar nerve in the forearm.

the forearm, the lacertus fibrosis is the likely site of compression. Pain in the proximal forearm, reproduced by resistance to flexion of the flexor digitorum superficialis of the long finger, helps to localize the pathology to the flexor superficialis arch.[24] When surgical release of a pronator syndrome is necessary, the median nerve is first identified proximal to the lacertus fibrosis and then followed distally through the flexor superficialis bridge. It is necessary to develop the plane between the lower border of the pronator teres and the proximal margin of the flexor carpi radialis.

The anterior interosseous nerve syndrome[14] is a result of compression of the anterior interosseous branch of the median nerve, usually at a site close to its branching.[13] The anterior interosseous nerve usually arises from the median nerve approximately 7 cm distal to the lateral epicondyle (Figure 7B). The anterior in-

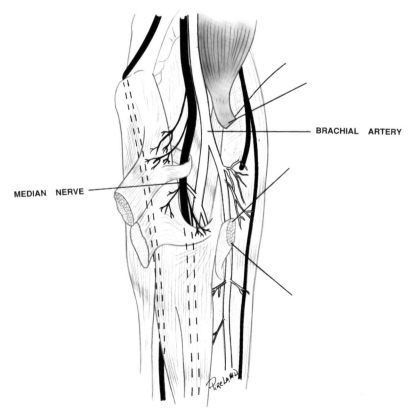

Figure 6. Anatomy of the anterior elbow. The pronator teres muscle and biceps tendon have been cut and retracted to expose the median nerve and brachial artery.

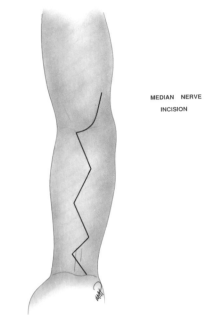

MEDIAN NERVE
INCISION

Figure 7A. Incision for the extensile exposure of the median nerve in the distal arm and forearm.

terosseous nerve syndrome is characterized by an inability to flex the terminal phalanges of the thumb, index, and long fingers. Sensation in the hand is undisturbed. The median nerve should be identified proximal to the lacertus fibrosis and traced distally through the pronator teres. The most common restraining structure is the tendinous origin of the deep head of the pronator teres.[26]

Combined Surgical Exposure of the Median and Ulnar Nerves

The exposure of the median and ulnar nerves in the region of the elbow may be performed through one incision by simply carrying the medial upper arm incision caudally in an S-shaped fashion, similar to that illustrated in Figure 7A. In the region of the elbow, the single incision approach is not often used because a

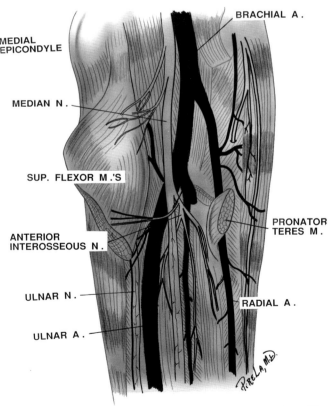

BRACHIAL A.

MEDIAL EPICONDYLE

MEDIAN N.

SUP. FLEXOR M.'S

PRONATOR TERES M.

ANTERIOR INTEROSSEOUS N.

ULNAR N.

RADIAL A.

ULNAR A.

Figure 7B. Anterior interosseous nerve coming off the median nerve in the proximal forearm.

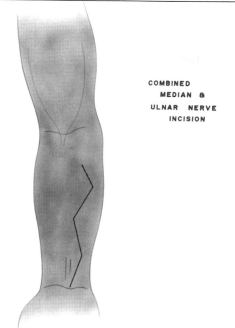

COMBINED
MEDIAN &
ULNAR NERVE
INCISION

Figure 8. Incision used to expose the median and ulnar nerves in the distal forearm.

more limited exposure to just one of the nerves is indicated. A limited exposure is used when appropriate. At the level of the elbow, the single incision gains access to the antecubital fossae and the cubital tunnel where the median and ulnar nerves, respectively, pass. Exposure of both of these nerves is straightforward in this region. If any difficulty is encountered in locating either of these nerves during a surgical exposure due to anatomic variation or scarring from previous injury or surgery, it would be prudent to find the nerve by a more aggressive and more proximal exposure.

Approximately 8 cm proximal to the medial epicondyle, the ulnar nerve normally passes from the anterior plane of the medial intermuscular septum to the posterior plane of the septum. The arcade of Struthers is formed by a thickening of the deep investing fascia of the distal part of the arm, by superficial muscular fibers of the medial head of the triceps, and by attachments of the internal brachial ligament. Its anterior border is the medial intermuscular septum.[10] Proximal to the elbow, the ulnar nerve should be freed for at least 8 cm from the

medial epicondyle to avoid potential compression in the arcade of Struthers.

If both the median and ulnar nerves require exposure in the distal forearm, a single incision may be used. (Figure 8). Inglis[10] recommends a longitudinal incision midway between the two nerves. This should be an "S-course" with angles 90 degrees or more. The antebrachial fascia is opened and the interval developed between the palmaris longus and flexor carpi ulnaris muscles. The ulnar nerve throughout the forearm is in the plane between the flexor carpi ulnaris and the flexor digitorum profundus muscles. The median nerve lies beneath the flexor digitorum superficialis. This incision can provide good exposure of both nerves in the distal two-thirds of the forearm.

Radial Nerve

The radial nerve, as it courses across the region of the elbow, follows a complex anatomic course. Reflection of the brachioradialis and the extensor radialis longus muscles allows the exposure of the radial nerve as it crosses the elbow and maintains its submuscular descent into the forearm. In the region of the elbow, it branches into a superficial and deep branch. The superficial branch descends into the forearm between and underneath the brachioradialis and extensor carpi radialis longus muscles. The deep branch (the posterior interosseous nerve) passes underneath the flexor carpi radialis longus muscle.

It is emphasized again that with careful dissection and retraction of the muscles under which the radial nerve passes, it can be safely followed (without significant nervous or other soft-tissue injury) over its entire course into the forearm. Protection of the motor branches and an understanding of the location of the complicated regions of its exposure (such as the intermuscular septum; as mentioned before and illustrated in Figures 3A,B) are critical.

Exposure of the radial nerve as it passes distally toward the elbow is performed with an incision along the medial border of the brachioradialis muscle (Figures 9A,B). Reflec-

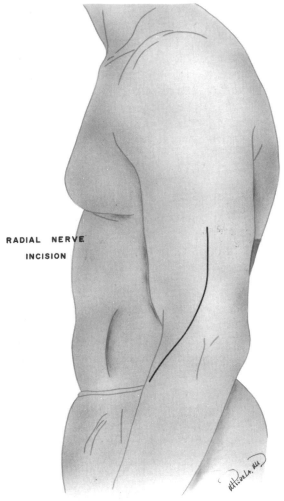

RADIAL NERVE
INCISION

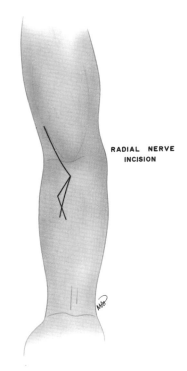

RADIAL NERVE
INCISION

Figure 9B. *Two options for exposing the radial nerve anteriorly.*

Figure 9A. Incision used to expose the radial nerve in the distal arm and proximal forearm. This incision can be extended proximally and distally as needed for additional exposure.

tion of the brachioradialis muscle laterally allows the reidentification of the radial nerve. Care must be taken to minimize lateral muscle dissection in this segment, which could injure motor branches to the muscle. Multiple motor branches, and the posterior antebrachial cutaneous nerve, branch from the radial nerve in this segment and can be visualized through this exposure.

The radial nerve as it passes across the region of the elbow is a similarly complex anatomic exposure. An anterolateral incision should ex-

tend from 8–10 cm proximal to the bi-epicondylar line and end about 5–6 cm distal to the line.[12] Lateral reflection of the brachioradialis and the extensor radialis longus muscles allows the exposure of the radial nerve as it crosses the elbow and maintains its submuscular descent into the forearm. The biceps tendon and muscle, together with the musculocutaneous nerve, are retracted medially. The musculocutaneous nerve lies at a more superficial level than the radial nerve. In the region of the elbow, the radial nerve branches into a superficial sensory branch and a deep motor branch, usually at the level of the radiocapitellar joint, but in a range of 5 cm proximal or distal to this point.[25] The superficial branch descends into the forearm between and underneath the brachioradialis and extensor carpi radialis muscles. The superficial radial nerve is a key to accurate exposure. It is traced proximally to the radial nerve and then distally to the posterior interosseous nerve. The deep

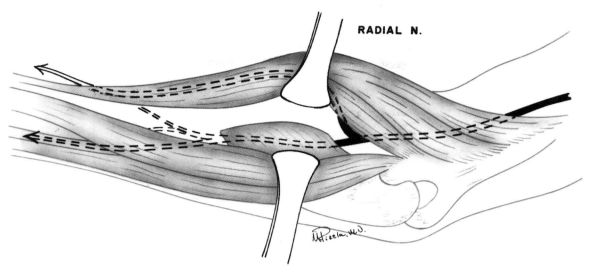

Figure 9C. *Dorsolateral exposure of the radial nerve as it branches into its superficial branch and the posterior interosseous nerve (P.I.N.). The relationship of the mobile wad and the supinator muscle is also observed.*

branch, the posterior interosseous nerve, passes underneath the flexor carpi radialis longus muscle and between the two heads of the supinator muscle. The nerve lies deep in the cubital fossa. The incision should be generous in order to obtain adequate visualization.

Common syndromes with radial nerve injury include one associated with the compression of the radial nerve as it passes through the intermuscular septum,[18] "Saturday night palsy" (caused by prolonged pressure exerted on the nerve as it passes around the proximal humerus), fracture of the proximal humerus (associated with injury to the closely approximated radial nerve), and injury to the nerve in the region of the radial tunnel (which comprises the tunnel under and around the brachioradialis and extensor carpi radialis longus muscles, the capitulum, the biceps tendon, the head of the radius, the pronator teres, the extensor carpi radialis brevis, and the superficial and deep heads of the supinator muscles in descending order). The latter region has been loosely referred to as the *radial tunnel*, and the syndrome associated with it as the *resistant tennis elbow syndrome* (see Chapter 4).

The superficial radial nerve in the forearm continues in its position beneath the extensor carpi radialis longus muscle to the junction of the middle and lower thirds of the forearm. It pierces the deep fascia and supplies cutaneous branches to the radial posterior aspect of the carpus, and the thumb, index, and middle fingers.[23] The point of superficial penetration is 8–9 cm proximal to the tip of the radial styloid process, or just above the junction of the middle and lower thirds of the forearm.[2] This nerve can be exposed by a longitudinal incision on the radiodorsal aspect of the distal upper arm (Figure 9A) or anteriorly on the proximal forearm (Figure 9B). The most serious complication of elective surgery in this area is a painful neuroma of one of the branches of the superficial radial nerve, which may follow laceration, retraction stretch, or blunt injury, and is termed *cheiralgia paresthetica*. This region is exposed to everyday activity-related trauma, while wrist movement is a further irritant. Therefore, multiple factors serve to prolong discomfort.

The radial nerve and its major branches at the elbow can be exposed in the lower arm and forearm through an incision that begins anteriorly between the brachialis and the brachioradialis muscles and extends dorsally into the forearm between the extensor carpi radialis

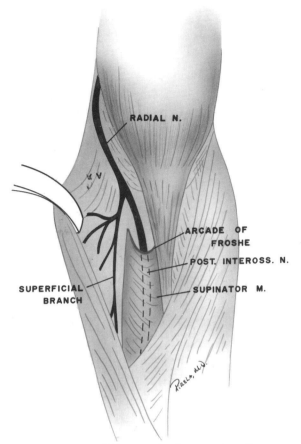

Figure 9D. Radial nerve in the anterior elbow region. The arcade of Frohse (fibrous arch of the supinator) is also shown.

brevis and the extensor digitorum communis muscle (Figure 9C).[25] The plane between the extensor carpi radialis brevis and the extensor digitorum communis muscle is defined distally and then dissected proximally to the lateral epicondyle. The supinator muscle is then visualized in the depth of the wound. At the lower end of the supinator, the terminal branches of the posterior interosseous nerve are observed. If the posterior interosseous nerve is identified on the proximal side of the supinator muscle, its path can be traced distally within the supinator. The extensor carpi radialis brevis, like the supinator, has a tendinous origin from the lateral epicondyle and may contribute to development of radial tunnel syndrome.[17]

In the average forearm, the posterior interosseous nerve enters the supinator muscle approximately 5 cm distal to the tip of the external condyle of the humerus. The relationship of the branches at the level of the supinator muscle is inconsistent; therefore, care must be exercised in identifying the branches during decompression of the posterior interosseous nerve as it enters the supinator muscle.[10] The posterior interosseous nerve enters the supinator muscle through an inverted fibrous arch formed by the tendinous-thickened edge of the proximal border of the superficial head of the supinator.[24,25] This arch was described in 1908 by the anatomist Frohse,[25] and is termed the *arcade of Frohse* (Figure 9D).

Palm and Wrist Region

Over the years, many incisions have been described to expose the median and ulnar nerves in the palm; however, before performing surgery on the palm, it is important that the surgeon be familiar with the anatomy and anatomic variations that may exist with respect to the median nerve. In addition, the course and territory of the palmar cutaneous branches of the median and ulnar nerves are important to know in order to avoid inadvertent injury, bearing in mind that even the slightest injury to a cutaneous nerve about the palm and wrist can cause severe morbidity and disuse of an extremity.[15] Carpal tunnel decompression is one of the most commonly performed surgical procedures today. It is therefore prudent that surgeons performing this procedure be aware of the complications as well as the treatment of the adverse effects (see Chapters 6 and 14).

General Principles

Surgical principles of importance regarding the median and ulnar nerves in the palm are:

1. Do not cross the flexor crease of the wrist with a straight incision, that is, at 90 degrees to the flexor crease. Violating this principle may cause severe scar formation, flexion contracture, and limited range of motion of the wrist.

2. Longitudinal incision(s) and not transverse incision(s) should be used to avoid injury to adjacent cutaneous nerves (please refer to the section on the palmar cutaneous nerve). With the recent development of endoscopic carpal tunnel release and the resurgence of the transverse incision placed at the level of the flexor crease of the wrist, it is anticipated that an increase in the number of complications due to cutaneous nerve injury will occur.[6]

3. At the level of the flexor crease of the wrist, the incision should not be on the radial side of the axis of the ring finger. As in principle 2, above, risk of injury to the palmar cutaneous nerve with the development of a symptomatic neuroma increases if the incision is placed on the radial side of the axis ("line of Taleisnik") (Figure 10).

4. The surgical exposure should perhaps be performed under exsanguination and tourniquet control to minimize bleeding and difficulty with visualization; however, some circumstances may contraindicate the use of a tourniquet. A typical example may be a patient with chronic renal failure with carpal tunnel syndrome requiring surgical decompression and having an arteriovenous access shunt on the symptomatic side. In this situation, meticulous hemostasis is essential.

5. Surgery can be facilitated by the use of magnification to identify peripheral branches, which at times may be very small. Loupe magnification of 3.5x is usually adequate. Procedures such as internal neurolysis, if indicated, are best performed with the aid of a surgical microscope.

6. The transverse carpal ligament should be incised under direct vision.

7. Opening of the carpal tunnel roof should be on the ulnar side of the transverse carpal ligament just radial to the hook of the hamate to avoid injury to the motor branch of the median nerve, which most commonly comes off on the radial side of the median nerve (see section on variations of the motor branch). Entry to Guyon's canal is also facilitated with this exposure.

8. After opening the carpal tunnel, always identify the motor branch and determine its relationship to the transverse carpal ligament. If there is a transligamentous course of the motor branch, the branch must be released in order to prevent a traction palsy of the motor branch (see next section). Similarly, if a fibrous band is anchored to the branch, this structure also must be sectioned to prevent tethering of the nerve.

9. Always inspect the contents of the carpal tunnel and check the floor for any pathology. Rarely, a tumor may be discovered.

10. In general, incisions in the creases of the palm should be avoided.

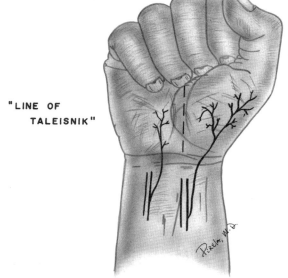

"LINE OF TALEISNIK"

Figure 10. "Line of Taleisnik" is shown on the palmar surface of the hand. This line is a useful landmark for avoiding injury to the palmar cutaneous branch of the median nerve.

Variations of the Median Nerve

From the surgical point of view, the most important anatomic variation of the median nerve relates to its motor branch that supplies the muscles of the thenar eminence. Lanz[16] classified the variations of the motor branch into four groups depending on the course of the branch, its position to the transverse carpal lig-

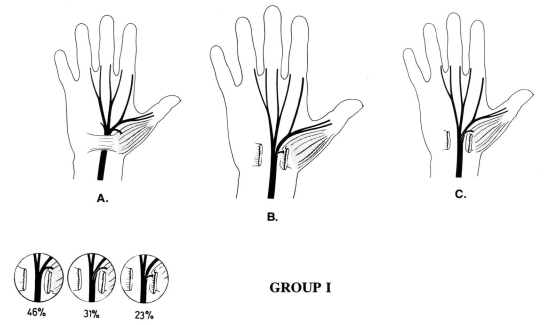

GROUP I

Figure 11. Lanz Group I variations of the median nerve include the most common anatomic variations of the motor branch of the median nerve. The extraligamentous route (A) is the most common. The subligamentous course (C) is the second most common variation followed by the transligamentous (B). Courtesy of the Mosby Publishing Company. Journal of Hand Surgery. 2:44–53, 1977. Reprinted with permission.

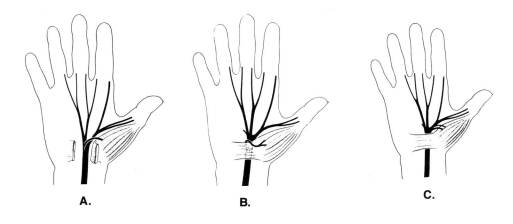

GROUP II

Figure 12. Lanz Group II variations of the motor branch of the median nerve, which includes the recurrent motor branch leaving from the ulnar aspect of the median nerve as well as double thenar motor branch variation. Courtesy of the Mosby Publishing Company. Journal of Hand Surgery. 2:44–53, 1977. Reprinted with permission.

ament, the presence of accessory nerves, and the relationship of the branch to the trunk of the median nerve. Group I (Figure 11) variations relate to the course of the motor branch. The three subtypes are: **(1)** The *extraligament-* *ous* recurrent course, which is, by far, the most common variation, occurring in 46% of all cases; **(2)** The *subligamentous* course occurs in 31% of all cases and is the second most common route of the motor branch. This branch is

GROUP III

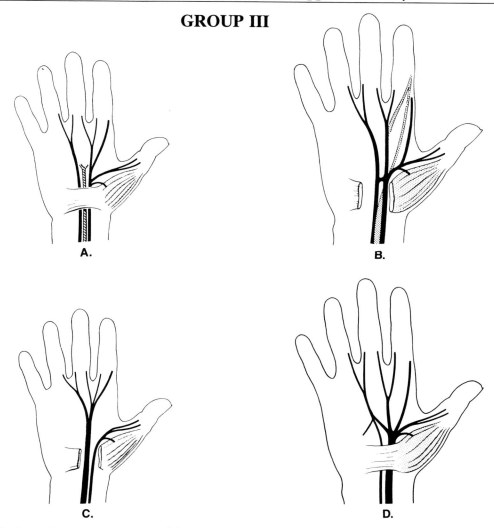

Figure 13. Lanz Group III variations of the recurrent nerve. This group is characterized by high division of the median nerve (proximal to the transverse carpal ligament). Courtesy of the Mosby Publishing Company. Journal of Hand Surgery. 2:44–53, 1977. Reprinted with permission.

given off beneath the transverse carpal ligament and then continues distally to gain access to the thenar musculature; **(3)** The *transligamentous* route for the motor branch is the third most common course, occurring in 23% of all cases. In this variation, the branch passes through the transverse carpal ligament to reach the muscles of the thenar eminence.

Group II (Figure 12) variations are composed of accessory branches at the level of the carpal tunnel. These variations are rare and may be given off the ulnar side of the median nerve.

The majority of these branches are sensory in nature and actually supply sensation to the skin. Lanz recommended preserving these branches for fear of developing painful neuromas. Group III (Figure 13) variations are categorized by high (proximal) division of the motor branch. A persistent median artery and an accessory lumbrical between the branches have been reported. Variability in the size of the branches also was reported in Lanz's study. Group IV (Figure 14) comprises accessory branches proximal to the carpal tunnel. There

GROUP IV

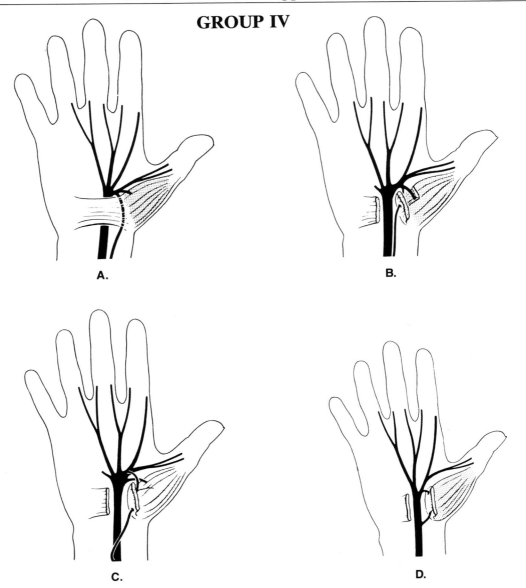

Figure 14. Lanz Group IV variations are characterized by an accessory branch to the thenar musculature that occurs proximal to the transverse carpal ligament. Courtesy of the Mosby Publishing Company. Journal of Hand Surgery. 2:44–53, 1977. Reprinted with permission.

is also a relatively small number of cases in this category.

Palmar Cutaneous Nerve

The course of the palmar cutaneous nerve of the median nerve and its relationship to surgical incisions has been documented by Taleisnik.[29] In a study consisting of 12 cadaveric limbs, the origin and course of the palmar cutaneous nerve were described. The palmar cutaneous nerve originates from the median nerve in the distal third of the forearm. Before its takeoff from the median nerve, a distinct bundle corresponding to the palmar cutaneous nerve can be identified on the palmar-radial aspect of the nerve according to Sunderland.[28] The nerve proceeds distally in the interval be-

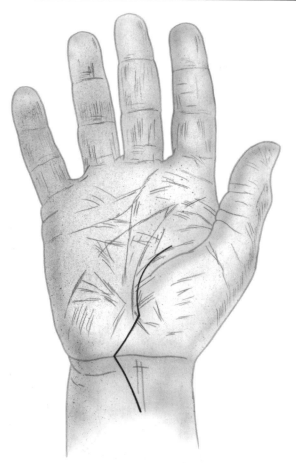

Figure 15A. Standard carpal tunnel incision. This incision allows inspection of the motor branch of the median nerve and carpal tunnel as well as access to Guyon's tunnel and ulnar nerve if necessary.

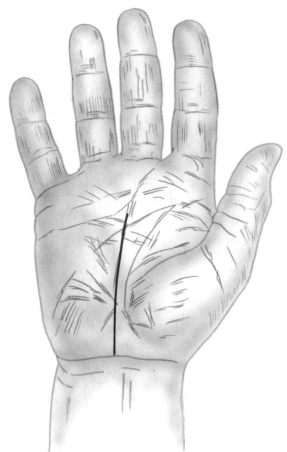

Figure 15B. Alternate incision for exposure of the carpal tunnel.

tween the palmaris longus and flexor carpi radialis tendons to enter its tunnel. The branch may surface from its deep position at either the antebrachial fascia or the transverse carpal ligament to later divide into a larger radial branch and a smaller ulnar branch. Taleisnik has shown that the palmar cutaneous nerve may be injured by either the transverse or longitudinal incisions during a carpal tunnel decompressive procedure and has therefore recommended an incision on the ulnar side of the axis of the ring finger at the level of the flexor crease of the wrist (see Figure 10). In addition to the more common iatrogenic complications, entrapment neuropathy of the palmar cutaneous nerve has been described by Stellbrink.[27]

Incisions and Exposure

Keeping in mind the surgical principles discussed earlier, the incision(s) for exposing the median and ulnar nerves of the palm that is consistent with these principles are described.

A commonly used incision to gain access to the carpal tunnel that has stood the test of time is one that begins in the midpalm just distal to the thenar eminence in line with the third ray and continues proximally parallel to the thenar eminence to about 2.5–3 cm distal to the flexor crease of the wrist. The incision continues in an ulnar direction making a sharp 50° turn toward the flexor crease of the wrist. This portion of the incision should end at a point that is in line with the axis of the ring finger ("line of Taleisnik"). The flexor crease of the wrist is crossed proceeding in a radially directed fashion with another sharp turn measuring approximately 100° with respect to the incision that was placed on the palm (Figure 15A). The distal forearm incision is continued proximally for approximately 3 cm.

The advantages of this exposure are: **(1)** The entire carpal tunnel region can be easily visualized; **(2)** The valley of the great pillars of the palm, which occasionally can be a cause of pain and discomfort after surgery, is avoided; **(3)** This incision helps to reduce the possibility of iatrogenic injury to the palmar cutaneous branch of the median nerve; **(4)** Access to Guyon's tunnel can be easily accomplished if so desired; **(5)** Release of the motor branch of the median nerve, particularly if it takes a transligamentous route, can also be easily accomplished as described above; **(6)** Additional surgical procedures that are at times necessary during a decompressive carpal tunnel surgery can be performed (i.e. internal neurolysis or epineurotomy of the median nerve, and an opponens plasty such as the Camitz procedure in cases where the median nerve has been compressed for a long period of time).

Another incision that has gained popularity over the years, particularly among surgeons who commonly perform carpal tunnel decompressive surgery, begins as described above and parallels the thenar eminence continuing to the flexor crease of the wrist and terminates (Figure 15B). The dissection is carried through the palmar fascia down to the transverse carpal tunnel ligament from a distal to proximal direction on the extreme ulnar side of the transverse carpal ligament. Special care is taken to protect the superficial palmar arch and the motor branch of the median nerve. The opening of the roof of the canal is facilitated with the aid of a hemostat slightly depressing the underlying structures. With this incision, the proximal portion of the transverse carpal ligament that is in continuity with the antebrachial fascia cannot be incised unless undermining on the palmar and dorsal sides of the ligament and fascia is performed. Once sufficient undermining is per-

formed, the surgeon places the wrist into maximal extension and places a retractor at the apex of the proximal incision lifting the palmar fascia. Another instrument such as a joker is placed into the carpal tunnel to protect the median nerve. At this point, the surgeon changes position to have an end-on (axial), direct view of the proximal incision. With this exposure and under *direct* vision, the remaining proximal portion of the transverse carpal ligament and the distal antebrachial fascia may be incised safely without extending the skin incision proximal to the flexor crease of the wrist. It is important to remember that this exposure should only be used for uncomplicated carpal tunnel decompression where a limited exposure of the median nerve is required.

A third incision is the transverse incision placed in the flexor crease of the wrist. This incision has regained popularity with the introduction of endoscopic carpal tunnel release. As stated before, care must be taken to protect branches of the palmar cutaneous nerve to avoid iatrogenic injury. The two-transverse incision technique, with the second incision placed in the midpalm, is stated to be safer than the single incision.[5] Complications, such as laceration of digital nerves and instrument failure, have occurred (personal communication, Agee, Oct. 1990). In the series by Agee et al[1], no complications with respect to iatrogenic nerve laceration occurred. Two patients, however, had persistent carpal tunnel syndrome requiring reoperation. Patients who had undergone unilateral endoscopic release returned to work 27 days sooner than the control group. In another study performed by Chow,[5] endoscopic carpal tunnel release was evaluated in 62 hands and 46 patients with a brief follow-up period. No complications were encountered. In this study it was found that a rapid recovery with decreased scarring and postoperative pain and no loss of grip or pinch strength was observed compared to the conventional method of carpal tunnel release. Time will tell if there is a place for this procedure in the surgeon's armamentarium.

The ulnar nerve can be exposed through the two longitudinal palmar incisions described

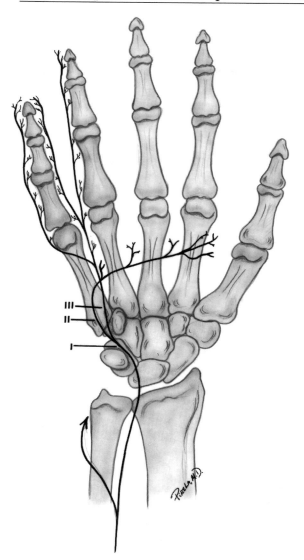

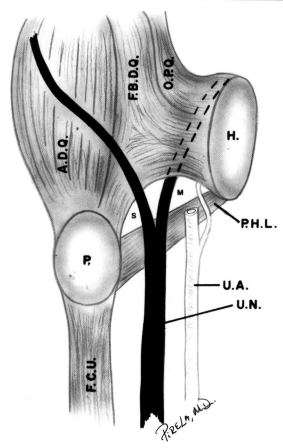

Figure 16B. *Ulnar nerve and its relationships in Guyon's tunnel. The sensory portion (S) and the motor portion (M) and their relationship to the pisohamate ligament (P.H.L.), the hamate (H.), and pisiform bones (P.) are emphasized. The ulnar artery (U.A.) is noted medial to the ulnar nerve (U.N.).*

Figure 16A. *Course and distribution of the ulnar nerve in the wrist, hand, and fingers. The dorsal sensory branch of the ulnar nerve (arrow) is observed as well as the main trunk of the ulnar nerve (I). The motor portion (II) is shown. The sensory portion of the ulnar nerve (III), supplying the ulnar one-and-a-half digits of the hand, is also demonstrated.*

previously. The ulnar nerve is palmar and ulnar to the median nerve in the hand. In addition, the ulnar nerve is located in its own tunnel and is on the ulnar side of the ulnar artery. Within Guyon's tunnel, the ulnar nerve separates into two branches: a sensory branch and a motor branch (Figures 16A,B,C). The sensory branch usually supplies the ulnar side of the ring finger and the ulnar and radial sides of the small finger. The motor branch continues underneath the pisohamate ligament to supply the intrinsic muscles of the hand—the abductor and flexor digiti minimi brevis, the opponens, the ulnar two lumbricals, all of the interossei, the adductor pollicis, and the deep head of the flexor pollicis brevis. If the dissection is carried out in a distal to proximal direction, the exposure is facilitated by locating the superficial palmar arch and tracing it proximally to Guyon's tunnel. With the aid of a blunt instrument inserted into

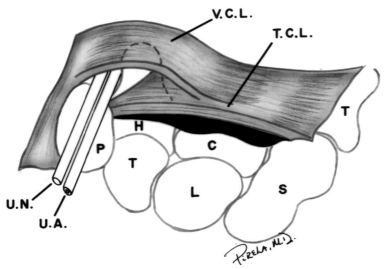

Figure 16C. Relationship of the ulnar artery (UA) and the ulnar nerve (UN) to the carpal tunnel to the carpal bones, the transverse carpal ligament (TCL) and the volar carpal ligament (VCL) is demonstrated.

the tunnel, the radial wall can be incised, exposing the ulnar artery and nerve. The tunnel should be opened completely; partial uncovering of the tunnel can result in a compressive neuropathy of the ulnar nerve.

Digits

To expose the digital nerves on the fingers, two incisions have withstood the test of time: Bruner's palmar zigzag incision and Bunnel's midaxial incision.[3,4] The former is more popular than the latter. The two incisions are designed to allow maximal exposure of the palmar structures of the finger, including the digital nerves, and to prevent postoperative flexion contracture, which can be very disabling. The Bruner incision is performed by connecting a point from the axilla of the base of the finger (proximal digital flexor crease) to the axilla of the opposite side of the finger distally on the middle digital flexor crease (proximal interphalangeal crease). The incision can be extended distally to the distal digital flexor crease (distal interphalangeal crease) if needed in a similar fashion (Figure 17A).

The midaxial or midlateral incision is performed by locating an imaginary plane located between the dorsal and palmar aspect of the finger. The incision is performed between the palmar and dorsal branches of the palmar digital nerve (Figure 17B). Care must be observed when extending the incision proximally in order to avoid injury to the dorsal digital branch.

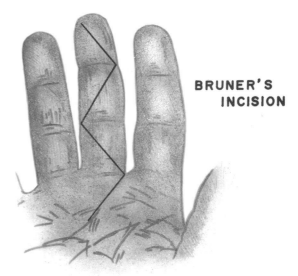

BRUNER'S INCISION

Figure 17A. Standard Bruner's incision for exposing the digital nerves in the fingers.

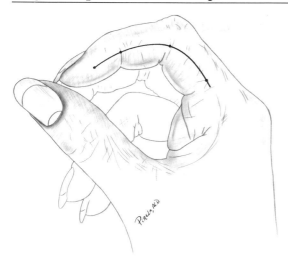

Figure 17B. *Standard midlateral (midaxial) incision for exposing the digital nerves in the fingers. Care should be taken when using this incision to protect the dorsal sensory branch of the digital nerve that courses from the palmar aspect of the finger to the base of the finger.*

References

1. Agee, JM, Tortosa R, Berry D, et al. Endoscopic release of the carpal tunnel: a randomized multicenter study. Presented at the 45th Annual meeting of the American Society for Surgery of the Hand; September 1990; Toronto, Canada.
2. Bateman JE. *Trauma to Nerves in Limbs.* Philadelphia, Pa; WB Saunders Co; 1962:31–55.
3. Bruner JM. Incisions for plastic and reconstructive (non-septic) surgery of the hand. *Br J Plast Surg.* 1951;4:48–55.
4. Bunnell S. *Surgery of the Hand,* 2nd ed. Philadelphia, Pa: JB Lippincott; 1948.
5. Chow JCY. Endoscopic release of the carpal ligament: a new technique for carpal tunnel syndrome. *Arthroscopy.* 1989;5:19–24.
6. Conolly WB. Minor surgical procedures and infections. In: McFarlane RM, ed. *Unsatisfactory Results in Hand Surgery.* New York, NY: Churchill Livingstone; 1987:41–64.
7. Grant JCB. *An Atlas of Anatomy.* Baltimore, Md: Williams and Wilkins; 1948;1:8–62.
8. Gray H; Lewis WH, ed. *Gray's Anatomy of the Human Body.* 24th ed. Philadelphia, Pa; Lea & Febiger; 1942:947–961.
9. Hollinshead WH. *Anatomy for Surgeons: The Back and Limbs.* 2nd ed. New York, NY: Hoeber Medical Division; 1969;3:349–574.
10. Inglis AE. Surgical exposure of peripheral nerves. In: Omer GE Jr, Spinner M, eds. *Management of Peripheral Nerve Problems,* Philadelphia, Pa: WB Saunders; 1980;317–350.
11. Johnson RK, Spinner M, Shrewsbury NM. Median nerve entrapment syndrome in the proximal forearm. *J Hand Surg.* 1979;4:48–51.
12. Kaplan EB. *Surgical Approaches to the Neck, Cervical Spine and Upper Extremity.* Philadelphia, Pa: WB Saunders Co; 1966:109.
13. Kemp LG. Surgery of peripheral nerves. In: Kempe LG, ed. *Operative Neurosurgery.* New York, NY: Springer Verlag; 1970;2:203–232.
14. Kiloh LG, Nevin S. Isolated neuritis of the anterior interosseous nerve. *Br Med J.* 1952;1:850–851.
15. Lankford LL. Reflex sympathetic dystrophy. In: Hunter JM, Schneider LH, Mackin EJ, et al, eds: *Rehabilitation of the Hand: Surgery and Therapy.* 3rd ed. St. Louis, Mo: Mosby-Yearbook;1990:763–786.
16. Lanz U. Anatomical variations of the median nerve in the carpal tunnel. *J Hand Surg.* 1977;2:44–53.
17. Lister GD, Belsole RB, Kleinert HE. The radial tunnel syndrome. *J Hand Surg.* 1979;4:52–59.
18. Lotem M, Fried A, Levy M, et al. Radial palsy following muscular effort. *J Bone Joint Surg Br.* 1971;53B:500–506.
19. Manske PR. Compression of the radial nerve by the triceps muscle. *J Bone Joint Surg Am.* 1977;59A:835–836.
20. Omer GE Jr. The ulnar nerve at the elbow. In: Strickland JW, Steichen JB, eds. *Difficult Problems in Hand Surgery.* Saint Louis, Mo: Mosby-Yearbook; 1982: 374–378.
21. Omer GE Jr. The cubital tunnel syndrome. In: Szabo RM, ed. *Nerve Compression Syndromes: Diagnosis and Treatment.* Thorofare, NJ: SLACK Inc; 1989: 163–175.
22. Seletz E. Anatomic surgical approaches to peripheral nerves. *Surg Clin N Am.* 1972;52:1211–1233.
23. Sobotta J, Mc Murrich J. *Atlas and Text-Book of Human Anatomy.* Philadelphia, Pa: WB Saunders Co; 1914.
24. Spinner M. The arcade of Frohse and its relationship to posterior interosseous nerve paralysis. *J Bone Joint Surg Br.* 1968;50B:809–812.
25. Spinner M. *Injuries to the Major Branches of Peripheral Nerves of the Forearm.* 2nd ed. Philadelphia, Pa: WB Saunders Co; 1978:80.
26. Spinner M. Management of nerve compression lesions of the upper extremity. In: Omer GE Jr, Spinner M, eds. *Management of Peripheral Nerve Problems.* Philadelphia, Pa: WB Saunders Co; 1980:569–592.
27. Stellbrink G. Compression of the palmar branch of the median nerve by atypical palmaris longus muscle. *Handchirurgie.* 1972; 4:155–157.
28. Sunderland S. *Nerves and Nerve Injuries.* London, England. E and S Livingstone Ltd; 1968.
29. Taleisnik J. The palmar cutaneous branch of the median nerve and the approach to the carpal tunnel. *J Bone Joint Surg Am.* September 1973; 55A:1212–1217.

CHAPTER 11

Surgical Exposure of the Lumbosacral Plexus and Proximal Sciatic Nerve

Edward C. Benzel, MD, FACS

Fortunately, lesions of the lumbar and sacral plexuses (heretofore collectively referred to as the lumbosacral plexus) and the proximal sciatic nerve are infrequent. Unfortunately, an inappropriately conservative approach is often undertaken in patients harboring these lesions because of the suspected degree of difficulty of the surgical approach. The bony and soft-tissue confines of the peritoneal cavity, retroperitoneum, pelvis, and gluteal region result in the application of the term "no-man's-land" to the region of the lumbosacral plexus and the proximal sciatic nerve.

Indications for surgery of nerves in this no-man's-land include tumors (usually nerve sheath tumors[4]), traumatic injuries (including penetrating, stretch, and injection injuries[14]), and, rarely, surgery for neural ablation.[3] Seven fundamental surgical approaches to the lumbosacral plexus and the proximal sciatic nerve exist. Any one or combination of these approaches may be used to expose a specific portion of this region. A combination of approaches (discussion follows sections on each of the seven approaches listed below) may be used when a long longitudinal exposure is indicated or when a lesion exists in a transition zone from one surgical approach to another. The seven surgical approaches are as follows:

1. A wide foraminotomy approach to the proximal nerve roots[7,12,17] (to gain access to the proximal nerve roots as they exit the dural sac and the spinal canal)

2. The lateral extracavitary approach to the spine[2,6,16] (to expose the nerve roots within the spinal canal, as well as approximately 4–6 cm lateral to the neuroforamina)

3. The anterolateral extraperitoneal approach to the spine[13,24] (to expose the proximal mid- to lower-retroperitoneal lumbar region)

4. The pelvic brim extraperitoneal approach[10,13,24] (to expose retroperitoneal lesions located in the low lumbar region)

5. The Pfannenstiel infraperitoneal approach[3,11,13] (to expose caudal infraperitoneal lesions within the pelvis)

6. The transperitoneal approach[1,13] (to expose, for the most part, the regions approached via approaches 3–5)

7. The extrapelvic infragluteal approach[3,4,9,14] (to expose the proximal sciatic nerve as it exits from the pelvis through the sciatic notch into the infragluteal space)

With an aggressive surgical approach, there is no absolute no-man's-land in the entire region of the lumbar and sacral plexuses and the proximal sciatic nerve, although regions that could be considered "relative no-man's-lands" do exist (i.e. the region of the sciatic nerve that is located within 2–3 cm of the sciatic notch). An understanding of the regional anatomy enhances one's ability to expose this region of the nervous system (several nicely done radiographic studies have enhanced the awareness

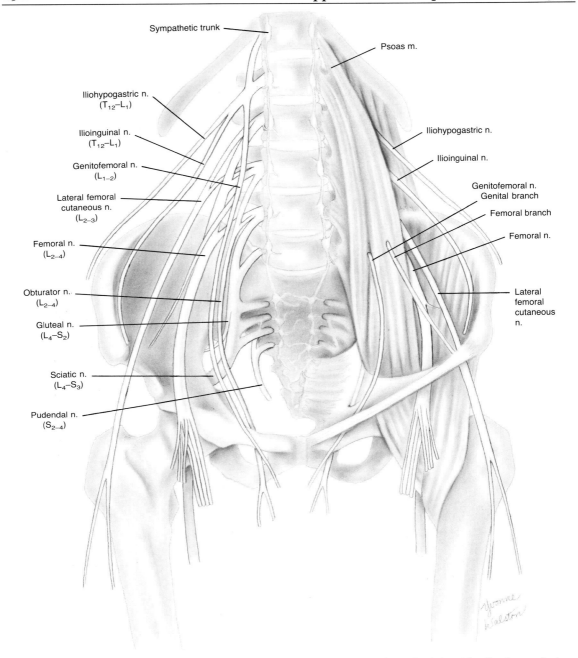

Figure 1. Lumbosacral plexus. Major neural pathways are illustrated on the left with all other soft tissue removed and on the right with retroperitoneal muscles left in place.

of clinicians with regard to the understanding of the anatomy[8,15,19,21,25–28]). In order to further enhance this understanding, the surgical approach to each of these seven regions will be discussed. A discussion of appropriate combined approaches and the indications for these surgical approaches will also be presented.

Figure 1 illustrates the lumbosacral plexus and its relationship to surrounding tissues. Figure 2 illustrates the axial anatomy of the lumbosacral plexus at a variety of levels. A correlation of Figures 1 and 2 should allow for an understanding of the three-dimensional anatomy of the lumbosacral plexus. The planes of dissec-

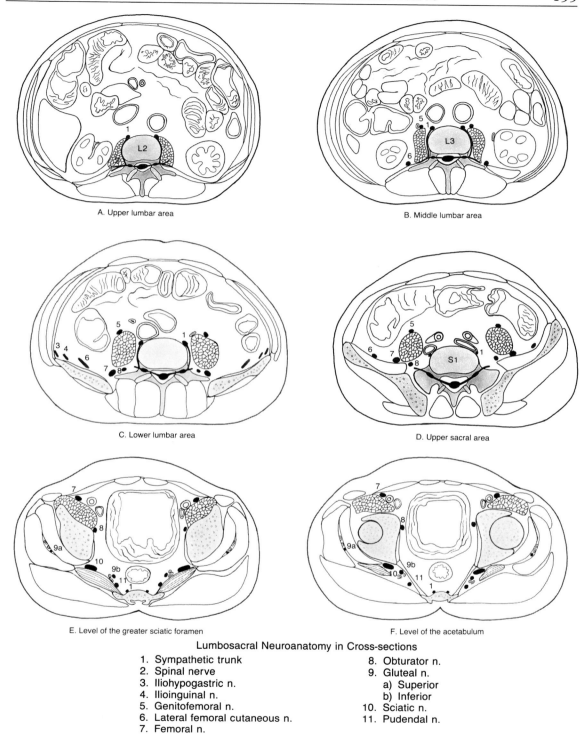

A. Upper lumbar area

B. Middle lumbar area

C. Lower lumbar area

D. Upper sacral area

E. Level of the greater sciatic foramen

F. Level of the acetabulum

Lumbosacral Neuroanatomy in Cross-sections

1. Sympathetic trunk
2. Spinal nerve
3. Iliohypogastric n.
4. Ilioinguinal n.
5. Genitofemoral n.
6. Lateral femoral cutaneous n.
7. Femoral n.
8. Obturator n.
9. Gluteal n.
   a) Superior
   b) Inferior
10. Sciatic n.
11. Pudendal n.

Figure 2. Illustration of the axial anatomy of the lumbosacral plexus and surrounding tissues at the L2 level (A); the L3 level (B); the L5 level (C); the S1 level (D); the S3,4 level (E); and the acetabulum level (F).

tion of several of the approaches for lumbosacral plexus exposure presented herein are illustrated in Figure 3, whereas Figure 4 illustrates the incisions used for the surgical exposures. A clear understanding of these planes is absolutely necessary before a surgical undertaking of any one of these approaches is entertained.

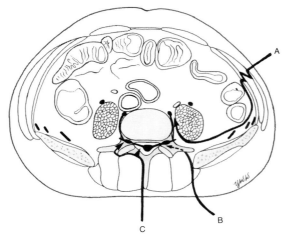

Figure 3. Planes of dissection of several of the operative approaches to the lumbosacral plexus: The anterolateral extraperitoneal and the pelvic brim approaches (A); the lateral extracavitary approach (B); and the wide foraminotomy approach (C).

Wide Foraminotomy Approach to the Proximal Nerve Roots

The midline exposure of the lumbar and upper sacral spine allows access to roughly the proximal 1–2 cm of the nerve roots as they exit the spinal canal, as well as the segment of the nerve root within the canal (Figure 5). One may approach this region with a lateral subperiosteal dissection, followed by a laminectomy or hemilaminectomy using standard spinal surgical techniques. The nerve root is then visualized within the spinal canal. Following further bone removal, the neuroforamina may be unroofed and the nerve root followed distally for approximately 1–2 cm.[7]

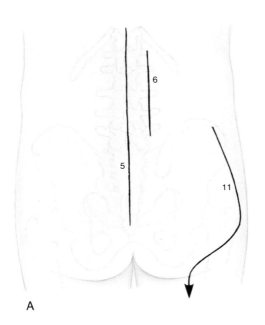

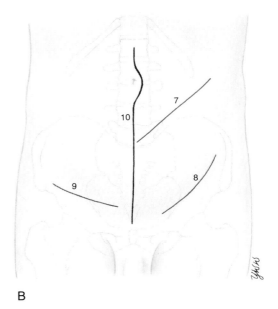

A   B

Figure 4. Some of the incisions used for surgical exposure of the lumbosacral plexus. A. The posterior incisions are illustrated: (5) the wide foraminotomy approach, (6) the lateral extracavitary approach, and (11) the extrapelvic infragluteal approach. B. The anterior incisions are illustrated: (7) the anterolateral extraperitoneal approach, (8) the pelvic brim extraperitoneal approach, (9) the Pfannenstiel infraperitoneal approach, and (10) the transperitoneal approach. Note: The numbering of each incision corresponds to the figure number in this chapter that describes the operation.

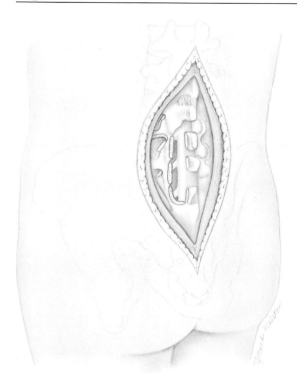

***Figure 5**. Illustration of the wide foraminotomy approach to the proximal nerve roots. A hemilaminectomy has been performed following a wide lateral soft-tissue retraction and dissection.*

A more lateral approach with extensive lateral paraspinous muscle retraction or splitting with soft-tissue dissection can be performed without the removal of the facet joint.[12,17] This gains access to the more distal aspect of the nerve root approachable from this operation.

The preservation of the integrity of the facet joint should be accomplished when possible. Subsequent degenerative changes, instability, and pain may be related to excessive bone removal in this region. If the facet joint is disrupted, the performance of a spinal fusion (either interbody or lateral) is a consideration.

The advantages of the wide foraminotomy approach to the posterior spine include the familiarity of the region to spine surgeons and the relatively uncomplicated nature of the surgical exposure. The disadvantages of this approach include its limited exposure. Only the very proximal portion of the nerve root is accessible by this approach.

Lateral Extracavitary Approach to the Proximal Lumbosacral Plexus

The lateral extracavitary approach to the spine, as originally described by Capener[6] and popularized by Larson et al,[16] can be used to gain access to the first 6 cm of the extradural lumbar nerve roots (Figure 6). All regions of the thoracic and lumbar spine can be approached with this operation, although surgical exposure of the lower lumbar region via the lateral extracavitary approach requires significant dorsal ilium resection. The three-quarter prone position is preferred by this author because it facilitates visualization of the surgical field by the surgeon. It simultaneously minimizes blood loss (due to lessened abdominal compression).[2]

The spine is approached as per Larson et al[16] and Benzel[2] through either a midline-oriented hockey-stick flap incision or through a paramedian longitudinal incision. A paramedian longitudinal incision is perhaps most appropriate for nerve exploration. Midline spinal exposure is not required for this operation; therefore, the creation of a cutaneous flap, with all its attendant risks, is not warranted. The thoracodorsal fascia is incised following its exposure. The erector spinae muscle is reflected medially following separation from the quadratus lumborum muscle. A well-defined plane exists between these two muscles (the middle layer of the thoracolumbar fascia). This plane is followed medially, allowing exposure of the transverse processes. Subperiosteal dissection along the underside of the transverse process allows one to follow the under surface of the transverse process, along the pedicle and the vertebral body, without fear of injury to the nerve roots as they exit the spinal canal. Following this exposure, the nerve roots can be isolated as they exit from the neuroforamina into the psoas muscle. This exposure is difficult due to the requisite muscle splitting. The nerves do not course between tissue planes in this region, thus necessitating the aforementioned muscle splitting. Further retraction laterally will allow access to the first 6 cm of the nerve after its exit from the spinal canal.

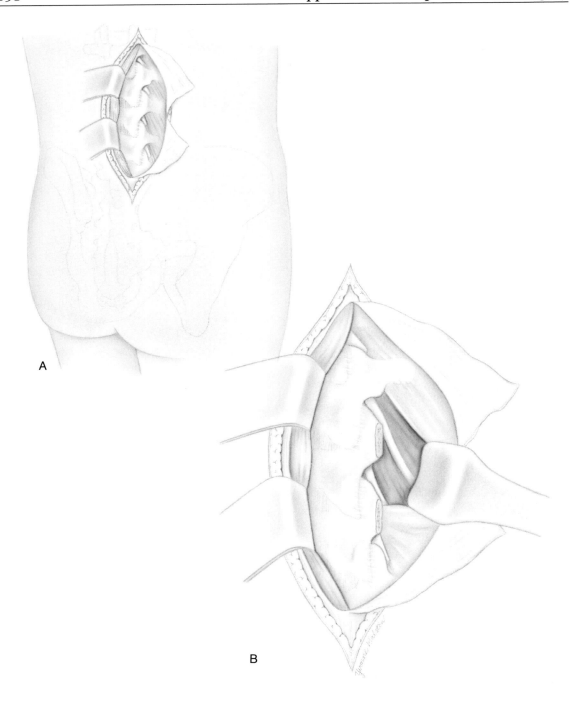

Figure 6. *Illustration of the exposure gained by the lateral extracavitary approach.* ***A.*** *The retraction of the erector spinae muscle medially allows visualization of the facet joints and transverse processes.* ***B.*** *Removal of the transverse processes and separation of the musculotendinous attachments to the vertebrae allow visualization of the proximal 5–6 cm of the nerve roots and plexus. Care must be taken to avoid injury to the nerve roots during the exposure. The oblique orientation of the nerve roots is emphasized.*

The advantages of this approach include the lack of intrapelvic dissection required and the ability to extend the dissection farther laterally than allowed with a wide foraminotomy approach. The disadvantages include the difficulties of dissecting across tissue planes and the resultant soft-tissue trauma incurred.

Anterolateral Extraperitoneal Approach

The anterolateral extraperitoneal approach to the upper lumbar spine is essentially the same approach used by surgeons to gain access to the sympathetic chain in the lumbar paravertebral region (see Figure 4).[13,24] This exposure (Figure 7) allows access to the L3–5 nerve roots from their exit point from the spinal canal to below the pelvic brim (although with greater difficulty, the upper lumbar nerve roots may be exposed). The patient is positioned so that the lumbar region is extended with a log roll and the patient rotated away from the side of the exposure. The incision courses from the lateral half of the twelfth rib in an anterior and medial direction. It is extended to below the level of the umbilicus, just lateral to midline and medial to the anterior superior iliac spine. Retraction is maintained with self-retaining and hand-held retractors. Retraction always should be performed with blunt instruments.

The dissection proceeds in an anatomic manner by muscle-splitting incisions through the external oblique, internal oblique, and transversalis muscles along the muscle fibers of each muscle layer. It must be kept in mind that as each anatomic layer is passed, the surgical field becomes smaller; therefore, the incision through each of the planes (especially the more superficial planes) should be longer than one might expect so that an adequate field of exposure is available when encountering the deep structures of concern. If exposure is of utmost importance, the internal oblique and transversus abdominus muscles may be incised across their muscle fibers in the same oblique direction as the skin incision.[13,24]

Following the entrance into the extraperitoneal space, the peritoneal contents are mobilized medially with the dissection remaining medial and posterior to the peritoneum and the renal fascia. Finger dissection or a sponge stick may be used to sweep the tissues away from the quadratus lumborum muscle, psoas muscle, and vertebral bodies. The lumbar veins and arteries may be obstacles to very medial dissection in the region of the neuroforamina. Their ligation may be necessary for adequate exposure. The preoperative performance of a spinal angiogram, in these circumstances, may be prudent.[2] The sacrifice of an important spinal radiculomedullary artery could be catastrophic.

If high lumbar exposure is necessary, the diaphragmatic crus may be separated from the anterior longitudinal ligament of the vertebral column. The sympathetic chain can be visualized in the groove between the psoas muscle and the vertebral body. The upper branches of the lumbosacral plexus can be visualized as they emerge from underneath or through the psoas muscle. The main branch of the lumbar plexus, the femoral nerve, rests between the psoas and iliacus muscle as it courses toward the pelvic floor. A number of the upper branches of the lumbar plexus also can be visualized in this region. These include the lateral femoral cutaneous, iliohypogastric, ilioinguinal, and genitofemoral nerves. The latter nerve is observed as it emerges medially through the psoas muscle belly. The lateral femoral cutaneous, iliohypogastric, and ilioinguinal nerves emerge either through the lateral aspect of or from underneath (and lateral to) the psoas muscle belly. These nerves may be followed proximally through the psoas muscle belly to the neuroforamina if necessary. Distal exposure is limited through this approach.

The advantages of this approach include the straightforward nature of the exposure, which is familiar to most spine and vascular surgeons; however, it offers a disappointingly narrow longitudinal exposure. This exposure is limited superiorly by the crus of the diaphragm and inferiorly by the pelvic brim. Through this approach, it is also difficult to expose the neuro-

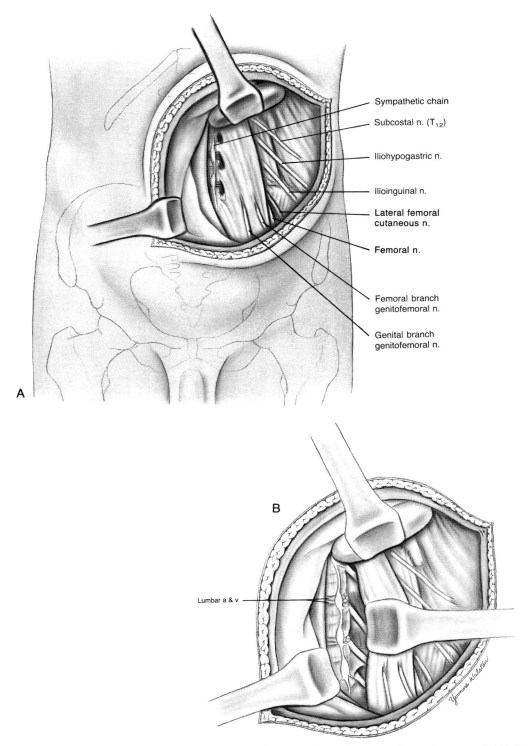

Sympathetic chain

Subcostal n. (T_{12})

Iliohypogastric n.

Ilioinguinal n.

**Lateral femoral
cutaneous n.**

Femoral n.

Femoral branch
genitofemoral n.

Genital branch
genitofemoral n.

Lumbar a & v

***Figure* 7.** *Illustration of the exposure gained by the anterolateral extraperitoneal approach (A). The perito-
neum is retracted medially. Musculotendinous attachments must be separated from the vertebrae in order
to visualize the nerve roots as they exit from the neuroforamina (B).*

foramina without psoas muscle retraction (which is difficult) or resection.

Pelvic Brim Extraperitoneal Approach

The approach to the intrapelvic portion of the lumbosacral plexus is challenging. As for most of the techniques already described, the exposure is defined in the spine literature for approaches to the spine and is adapted for exposure of the lumbosacral plexus (Figure 8).[10,13] The patient is positioned in an extended position with the log roll placed under the lower lumbar region on the side of surgery. This extends the lumbopelvic region and thrusts the anterior pelvic brim on the affected side forward. It therefore increases the visualization gained by the exposure and places the lumbosacral plexus in closer proximity to the surgeon. An incision beginning lateral to and slightly above the anterior superior iliac spine can be carried medially and inferiorly, and parallel and cephalad to the iliac crest and inguinal ligament. This gains access to the muscular plane below this level. An incision along the external oblique muscle fibers and across the internal oblique and transversus abdominus muscle fibers, in turn, gains access to the extraperitoneal pelvic structures. Extraperitoneal structures are swept from the pelvic floor posterior to the peritoneum and renal fascia. The nerves of the lumbar plexus are observed emerging from between the psoas and iliacus muscles (lateral femoral cutaneous, ilioinguinal, iliohypogastric, and femoral nerves) and medial to the psoas muscle (genitofemoral and obturator nerves). The obturator nerve may be located distally by palpation at its point of exit from the pelvis through the obturator foramen and more proximally by medial retraction of the iliac vessels. The proximal sacral plexus (i.e. L4 and L5 nerve root contributions) may be visualized following lateral psoas muscle retraction and medial iliac vessel retraction. More superficially and laterally, the lateral femoral cutaneous nerve may be visualized. Exposure of this nerve in this region may be required for

the surgical treatment of meralgia paresthetica.[29]

The advantages of this approach include the relatively good exposure of the intrapelvic lumbar plexus from an anterior and lateral orientation. On the other hand, it offers a limited overall exposure, and the intrapelvic sciatic nerve and lower sacral plexus are difficult, if not impossible, to adequately visualize through this approach.

Pfannenstiel Infraperitoneal Approach

The Pfannenstiel approach gains access to the lower pelvic lumbosacral plexus as the femoral, obturator, and sciatic nerves exit from the pelvis. The approach is illustrated in Figure 9. It is a very demanding approach with limited exposure often realized.[3,11,13] An 8 cm horizontal paramedian excision is made in the suprapubic region. It starts at the midline and extends laterally. The lateral aspect of the rectus abdominus muscle is isolated through a ventral incision in the sheath of the rectus. The rectus abdominus muscle is retracted medially. The posterior aspect of its sheath is then incised. This incision is extended laterally, gaining access to infraperitoneal structures. The sweeping of the soft tissues of the lower pelvis is performed in a similar manner as previously described with blunt retractors used to assist in obtaining and maintaining the exposure. Care is taken to protect the ureter and bladder. Obviously the bladder needs to be decompressed with a Foley catheter prior to this surgical procedure in order to facilitate exposure. Similarly, complete muscular relaxation is mandatory. The sciatic nerve, as it exits the pelvis, can be isolated underneath the psoas muscle (psoas muscle resection may be required as discussed in the previous section). The femoral nerve, likewise, is visualized as it rests between the psoas and iliacus muscles. The obturator nerve can be visualized as it passes toward the obturator foramen medial to the psoas muscle and lateral to the iliac vessels, through this exposure.

Primary nerve repair of branches of the lum-

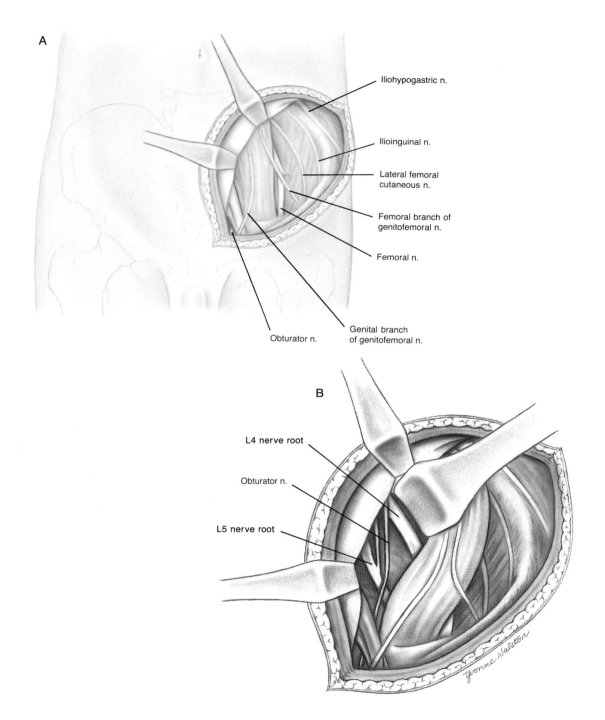

Figure 8. *Illustration of the pelvic brim extraperitoneal approach. A. A slightly exaggerated exposure is depicted. B. A close-up view of a deeper exposure following lateral retraction of the psoas muscle, which allows visualization of the L4 and L5 nerve roots as well as the obturator nerve, is illustrated. The peritoneum is retracted medially.*

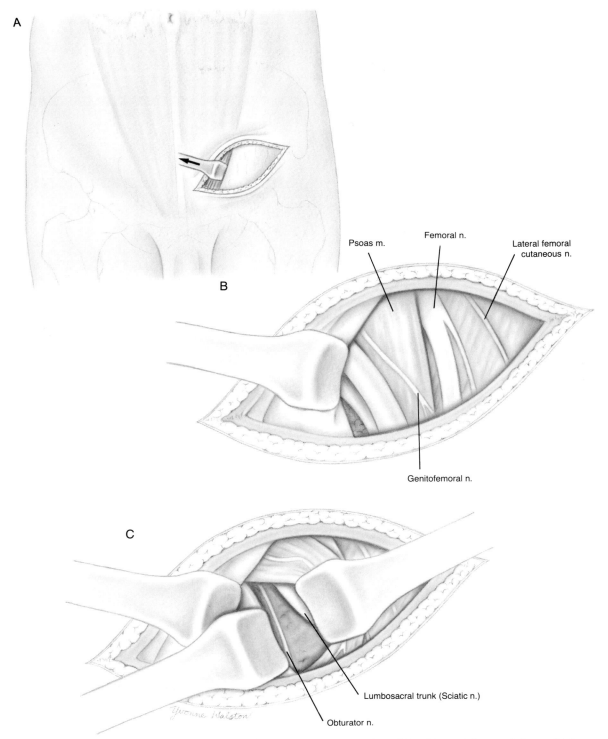

Figure 9. *Illustration of the Pfannenstiel infraperitoneal approach. A. The skin incision and the medial retraction of the rectus abdominus muscle are illustrated. B. Following deeper retraction, the retroperitoneal structures are visualized C. Medial retraction of the external iliac vessels and lateral retraction of the psoas muscle expose the obturator nerve and the proximal sciatic nerve.*

bar plexus is difficult and the sacral plexus impossible in this region because of the limited and deep exposure. Ablative procedures, such as obturator and femoral nerve neurectomies,[3] as well as the resection of nerve sheath tumors, however, are reasonably approached through this exposure.

This approach offers access to the deep pelvic paramedian structures. Its disadvantages are obviously the degree of difficulty associated with this exposure and the limited visualization gained. The farther one delves into the lower limits of this exposure, the greater the demands on the surgeon become.

Transperitoneal Approach

Much of the exposure achieved by the previous three techniques may be realized via the transperitoneal approach (Figure 10).[1,13] Following the performance of a standard midline laparotomy incision and entry into the peritoneal cavity, the small intestine is packed in the upper abdomen and retracted to the right. The sigmoid colon is retracted laterally and a longitudinal incision is made in the posterior peritoneum in the midline so as to expose the desired aspect of the retroperitoneal space. Occasionally the left nerve roots cannot be seen easily in this manner, and the colon may be retracted medially and mobilized from left to right after incision along the line of Toldt. Care should be taken to avoid injury to the ureters.

A horizontal low abdominal incision also may be used. This incision extends from just medial to one anterior superior iliac spine to just medial to the other. This incision should arc slightly inferiorly and then rise to its terminus on the opposite side (concave cephalad). The rectus abdominus muscles are transected transversely. This incision may give a slightly wider exposure to caudal structures. The sacral promontory is a consistent, easily identifiable landmark that should be used to identify the L5–S1 interspace.

An excellent exposure of the retroperitoneal space is achieved through the transperitoneal approach. Lower retroperitoneal structures are more accessible than the more proximal structures (especially those on the right due to the limitations created by the presence of the sigmoid colon), such as the proximal ilioinguinal, iliohypogastric, or genitofemoral nerves. The disadvantages include the requirement for a laparotomy and the potential for neural and vascular injury. The approach, however, is very useful when a wide exposure is needed such as for tumors of neural origin.[1]

Extrapelvic Infragluteal Approach

The extrapelvic proximal sciatic nerve can be approached easily utilizing the surgical exposure described by Henry[9] and illustrated in Figure 11. The patient is placed in the prone, semi-flexed position. A question mark or reversed question mark incision along the lateral aspect of the gluteus maximus muscle is made, is extended to midline underneath the inferior aspect of the muscle, and then is extended distally along the posterior midline of the thigh (as dictated by the length of exposure of the nerve required).[3,4,9,14] The skin and gluteus muscles (gluteal lid[9]) are then elevated as a unit (without separating the skin from the gluteus muscles). In order to elevate the flap, the gluteus muscle attachments to the femur must be incised. This incision is performed close to the femur itself, leaving enough length of the ligamentous attachments to the bone so that closure is facilitated. The extent of the reflection of the gluteus muscles from their femur attachments is again dictated by the proximal extent of the lesion being approached. The sciatic nerve lies deeply within the folds between the hamstring muscles. After the isolation of the nerve, the nerve is followed proximally. This is assisted greatly by the reflection of the gluteal lid medially. The nerve is followed proximally, with care taken to avoid injury to the inferior gluteal artery. This can result not only in ischemic complications but can be an extremely annoying intraoperative problem. This nerve is then followed as it passes under the piriformis muscle. The muscle may be incised to gain additional cephalad ex-

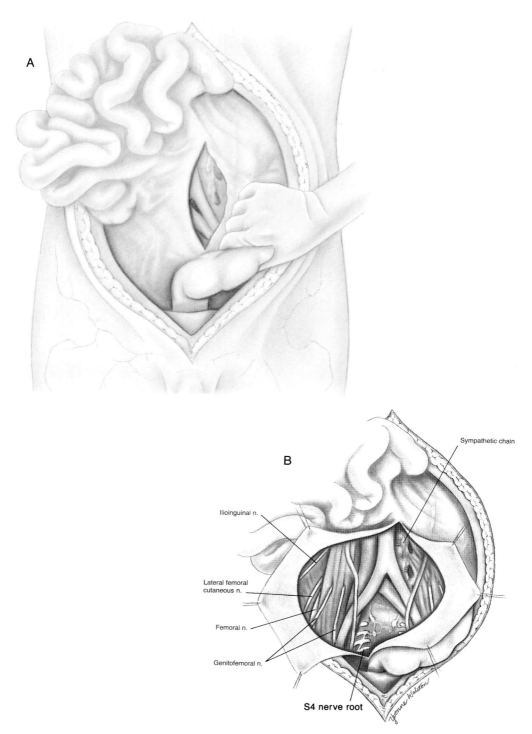

Figure 10. Illustration of the transperitoneal approach. A. The sigmoid colon is retracted laterally and caudally and the small intestines retracted rostrally. An incision in the posterior peritoneum has been made. B. Reflection of the posterior peritoneum gains access to the deep pelvic and retroperitoneal structures.

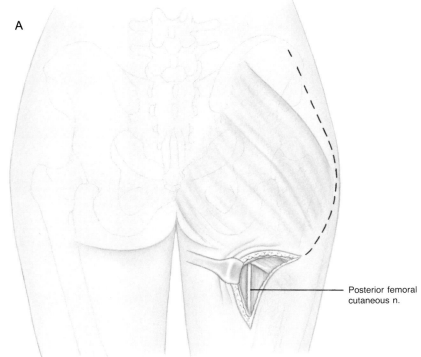

A

Posterior femoral
cutaneous n.

Figure 11A. Illustration of the extrapelvic infragluteal approach. A question mark incision is made, the length of which is determined by the extent of exposure required. The posterior femoral cutaneous nerve is encountered superficially. One should not confuse this with the sciatic nerve. Following elevation of the gluteal lid and separation of the hamstring muscles (the long head of the biceps femorus and the semitendinous muscles), the proximal sciatic nerve is exposed.

posture.[18] The surgeon must be aware that the nerve may pass through the piriformis muscle. Further dissection immediately dorsal and adjacent to the nerve can expose the nerve more proximally as it passes into the pelvis.

The cephalad portion of the sciatic nerve is extremely difficult to expose for nerve repair purposes. Surgical treatment of the piriformis syndrome,[5,18,20] sciatic nerve entrapment,[23] tumors,[4,22] and nerve repair[14] is facilitated by this approach. A combined approach for tumor resection at the superior extent of exposure of this procedure and the inferior extent of the exposure from the Pfannenstiel infraperitoneal or the anterior transabdominal laparotomy exposure will allow access to most lesions in this region (see next section).

The advantages of this approach are its wide exposure of the proximal extrapelvic sciatic nerve. Proximal to the piriformis muscle, however, the exposure is prohibitively difficult.

Combined Approaches

The combined approach using the Pfannenstiel infraperitoneal and the extrapelvic infragluteal approaches can be used to gain access to the "relative no-man's-land" existing in the lower pelvis. This requires, however, two different surgical procedures and two different patient positionings; therefore, simultaneous exposure cannot be entertained. Obviously, this is associated with significant problems if, for example, the pull-through of a nerve graft is desired. This should rarely, if ever, be required because primary nerve anastomoses or cable graft anastomoses for the proximal sciatic nerve are associated with a very low success rate. This, therefore, leaves only tumor resection, ablative procedures, and neurolysis procedures as indications for exposure of this relatively difficult-to-expose area of the nervous system.

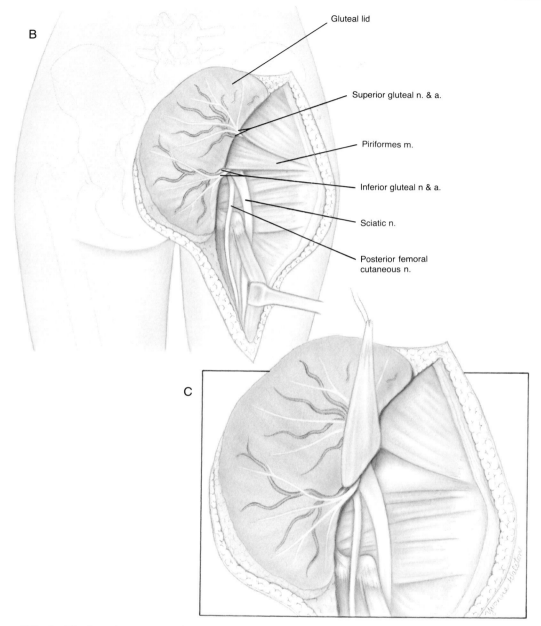

Figure 11B, C. *The long head of the biceps femorus muscle is held laterally by a retractor (B). Incision or reflection of the piriformis muscle allows exposure of the sciatic nerve to the level of the sciatic notch (C).*

The Pfannenstiel infraperitoneal and the pelvic brim extraperitoneal approaches can be used in combination and at the same time in order to gain access to deep pelvic lesions. The exposure in this region, although not as difficult as the exit zone of the sciatic nerve from the pelvis, is nevertheless challenging. Fortunately, exposure of the nerves in this region is limited almost solely to neurolysis procedures, tumor resections, and ablative procedures.

The combination of the anterolateral extraperitoneal and the pelvic brim extraperitoneal approaches would be appropriate for pathology traversing the boundaries of these two surgical approaches. The longitudinal exposure obtainable with the combination of these approaches is substantial. Such an extensive exposure, however, seldom would be necessary.

Similarly, the overlap between the proximal exposure of the anterolateral approach and the lateral extracavitary approach is extensive. A combination of these two approaches, therefore, seldom would be indicated. This is especially fortunate since two separate incisions with two separate surgical positionings would be required (as is the case with the extrapelvic infragluteal and Pfannenstiel infraperitoneal approaches).

For proximal lesions (especially those involving the spinal canal or intradural structures), a combined approach using the wide foraminotomy and the lateral extracavitary approaches is indicated. The combination of these two approaches is easily facilitated by the flap incision as described by Larson et al,[16] or perhaps, more appropriately, by a paramedian vertical incision. The paramedian vertical incision diminishes the chance of skin-flap vascular complications and healing problems while allowing ready access to both regions. Another advantage of the combined approach is that the facet joint usually can be left intact if an aggressive distal exposure via the lateral extracavitary approach and a proximal exposure via a wide foraminotomy are performed.

The transperitoneal approach alone offers a wide anterior midline expousre as well as many of the advantages of some of the combined approaches mentioned previously. If the risks associated with this technique offset the combined risks of the two or more individual approaches used in a combined approach, then the transperitoneal approach may be the best option.

Complications

The complications that may be encountered during or following the surgical approaches to the lumbosacral plexus are numerous. Perforation of the vena cava, aorta, iliac vessels, or lumbar arteries and veins may be catastrophic or, at the very least, a significant nuisance. Singultus secondary to intraoperative dia-

phragm manipulation may be disconcerting to both the patient and physician. Similarly, wound dehiscence or hernia may cause significant morbidity.

Retroperitoneal dissection may result in disruption of vital structures located in this space, such as vascular structures (as mentioned before) and urogenital structures. A knowledge of the whereabouts of important structures, such as the ureter, is of paramount importance during exposure of anatomic regions where these structures may be injured. In cases where the dissection is complicated by extenuating factors, such as prior radiation therapy, surgery, or extensive tumor bulk, the preoperative placement of a ureteral stint by an urologist may allow the intraoperative identification of the ureter. This may prevent a potentially catastrophic ureteral injury.

Finally, injury to radiculomedullary spinal arteries may result in paraplegia. Appropriate diagnostic avenues (such as angiography) must be used when such an injury may result from the surgical exposure. Alterations of surgical technique must be entertained if angiography demonstrates the presence of a radiculomedullary spinal artery in the region of planned dissection.[2,13]

References

1. Abernathey CD, Onofrio BM, Scheithauer B, et al. Surgical management of giant sacral schwannomas. *J Neurosurg.* 1986;65:286–295.
2. Benzel EC. The lateral extracavitary approach to the spine using the three-quarter prone position. *J Neurosurg.* 1989;71:837–841.
3. Benzel EC, Barolat-Romana G, Larson SJ. Femoral obturator and sciatic neurectomy with iliacus and psoas muscle section for spasticity following spinal cord injury. *Spine.* 1988;13:905–908.
4. Benzel EC, Morris DM, Fowler MR. Nerve sheath tumors of the sciatic nerve and sacral plexus. *J Surg Oncol.* 1988;39:8–16.
5. Brown JA, Braun MA, Namey TC. Pyriformis syndrome in a 10-year-old boy as a complication of operation with the patient in the sitting position. *Neurosurgery.* 1988;23:117–119.
6. Capener N. The evolution of lateral rhachotomy. *J Bone Joint Surg Br.* 1954;36B:173–179.
7. Fager CA. Surgery of ruptured lumbar intervertebral disk. In: Fager CA, ed. *Atlas of Spinal Surgery.* Philadelphia, Pa: Lea and Febiger; 1989:21–90.

8. Gebarski KS, Gebarski SS, Glazer GM, et al. The lumbosacral plexus: anatomic-radiologic-pathologic correlation using CT. *Radiographics.* 1986;6:401–425.

9. Henry AK. Exposures in the lower limb. In: Henry AK, ed. *Extensile Exposure.* 2nd ed. Edinburgh, Scotland, Churchill Livingstone; 1973;180–196.

10. Hodgson MB, Wong SK. A description of a technic and evaluation of results in anterior spinal fusion for deranged intervertebral disk and spondylolisthesis. *Clin Orthop.* 1968;56:133–162.

11. Ingram AV. Miscellaneous affections of the nervous system. In: Edmonson AS, Crenshaw AH, eds. *Campbell's Operative Orthopaedics.* 6th ed. St. Louis, Mo: Mosby-Yearbook; 1980;2:1567–1641.

12. Jane HA, Haworth CS, Broaddus WC, et al. A neurosurgical approach to far-lateral disc herniation. *J Neurosurg.* 1990;72:143–144.

13. Johnson RM, Southwick WO. Surgical approaches to the lumbosacral spine. In: Rothman RH, Simeone FA, eds. *The Spine.* 2nd ed. Philadelphia, Pa: WB Saunders Co; 1982;1:171–187.

14. Kline DG. Operative management of major nerve lesions of the lower extremity. *Surg Clin North Am.* 1972;52:1247–1265.

15. Lanzieri CF, Hilal SK. Computed tomography of the sacral plexus and sciatic nerve in the greater sciatic foramen. *AJR.* 1984;143:165–168.

16. Larson SJ, Holst RA, Hemmy DC, et al. Lateral extracavitary approach to traumatic lesions of the thoracic and lumbar spine. *J Neurosurg.* 1976;45:628–637.

17. Maroon JC, Kopitnik TA, Schulhof LA, et al. Diagnosis and microsurgical approach to far-lateral disc herniation in the lumbar spine. *J Neurosurg* 1990;72:378–382.

18. Mizuguchi T. Division of the pyriformis muscle for the treatment of sciatica: postlaminectomy syndrome and osetoarthritis of the spine. *Arch Surg.* 1976;111:719–722.

19. Pech P, Haughton V. A correlative CT and anatomic study of the sciatic nerve. *AJR.* 1985;144:1037–1041.

20. Pecina M. Contribution to the etiological explanation of the piriformis syndrome. *Acta Anat (Basel).* 1979;105:181–187.

21. Powers SK, Norman D, Edwards MSB. Computerized tomography of peripheral nerve lesions. *J Neurosurg.* 1983;59:131–136.

22. Robertson JH, Gropper GR, Dalrymple BS, et al. Sacral plexus nerve sheath tumor: case report. *Neurosurgery.* 1983;13:78–81.

23. Søgaard I. Sciatic nerve entrapment. *J Neurosurg.* 1983;58:275–276.

24. Southwick WO, Robinson RA. Surgical approaches to the vertebral bodies in the cervical and lumbar regions. *J Bone Joint Surg Am.* 1957;39A:631–644.

25. Vock P, Mattle H, Studer M, et al. Lumbosacral plexus lesions: correlation of clinical signs and computed tomography. *J Neurol Neurosurg Psychiatry.* 1988;51:72–79.

26. Wechsler RJ, Schilling JF. CT of the gluteal region. *AJR.* 1985;144:185–190.

27. Whelan MA, Gold RP. Computed tomography of the sacrum, I: normal anatomy. *AJR.* 1982;139:1183–1190.

28. Whelan MA, Hilal SK, Gold RP, et al. Computed tomography of the sacrum: II: pathology. *AJR.* 1982;139:1191–1195.

29. Williams PH, Trzil KP. Management of meralgia paresthetica. *J Neurosurg* 1991;74:76–80.

CHAPTER 12

Surgical Exposure of the Peripheral Nerves of the Lower Extremity

Thomas Ducker, MD

Surgical exposure of the peripheral nerves of the lower extremity is required less frequently than exposure of the nerves of the upper extremity. The surgical techniques employed are, therefore, often somewhat foreign to most surgeons. This chapter discusses the regional anatomy as it pertains to surgical techniques, calling upon selected specific references[1,2,4,5,7,8,9] and general references that may also be useful.[3,6]

Anterior Thigh

In the anterior aspect of the thigh, two nerves of clinical importance are the lateral femoral cutaneous and the femoral nerves. The anatomical relationships and the surgical exposure of both of these nerves is relatively straightforward.

Lateral Femoral Cutaneous Nerve

The lateral femoral cutaneous nerve is commonly entrapped as it exits the pelvis.[1,2,9] It typically courses through the pelvis along the lateral border of the psoas major muscle and then runs across the iliacus muscle obliquely toward the anterior superior iliac spine (see Chapter 12). At the anterior superior iliac spine it passes under the inguinal ligament and over the sartorius muscle. It then branches into a distinct mid-anterior and posterior branch.

As the nerve courses around the anterior superior iliac spine, in the vicinity of the strong inguinal ligament, it can be entrapped and compressed. This is usually associated with swelling and/or neuroma formation, which may lead to the clinical syndrome meralgia paresthetica, consisting of pain, dysesthesia, and often hypalgesia. These symptoms occur more often in the distribution of the midanterior branch than the posterior branch. Both, however, may be involved. More than 90% of symptomatic patients with this condition are best managed by conservative means.

Lateral femoral cutaneous neuropathy should be differentiated from far lateral disc herniation at the Ll–2 or L2–3 level. Disc herniation, however, is associated with muscle dysfunction. Electromyelography (EMG) is helpful in differentiation since meralgia paresthetica is purely a sensory phenomenon.

Operative exposure of the lateral femoral cutaneous nerve is usually accomplished under local anesthesia. A 6–8 cm skin incision along the skin lines beneath the lateral extent of the inguinal ligament and the anterior superior iliac spine is carried down to fascia lata (the lateral aspect of the exposure depicted in Figure 1). A self-retaining retractor is placed in the wound. The fascia lata is then incised in the same direction as the skin incision.

By dissecting bluntly beneath fascia lata, the nerve is identified. The most common site of nerve entrapment is at the level of the inguinal ligament. A rongeur is used to remove the medial edge of the iliac bone in order to create a tunnel for the nerve. The superior aspect of the inguinal ligament is preserved.

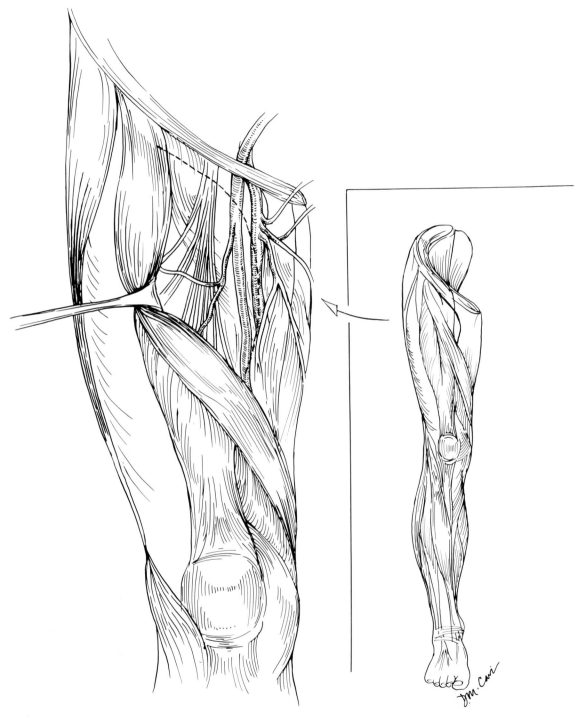

Figure 1. *The incision for exposing the lateral femoral cutaneous and femoral nerves begins approximately 2.0 cm below the anterior superior iliac spine. The proximal aspect of the incision is used to expose the lateral femoral cutaneous nerve. For the femoral nerve, the incision starts just below the anterior iliac spine and then curves down over the thigh to cross over the sartorius muscle. By gently retracting the muscles laterally, the femoral nerve with its branches is easily identified. The saphenous nerve is usually identified as the largest (and most medial) superficial branch.*

The nerve occasionally divides proximal to the inguinal ligament. Most commonly, however, it branches in the leg. These variations may be important at the time of surgery. Rarely, the nerve may pass between the two leaves of the inguinal ligament which may cause similar symptomatology and may respond as well to surgery.

Surgical treatment of meralgia paresthetica is controversial. Simple section of the nerve has been suggested as the best treatment. Good results have been reported from exposing the nerve, pulling it down, and transecting it above the neuroma.

Transecting the nerve is not required in all cases. If one simply provides a bony decompression in the path of the nerve as it courses around the anterior superior iliac spine, the continuity of the nerve can be preserved. The neuroma will often resolve and the patient's symptoms subside. The results are not instantaneous, however. Bone wax may be used to discourage local bone regrowth.

The Femoral Nerve

The femoral nerve[4] is the largest branch of the lumbar plexus. It provides considerable sensory innervation to the anterior aspect of the thigh and knee, and motor innervation to the quadriceps muscles. As it emerges from the pelvis in a groove between the psoas and the iliacus muscles, it closely approximates the external iliac artery. Together with the artery, the nerve passes beneath the inguinal ligament in the femoral triangle. The vein and lymphatics are located further medially.

High in the inguinal region, it gives a branch to the sartorius muscle. Clinically, it is sometimes difficult to ascertain sartorius muscle weakness. EMG studies may be helpful. If sartorius muscle dysfunction is demonstrated, a high femoral nerve injury is likely.

Within 2–3 cm below the inguinal ligament, the femoral nerve divides into many branches. Superficially, the cutaneous branches may be divided into anterior, intermediate, and medial components, the most medial of which is the saphenous nerve that supplies cutaneous sensory innervation to the medial aspect of the

lower leg. The saphenous nerve passes deep to the sartorius muscle and accompanies the femoral artery.

The major motor branches of the femoral nerve lie directly adjacent to or beneath the target muscles, starting with the sizeable branch to the rectus femoris and vastus medialis muscles. Approximately 10 cm further along its course, the nerve divides into multiple branches. Due to this anatomical relationship, it is practically impossible to distinguish the neural anatomy following deep devitalizing injuries to the terminal region of the femoral nerve.

The surgical approach to the proximal portion of the femoral nerve is achieved by using either a vertical incision or the preferred 'skin line' incision which is parallel to (and 2 cm below) the inguinal ligament (Figure 1). The latter is curved downward over the sartorius muscle. A small branch of the genitofemoral nerve may also be identified and dissected.

Once the skin and subcutaneous tissues are divided, fascia lata is identified, incised and retracted widely. The deeper fascia is then incised over the femoral triangle. This fascial layer is an extension of fascia lata. The incision over fascia lata should run parallel to the medial margin of the sartorius muscle. Upon retracting this fascia, the femoral nerve, artery, and vein are visible. The femoral artery then can be dissected, freed and retracted medially.

A vertical incision is made over the final fascial layer, the iliacus fascia. Extension and exposure of the femoral nerve between the iliacus and psoas muscles is performed proximally toward and underneath the inguinal ligament. The nerve then can be easily dissected distally to its multiple branches where the cutaneous branches tend to be more superficial and the muscle branches tend to be deeper.

The distal saphenous nerve may be used for nerve grafting. It is harvested by tracing it distally to the medial aspect of the knee. The sural nerve may be used if the available saphenous nerve is inadequate.

If the femoral nerve has been sharply transected, a single anastomosis can be achieved. Nerve length is gained by dissecting the nerve proximally underneath the inguinal ligament and distally to past its branching point. A primary anastomosis is then performed. Postoperatively, the patient should be placed in a hip spica orthosis with the leg flexed approximately 70°.

It is difficult to differentiate between motor and sensory branches in extensively injured nerves. The most superficial branches tend to be sensory, and the deeper branches tend to be motor. In the author's experience, the major branches to the vastus medialis and vastus lateralis can be successfully anastomosed with cable grafts, facilitating return of a near normal gait. Distal sensory loss from permanent changes in the saphenous nerve is not a handicap.

Posterior Buttocks and Posterior Thigh

Injury to the sciatic nerve is common and is often associated with a proximal neurologic deficit.[5] Associated vascular injury is uncommon due to the lack of anatomically close vascular relationships. The goal of therapy is to restore muscle function if possible, and to obtain protective sensation.

The sciatic nerve arises from the lumbosacral plexus, from the fifth lumbar, first sacral, and second sacral nerves. The more superior and lateral aspect of the lumbosacral plexus gives rise to the common peroneal nerve, while the more medial and inferior aspect of the plexus contributes to the tibial nerve. Often, these two segments can be identified through nearly the entire length of the thigh. The common peroneal portion of the sciatic nerve is positioned laterally.

The sciatic nerve exits the pelvis through the great sciatic foramen. Once it has left the confines of the pelvic structures, it is easily identified and dissected. Figure 2 illustrates the anatomy for the proximal exposure of the sciatic nerve.

To achieve exposure of the sciatic nerve at the level of the sciatic notch, the patient is placed in a prone position. A line from the posterior iliac spine toward the greater trochanter is imagined. The incision is made along the distal aspect of this line and curved underneath the crease of the gluteus maximus muscle. It is carried through the soft tissue to the muscle itself. The gluteus maximus muscle may be partly transected close to its insertion onto the femur, iliotibial band, and fascia lata. The gluteus maximus muscle is then retracted superiorly and hinged medially to expose the sciatic nerve as it exits beneath the piriformis muscle and leaves the pelvis (Figure 2). See Chapter 11 for additional discussion.

The sciatic nerve is identified by carrying the incision distally and following the nerve proximally. Many variations occur in the sciatic nerve's relationship to the piriformis muscle: the piriformis muscle occasionally passes between the two divisions of the nerve, but most commonly the nerve courses below this muscle. The inferior gluteal artery should be identified and protected because it contributes to the blood supply of the sciatic nerve.

In the posterior thigh, the sciatic nerve is easily exposed with a vertical incision. In the mid-thigh, the biceps femoris muscle passes over the nerve. The integrity of this muscle should be preserved. In the distal aspect of the thigh, the biceps femoris muscle is retracted laterally (Figure 3). More proximally, the biceps muscle is retracted medially (Figure 2). The posterior femoral cutaneous nerve (see Chapter 11) is maintained by medial biceps femoris muscle retraction, thus leading to no additional sensory loss.

Once the sciatic nerve is dissected, the author usually attempts to divide its two major branches, the common peroneal and tibial nerves. This facilitates repair by allowing for two separate anastomoses. In many cases, only one part of the nerve requires repair, while the other simply requires a careful neurolysis. By using the techniques of intraoperative nerve action potential recording described in Chapter 3, intraoperative decision-making is facilitated.

The more distal aspect of the sciatic nerve in the thigh is easily exposed through a curvilinear incision over the popliteal fossa (Figure 2). The common peroneal and tibial branches are readily identified between the biceps femoris muscle laterally and the semitendinosus and

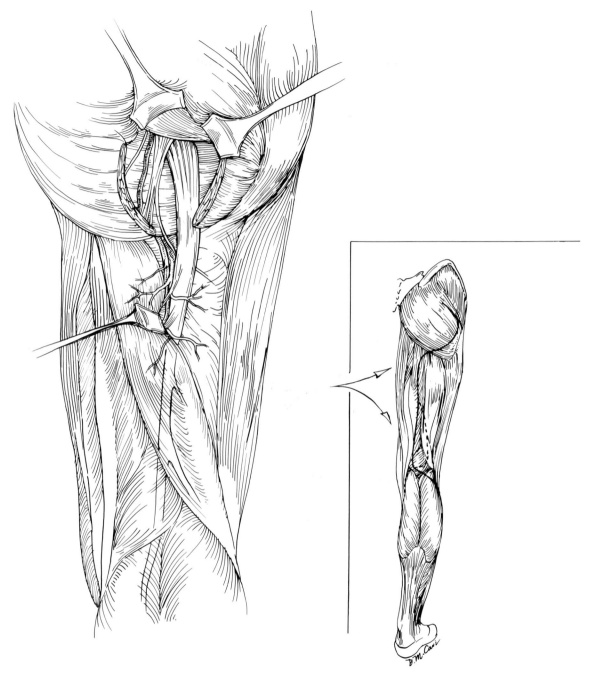

Figure 2. *To expose the proximal sciatic nerve, an imaginary line is drawn from the posterior superior iliac spine toward the greater trochanter, so that the incision can be curved caudally toward the greater trochanter and then curved back toward the middle of the thigh. An incision of at least half if not more of the insertion onto the iliotibial band of the gluteal muscle is required in order to reflect it superiorly to the level of the piriformis muscle. For proximal sciatic nerve exposure, the biceps femoris muscle is retracted medially. A distal sciatic (tibial) nerve exposure is gained by making a curvilinear incision over the popliteal fossa (dotted line in inset). A proximal peroneal nerve exposure is facilitated by using the distal aspect of the incision marked by the solid line in the inset.*

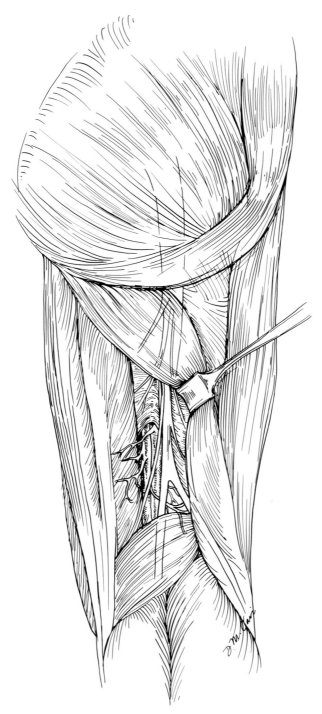

Figure 3. *The sciatic nerve in the midthigh is exposed through a medial midline incision. The biceps femoris muscle is retracted laterally. An important point to remember is that this muscle passes over the sciatic nerve more proximally. The sciatic nerve divides into its two major branches between the mid and lower third of the thigh. For exposure of the tibial and peroneal nerves in the popliteal fossa, a curvilinear and/or Z-plasty incision is used so that the joint is not crossed directly (see Figure 2).*

semimembranosus muscles medially (Figure 3). By dissecting under the biceps femoris muscle and working proximally, the nerve can be completely freed from surrounding tissue. The femur in this region is directly below the nerve and can be readily palpated.

Distal Posterior Leg

In the distal leg, the common peroneal[7] and tibial[8] nerves have already divided. The common peroneal nerve hugs the border of the biceps femoris muscle as it descends on the fascial attachments next to the fibula. The nerve then passes around to the lateral aspect of the proximal fibula. The common peroneal nerve is palpable just below the prominence of the fibular head. It passes below the extensor digitorum longus and the peroneus muscles. The superficial branch maintains a lateral course and innervates the cutaneous aspect of the dorsum of the foot.

The deep peroneal nerve is the more important branch. It innervates the extensors of the toes. The tibial nerve descends through the midportion of the popliteal fossa between the heads of the gastrocnemius muscle into the back of the leg (Figure 4).

Two important cutaneous branches are found at the point of bifurcation of the sciatic nerve into distinct entities of the common peroneal nerve and the tibial nerve. The lateral cutaneous sural nerve arises from the common peroneal nerve, and the medial cutaneous sural nerve arises from the tibial nerve. Often these two branches will rejoin as the common sural nerve. If these branches are observed to be intact during the exposure of this region, they should be preserved.

Lateral Calf

Exposure of the common peroneal nerve in the popliteal fossa is accomplished with a curvilinear incision.[2] In this manner, the incision does not directly cross the region of the popliteal fossa. The nerve's course, once the subcutaneous tissue is penetrated and flaps are raised,

is easily identified on the medial and inferior aspect of the biceps femoris muscle. It then passes lateral to the lateral head of the gastrocnemius muscle. Once beneath the fibular head, a small recurrent articular branch is observed. It then divides into its two major branches: **(1)** the deep peroneal nerve supplies the tibialis anterior muscle and the extensors of the toes; **(2)** the superficial peroneal nerve provides two small branches to the peroneus longus and brevis muscles and is responsible for sensation on the dorsum of the foot.

The most common location for peroneal nerve injury is just below the fibular head and below the large attachment for the biceps femoris muscle. Beneath the fibular head, there is a groove under which the common peroneal nerve passes. It is in this groove that the nerve is commonly injured. The injury may be as trivial as a minor blow, may be caused by squatting for a prolonged period of time, or may be a result of cast compression. The common peroneal nerve is very vulnerable to injury as it passes over (around) the fibular head.

The most frequent operation on the common peroneal nerve in this area is a release of the distal fascia over the nerve with an accompanying external neurolysis. A curvilinear incision is used for the exposure of the nerve, beginning in the popliteal fossa. It is curved downward on the lateral aspect of the thigh (Figure 5). A cutaneous flap is raised. An external neurolysis may then be performed distally to where it branches into its deep and superficial components.

The common peroneal nerve is essential for dorsiflexion of the foot. While foot drop can be treated with a cock-up splint and brace, aggressive attempts at the restoration of nerve function is desirable in younger patients.

A more distal exposure is needed for anastomotic repair of the common peroneal nerve. The knee joint can be flexed to as much as 70°–80° in order to obtain a relaxed nerve. The leg is casted for 3 weeks in this position. The cast is then removed and a splint applied so that the leg is not overextended for the next 2–3 weeks. Physical therapy is used in order to obtain full mobility of the knee.

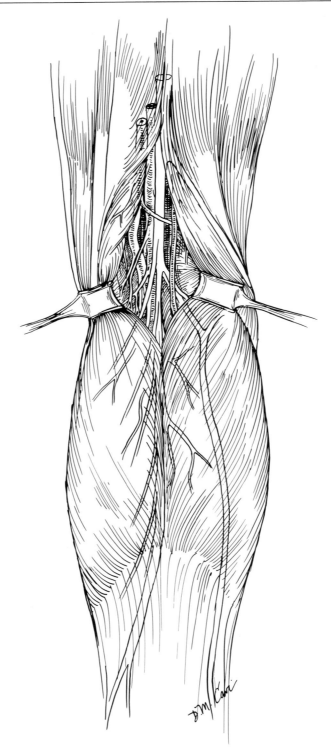

Figure 4. *The distal tibial nerve (distal to the popliteal fossa) is a direct extension of the sciatic nerve. In this region, it courses adjacent to the popliteal artery and deep to the arch of the soleus muscle.*

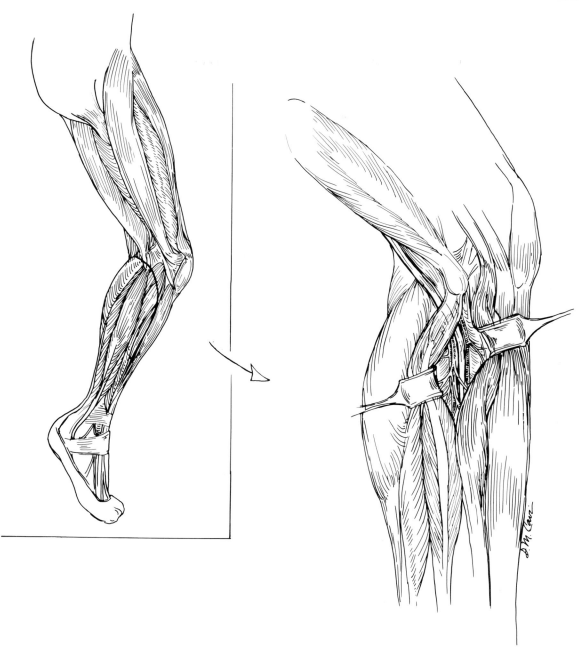

Figure 5. *The peroneal nerve is commonly injured as it courses around the rostral portion of the fibula, below the fibular head. Exposure of this region is illustrated. The nerve can be traced from the insertion of the biceps femoris muscle to the attachments of the gastrocnemius and soleus muscles. The common peroneal nerve bifurcates into its deep and superficial branches, just after it passes around the fibula. The deep peroneal branches pass obliquely forward, deep into the extensor digitorum longus muscle. It terminates anterior to the interosseous membrane where it lies adjacent to the anterior tibial artery. The superficial branch initially lies deep to the peroneus longus muscle. It then passes forward and downward between the peroneus longus and extensor digitorum longus muscles. It pierces the deep fascia in the distal third of the leg.*

On rare occasion, the deep peroneal nerve can be injured focally. This nerve is located on the lateral border of the fibula and adjacent to the extensor digitorum longus muscle. At this point the anterior compartment of the leg is vulnerable to pressure and compression. A syndrome of anterior tibial compartment compression is characterized by severe pain, swelling, and discoloration over the anterior aspect of the leg and over the foot with strenuous activity. Weakness of foot dorsiflexion may be present. The treatment of this condition it to enlarge the osseous fascial compartment where the nerve is entrapped along with the artery. Following decompression, the patient should be relieved of the symptoms of the so-called "shin splints".

The incision for this exposure is over the palpable tibialis anterior muscle. The dissection is carried distally between the tibialis anterior and the extensor hallucis longus muscles. Once the deep peroneal nerve is exposed, the anterior tibial artery and vein are visualized. By simply separating the strong fascial planes in this area, a neurolysis can be achieved.

Medial Calf

The tibial nerve lies directly in the midline of the popliteal fossa. It courses between the two heads of the gastrocnemius muscle to lie between the flexor digitorum longus and the flexor hallucis longus muscles (Figure 4). Just distal to the knee posteriorly, the tibial nerve divides into many branches. These include two branches to the gastrocnemius muscle and branches to the popliteus muscle and the plantar flexors of the foot. Further distally, the branches to the flexor digitorum longus and hallucis longus muscles become apparent. The deep aspect of the tibial nerve continues distally. Near the ankle, it may be entrapped in a similar manner to median nerve entrapment in the carpal tunnel syndrome.

The approach to the tibial nerve in the popliteal fossa is best made through a Z-plasty type of exposure. Further distally, an incision along the medial border of the gastrocnemius muscle can be used for exposure of the tibial nerve in

the dorsal midline. Once the incision is carried through the fascia, the medial border of the gastrocnemius muscle can be retracted to expose the popliteus and soleus muscles. It is necessary to dissect through some of the fibers of the soleus muscle to visualize the medial aspect of the transverse intermuscular septum. Once this fascial layer is opened vertically, the tibial nerve is easily exposed directly behind the tibia (Figure 6). Following its exposure, distal dissection of the tibial nerve is carried out with ease.

At the level of the ankle, the tibial nerve can be entrapped in the "tarsal tunnel." The nerve is simply exposed around the medial malleolus through the thick fascial planes which support the ankle. The strong flexor retinaculum on the medial aspect of the ankle needs to be opened in order to fully decompress the nerve in this area.

Rarely is it necessary to take down the muscular attachments of the gastrocnemius muscle in order to obtain exposure of the nerve in the popliteal fossa and in the more medial aspect of the leg itself. The tibial nerve, as it leaves the popliteal fossa, passes under a tendinous arch of the soleus muscle. This should be opened. The nerve then descends beneath the transverse intermuscular septum where it overlies the tibialis posterior muscle proceeding toward the medial malleolus.

The distal aspect of the tibial nerve can be entrapped under the retinaculum beneath the medial malleolus. This causes a distal entrapment syndrome described in Chapter 7.

Summary

There are many anatomical variations of peripheral nerves of the lower extremity. Only by studying a variety of textbooks, both old and new, can the patient's particular problems often be appreciated. This allows for the best possible patient care.

References

1. Aldrich EF, Van den Heever CM. Suprainguinal ligament approach for surgical treatment of meralgia paresthetica: technical note. *J Neurosurg*. 1989; 70:492–494.

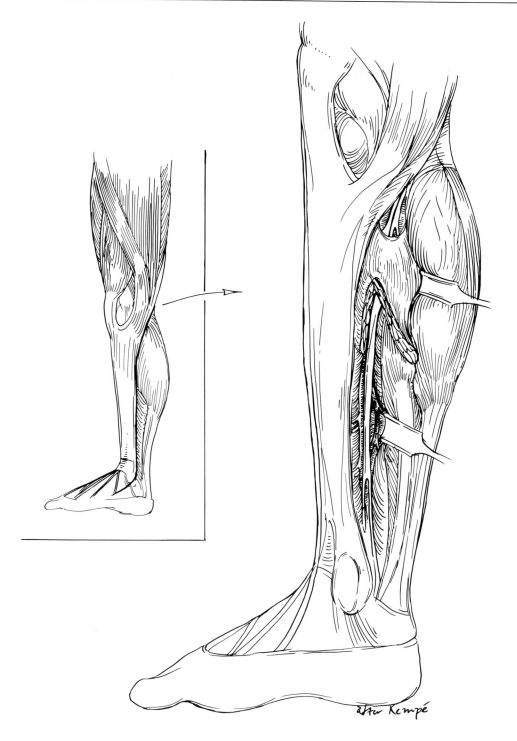

Figure 6. *Caudal to the popliteal fossa, the tibial nerve is most easily exposed from a medial orientation. Once the nerve courses deep to the soleus muscle, the nerve and artery are in close proximity to the posterior surface of the tibia itself. Consequently, the distal aspects of the gastrocnemius and soleus muscles can be retracted posteriorly, while the small flexor digitorum longus muscle are retracted anteriorly in order to expose the nerve.*

2. Keegan JJ, Holyoke EA. Meralgia paresthetica: an anatomical and surgical study. *J Neurosurg.* 1962;19:341–345.

3. Kempe LG. Surgery of peripheral nerves. In: Kempe LG, ed. *Operative Neurosurgery.* New York, NY: Springer-Verlag; 1970:2:203–232.

4. Seletz E. The femoral nerve. In: Seletz E, ed. *Surgery of Peripheral Nerves.* Springfield, Ill: Charles C. Thomas; 1951:114–118.

5. Seletz E. The sciatic nerve. In: Seletz E, ed. *Surgery of Peripheral Nerves.* Springfield, Ill: Charles C. Thomas; 1951:119–117.

6. Seletz E. The foot. In: Seletz E, ed. *Surgery of Peripheral Nerves.* Springfield, Ill: Charles C. Thomas; 1951:138-144.

7. Seletz E. The peroneal nerve. In: Seletz E, ed. *Surgery of Peripheral Nerves.* Springfield, Ill: Charles C. Thomas; 1951:145–154.

8. Seletz E. The tibial nerve. In: Seletz E, ed. *Surgery of Peripheral Nerves.* Springfield, Ill: Charles C. Thomas; 1951:155–170.

9. Williams PH, Trzil KP. Management of meralgia paresthetica. *J Neurosurg.* 1991;74:76–80.

PART V

SPECIAL CONSIDERATIONS

CHAPTER 13

Diagnosis and Treatment of Pain Associated with Nerve Injury

James N. Campbell, MD

Whereas loss of sensory and motor function are important manifestations of nerve injury, often one of the most troublesome complications is pain. In evaluating this problem, it is well to begin with considering how nerves cause pain.

Etiology of Pain

Pain normally arises from activity in specialized nerve fibers, termed *nociceptors*.[4] The question arises, does nerve injury pain represent an activation of nociceptors (an active process), or does nerve injury pain arise from loss of afferent input to the spinal cord (a release mechanism, i.e. a passive process)[6]? Prevailing evidence favors the first mechanism in most situations. Namely, the nerve injury somehow leads to activity in nociceptive fibers and thus induces the painful condition. This has important therapeutic implications: *The first and foremost goal of therapy is to eliminate the nociceptive input arising from the nerve injury.*

An important feature of nerve injury pain is hyperalgesia (hypersensitivity).[5,6] In hyperalgesic states, the normal relationship between stimulus intensity and neural response is enhanced. Stimuli that ordinarily are considered nonpainful cause pain. Nociceptors in the periphery can be sensitized (i.e. develop an enhanced response to natural stimuli). This sensitization provides a basis for certain aspects of hyperalgesia due to inflammation. When nociceptors activate certain central cells, a central form of sensitization occurs such that input from receptors other than nociceptors induces pain. Thus, patients with nerve injury may have what is termed "touch evoked pain" (lightly touching the skin hurts; sometimes termed *allodynia*). The region wherein this mechanical hyperalgesia occurs typically includes the area innervated by the nerve but may also extend far outside this area. In some cases, cooling, as well as mechanical stimuli, induces excessive pain. As will be described subsequently, this phenomenon of cooling hyperalgesia is a clue that the sympathetic nervous system may play a role in the pain.

Pain and the Electrophysiology of Nerve Injury

Nerve injury pain is a positive phenomenon—there must be activity in nociceptive fibers. This can occur in one of several ways.[8] One mechanism concerns the capacity, in some patients, of the sympathetic nervous system to induce activity in nociceptive fibers.[12,20] Nerve injury can also induce neural activity by causing ectopic generation of action potentials (*ectopic generators*). That is, fibers of passage at the injury site can generate neural activity spontaneously. Surprisingly, electrophysiologic data from nerve fibers that end in a neuroma suggest that ectopic generators are of equivocal importance in nerve injury pain. In many studies few fibers that end in a neuroma created by nerve ligation are spontaneously active.

Another related mechanism is that of *ectopic excitability*. This refers to the capacity of the fibers to be activated by stimuli applied to the nerve trunk. Thus, when there is ectopic excitability to mechanical stimuli, fibers may be activated in the region of injury either by endogenously or exogenously generated mechanical stimuli. Electrophysiologic evidence suggests that ectopic excitability is an important mechanism of pain in nerve injury.

A third mechanism refers to the compelling clinical evidence that nociceptive fibers innervate the nerve trunks themselves. Thus, at a compression or injury site, the nerve is quite often tender. Pain is therefore described as originating at the compression site (rather than the area innervated by the involved nerve). This is likely due to nociceptive fibers that constitute the *nervi nervorum*. The nervi nervorum fibers, which innervate the epineurium of the nerve, are activated by the entrapment or by other mechanical factors that induce traction on the nerve trunk.

Yet another mechanism for pain from nerve injury involves the phenomenon of *cross talk*. Cross talk refers to cross activation of nerve fibers within the nerve trunk. Evidence suggests that cross talk occurs at nerve injury sites. The importance of cross talk however, as a mechanism for pain is far from clear.

Nerve Injury Milieu

As noted previously, entrapment of a nerve may activate the nervi nervorum fibers and cause pain. When this happens, the nerve is locally tender. Thus local tenderness may be a harbinger of nerve entrapment. Entrapment is likely the most common manner in which a nerve injury causes pain. Recently, an animal model of nerve injury pain was introduced, whereby ligatures are placed loosely around the sciatic nerve in rats. The animals display behavioral signs of hyperalgesia similar to what is observed in humans. This model will provide investigators a potent means to investigate further the mechanisms for pain, both peripherally and centrally. In addition, there is great promise that this model will lead to more effective treatments for neuropathic pain.[2]

When a nerve is entrapped, axonal transport is blocked. This leads to the so-called Tinel's sign. Tinel's sign results when the nerve is ectopically sensitive (ectopic excitability). When the skin is tapped briskly over the entrapment site, the patient reports paresthesias in the area served by the sensory fibers in the nerve. Tinel's sign combined with local tenderness constitutes strong evidence for nerve entrapment, irrespective of other data.

Of course, in many instances nerve entrapment leads to neurologic impairment. Sensory loss can be assessed along with motor impairment. Sensory deficit, atrophy, and muscle weakness, therefore, can also serve as indicators of nerve entrapment.

Electrophysiologic studies supplement the diagnosis of nerve entrapment syndromes. Slowed conduction often can be demonstrated at the point of entrapment. In advanced cases the electromyographic study will reveal denervation in the relevant muscles. A negative electromyogram and nerve conduction study do not exclude the diagnosis of nerve entrapment.

Structural Nerve Injuries

Neuromas

When a nerve is severed and the proximal axons are still in continuity with the dorsal root ganglion, neuromas will form. A *neuroma* is a densely packed cluster of regenerative sprouts that arise when there is discontinuity of the nerve, usually secondary to trauma. In addition, fibrous tissues proliferate at the point of nerve injury. The fibrous tissue may contribute to the blockage of successful regeneration.

Some neuromas are painful and others are not.[6] Why is this? The key to understanding this inconsistency emerges from consideration of the electrophysiologic data noted previously. Ectopic excitability rather than ectopic spontaneous generation of action potentials emerges as the dominant finding in electrophysiologic recordings from traumatically injured nerves. The clinical corollary is that the milieu of a neuroma rather than the neuroma itself determines whether pain develops. Thus, in many, and perhaps the majority of cases, pain results due to the location of the nerve. Neuromas tend to be painful in locations where the severed nerves are subjected to excessive mechanical forces. This is particularly the case with nerve injuries in the hand and foot.

Many surgical techniques that are used to treat neuromas have been described. Simply excising the neuroma does not permanently eliminate the neuroma. As long as the nerve fiber has a viable cell body in the dorsal root ganglion and distal regeneration does not occur, a neuroma will form. The goal of surgical therapy, in these cases, is to relocate the neuroma to a different site. This site should be away from scar tissue, moving structures such as tendons, and joints. In addition, the neuroma bed should be protected from external stimuli. These objectives can be achieved in a number of ways. One is to put the severed nerve into deep muscle that has limited excursion. In certain instances it may be worthwhile to consider a nerve graft repair, if only to prevent the neuroma from reforming.

Painful Nerve Lesions in Continuity

In certain instances the nerve is injured but still in continuity. Perhaps some of the axons are severed, but the nerve is still functional. As with neuromas, pain may or may not be a problem. Where pain is present, the external milieu of the nerve may be responsible. In other cases the internal matrix of scar in the nerve may somehow promote activity in nociceptive fibers. The relative role of these two mechanisms may be difficult to discern on clinical grounds.

The first issue to consider is whether the nerve is entrapped. The nerve may be bound to adjacent tendons and scar, such that movement of the extremity results in the application of

shearing forces to the nerve. Muscle flaps may be rotated to protect the nerve. This technique has been applied most frequently with the median nerve at the wrist, where the abductor digiti muscle may be rotated over the nerve. The muscle may provide a useful cushion and may help keep the nerve from becoming stuck to the overlying skin. The long-term role of this procedure in relieving pain, however, is unsubstantiated.

In some cases nerve graft repair has been successful. In these cases the nerve is not entrapped and yet pain is severe. There have been several cases where the author has grafted the injured nerve to achieve pain control, even when the nerve had some function. Grafting may work by lengthening the nerve (thus eliminating tension), by removing the scarred focus, or by facilitating successful regeneration.

Neurotomy (proximal nerve resection) may be the treatment of choice in many circumstances. For example, during inguinal herniorrhaphy, the ilioinguinal or genitofemoral nerves or both may be injured. Whether the nerves are directly injured, entrapped, or severed is seldom clear. These patients have persistent pain in the inguinal area that often spreads to the labia or testicle with or without a sensory deficit. If the pain is temporarily abated with anesthetic blocks of the ilioinguinal and genitofemoral nerves, the ilioinguinal nerve is severed near the anterior superior iliac spine, and at the same session, the genitofemoral nerve may be severed in the retroperitoneal space as it courses longitudinally on the psoas muscle.

Another example is an injury to the palmar cutaneous nerve. This nerve may be injured in the course of carpal tunnel surgery. Patients with this injury present with pain over the palmar surface, perhaps with profound hyperalgesia, with or without an obvious sensory deficit. Often there will be tenderness at the wrist crease. The problem can be solved with resection of the palmar cutaneous nerve at its origin from the median nerve 6–7 cm proximal to the wrist crease.

The principle involved in each of these examples is the same: Find a different milieu for the nerve; one free of tension, scar, tethering, motion, and excessive external mechanical stimuli. Neurotomy is particularly applicable when the nerve involved does not serve an important function. With major nerves this must be done only after extended deliberation with the patient. When a neurotomy is performed, a proximal nerve block (regional anesthesia) may help prevent pain from recurring (see discussion of phantom pain).

Palliative Measures for Controlling Nerve Injury Pain

Antidepressants

In some cases of nerve injury, despite a diligent effort, the pain cannot be solved by direct surgery. In these cases pharmacologic management may be indicated. Several drugs are worthy of consideration. Tricyclic antidepressants are of proven, though modest, value in this regard. Amitriptyline is most frequently used, though sedation can be an unacceptable side effect. Nortriptyline is much less sedating and appears to offer comparable results.

Anticonvulsants

Initial experience with clonazepam suggests that this benzodiazepine agonist, used often as an anticonvulsant drug, also may be of value. Sedation again is a limiting side effect. Occasionally other anticonvulsants, such as carbamazepine, are effective. Some believe that clonazepam is particularly useful for shooting or stabbing pain.

Narcotics

Narcotics have a role in the treatment of nerve injury pain. The approach is similar to that used for treating cancer pain. The goal is to maximize quality of life. Clearly there will be a trade-off between side effects and pain relief. Striking a balance is sometimes a daunting task. Patients with a history of substance abuse prob-

ably should not be given trials of narcotic therapy. Short-acting narcotics (e.g. oxycodone) have a limited role. One should use drugs, such as morphine or methadone, which have a relatively long serum half-life. The intrathecal delivery of narcotics is currently undergoing evaluation in many centers. Too little experience exists to draw conclusions regarding long-term efficacy of this technique of drug delivery.

Electrical Stimulation

Electrical stimulation also plays a role in the treatment of chronic pain from nerve injury. In some cases the stimulation can be applied directly to the involved nerve (usually proximal to the lesion), and in other cases spinal cord stimulation is technically more appropriate. In either case, a trial of stimulation before implantation is appropriate. A presurgical trial of transcutaneous electrical stimulation is also appropriate. Failure of this modality, however, does not preclude the success of an implanted system.

DREZ Operation for Brachial Plexus Avulsion

Avulsion injury of the brachial plexus deserves special mention. Avulsion injuries involve a severe stretch of the brachial plexus, such that the roots are torn from the spinal cord. Three types of brachial plexus avulsion injuries have been defined: upper plexus avulsion, lower plexus avulsion, and avulsion of the entire plexus. Severe, disabling pain frequently results. The mechanism is not understood; however, one compellingly simple explanation is that an epileptic focus occurs in the injured dorsal horn. Since one of the primary functions of the dorsal horn relates to pain sensation, the outcome of this epileptic discharge is pain.

In these cases the elimination of the epileptic focus is an appropriate goal of therapy. This can be accomplished via the so-called DREZ (dorsal root entry zone) operation.[15] A series of microlesions are placed in the dorsal horn area from where the roots were avulsed. In the author's series, pain relief was observed in 85% of the cases with a mean follow-up period of 2 years.[7] The operation, however, is a serious undertaking. It entails risks of injury to the subjacent corticospinal tract.

DREZ Operation for Nonbrachial Plexus Avulsion

The success of the DREZ operation for brachial plexus avulsion has encouraged trials for other conditions. Some successes have been reported with postherpetic neuralgia, but the morbidity associated with treatment, particularly in older patients, is high. In addition, efficacy appears to be substantially less than that associated with similar surgery for postbrachial plexus avulsion pain. In paraplegics the DREZ operation seems helpful in cases where patients have particular problems with radicular pain referable to the level of spinal cord injury.

The role of the DREZ operation to treat pain from lesions of nerves distal to the dorsal root ganglion is unclear. The author has not observed the DREZ operation to be associated with clear success in this patient population. Furthermore, for reasons that are unclear, some patients seem (at least temporarily) to have worse pain after a DREZ operation.

Prevention and Treatment of Stump Pain and Phantom Pain

The origin of the pain in some cases of nerve injury is central. Anesthetic blockade of the injured nerves in these cases does not relieve the pain. The origin of this pain is based on neural events that are generated within the central nervous system (CNS) and that are independent, at least to some extent, of peripheral nervous system input. Such a scenario occurs in the context of phantom pain, with or without accompanying stump pain. Stump pain by itself sometimes can be helped by proximal neurotomy, though at a price, if the stump is rendered insensible. Proximal neurectomy is

not generally helpful in the case of phantom pain.

The presence of pain at the time of neurotomy (done as part of the limb amputation) increases the chance that phantom pain will occur. If the amputation is performed under regional anesthesia, the occurrence of phantom pain appears to be less prevalent. It is as if to suggest that noxious inputs into the CNS establish a sustained CNS pain engram that persists if a neurotomy is done in this circumstance. This suggests that it may well be prudent to block peripheral nervous system input to the CNS at the time of an operation that entails a peripheral nerve section, particularly if that nerve is the source of pain.

Regeneration Pain

Sometimes quite severe pain can arise from a nerve injury in the context of nerve regeneration. Presumably the nociceptive fibers in the process of regeneration in some patients become ectopically active. The problem is self-limited. As the regeneration is completed, the pain abates. It is extremely important to recognize the potential for this occurrence. Surgery is obviously most inappropriate and can threaten the regenerative process. The clinician must assess whether the pain is occurring in the context of a nerve lesion that is getting better or in the context of a nerve lesion where regeneration is not proceeding satisfactorily.

Pain and the Sympathetic Nervous System

In all cases where pain is associated with nerve injury (and other situations as well), one must consider whether the pain is sympathetically maintained (sympathetically maintained pain [SMP]). Patients with SMP have pain that is dependent on sympathetic efferent function. This disorder is sometimes referred to as *reflex sympathetic dystrophy* or *causalgia*.[3] These terms are avoided here because the linkage to the function of the sympathetic nervous system with these designations is not clear.

Mechanism of SMP

We are very close to understanding SMP at the molecular level. Several observations are noteworthy: (1) Walker and Nulson[19] noted that stimulation of the peripheral, but not central, cut end of the sympathetic chain reproduces pain in SMP patients after sympathectomy. (2) Local anesthetic blockade of the appropriate sympathetic ganglia (by definition) rapidly abolishes SMP (a series of blocks may do so permanently). (3) Depletion of peripheral norepinephrine by regional intravenous guanethidine[11] abolishes SMP (again, a series of such blocks may achieve sustained relief). (4) Intradermal injection of norepinephrine rekindles the pain and hyperalgesia previously relieved by a sympathetic block. Norepinephrine does not cause pain in normal individuals. (5) Anecdotal reports suggest that alpha-adrenergic antagonists,[18] including phenoxybenzamine,[10] and the alpha$_1$-adrenergic antagonist, prazosin,[1] may be effective in relieving pain in patients with SMP. (6) The skin in the area affected by pain may be abnormally cold in patients with SMP. Cold skin in a patient with pain, however, does not indicate in and of itself that the patient has SMP. Signs of increased sympathetic discharge do not provide a sufficient basis establishing the diagnosis of SMP.

Taken collectively, these observations suggest that SMP is an alpha-adrenergic receptor disease. Moreover, activation of these adrenergic receptors in patients with SMP evokes pain via activation of nociceptors. It may be that the adrenergic receptors are expressed directly on the nociceptors themselves. One conjecture is that nerve injury evokes a genetic signal in the dorsal root ganglion (as a consequence of neural activity), such that alpha receptors are sensitized and transferred to the peripheral terminals of the nociceptive fibers, i.e. the signal for the production of alpha$_1$-adrenergic receptors in nociceptive afferents is a nerve injury. It is hypothesized that injury produces neural activity in the nociceptive fibers, and this is a genetic signal in the dorsal root ganglion cell such that alpha$_1$ receptors are synthesized in abundance. After synthesis, the receptors are transported to the peripheral terminals of the nociceptive fibers and they thus make the nociceptors vulnerable to excitation via the local release of norepinephrine. The underlying disease heals. That is, the initial injury that incited the activity in the nociceptors goes away. The nociceptors remain active, however, as a consequence of the sympathetic activity in the region of the nociceptors. Further activity in the nociceptors serves as an ongoing genetic signal providing a further impetus for production of alpha$_1$-adrenergic receptors. Thus, a vicious cycle results.

This scenario helps explain the remarkable finding that one or a series of sympathetic blocks sometimes leads to a sustained relief of SMP.[13] By blocking the activation of the alpha$_1$ receptors via a sympathetic block or other sympatholytic therapy, the excitation of the nociceptors is eliminated, and the genetic signal conveyed via the neural activity in the nociceptive fibers in the dorsal root ganglion cells is eliminated.

A key component of this hypothesis is that alpha$_1$ receptors in the skin and in adjacent tissues become linked to the activation of nociceptors. Alpha receptors are of two types: the alpha$_1$ and alpha$_2$ receptors.[17] In a recent study it was determined that the topical application of the alpha$_2$-adrenergic agonist, clonidine, eliminates the hyperalgesia in the region of the application. The author has evaluated two patients in whom the topical application of clonidine eliminated nearly all of the pain experienced by the patient. It is reasoned that clonidine relieves pain in the vicinity of the application by locally blocking the release of norepinephrine via activation of alpha$_2$ receptors located on the terminals of the sympathetic efferent fibers. The administration of the alpha$_1$-selective agonist, phenylephrine, in the clonidine-treated area rekindled the pain previously extinguished by the topical clonidine. This evidence, therefore, supports the concept that SMP is an alpha$_1$-adrenergic disease. Topical treatment with clonidine in the hyperalgesia zone may be a useful treatment in some patients, in particular when the area of pain is very small.

Diagnosis of SMP

The ideal test in medicine is characterized by the following features: sensitivity, specificity, and safety. The traditional techniques for diagnosis of SMP are the local anesthetic sympathetic ganglion block (LAB) and the regional infusion of guanethidine (RIG). Both of these tests have problems with regard to sensitivity, specificity, and safety.

The LAB may fail to block properly the ganglion. When fluoroscopy is used as an adjunct to the performance of the LAB, the likelihood of missing the ganglion with the anesthetic is lessened; however, problems may still arise with respect to target localization. It is well to recall that in performing a stellate ganglion block, the desired target is the T2 ganglion, since the T2 ganglion supplies the sympathetic innervation to the hand.

Specificity is a problem with both the LAB and the RIG. No mechanism exists for interpreting the placebo response with either test. The existence of the placebo response is a most important point to consider when interpreting a test that concerns pain relief. Also, with the LAB procedure it is well to keep in mind that lidocaine and its analogues may attenuate, via a systemic effect, neuropathic pain. Similarly, lidocaine is usually given with the RIG in order to decrease pain from the initial norepinephrine release. This compromises interpretation of the test. Likewise, the tourniquet inflation applied during the RIG blocks conduction in sensory fibers and may, in and of itself, affect pain. An important and frequent problem with LAB is that the somatic roots that serve the painful area are very near the sympathetic chain. It may be difficult to determine whether the pain relief that is achieved from LAB is from the sympathetic block or from somatic blockade.

Although generally safe, both the RIG and LAB have been associated with several complications. These include injury to the recurrent laryngeal nerve, pneumothorax, inadvertent vascular injection, puncture of the kidney, and leakage of guanethidine into the systemic circulation. In addition, both tests are considered unpleasant and frequently are poorly tolerated by the patient.

Alternative Test for SMP: Systemic Infusion of Phentolamine

If SMP is an alpha$_1$-adrenergic receptor disease, then a logical test for the diagnosis of this disorder would be to administer a short-acting alpha-adrenergic blocking drug such as phentolamine. Patients with SMP should derive at least short-term benefit from an intravenous infusion of phentolamine.

To study this, the effects of systemic intravenous phentolamine with a local anesthetic ganglion block in patients suspected of having SMP were compared.[16] The pain relief obtained from the two tests was highly correlated.

Phentolamine infusion has a number of advantages over LAB: **(1)** It is essentially a painless test. It requires only an intravenous line through which the medications are given. **(2)** It is conducive to placebo controls. The patient has no knowledge as to when the phentolamine is administered. Thus, the effects of saline infusion can be tested prior to or following the administration of phentolamine. **(3)** It is likely to be more specific than other tests in that it targets specifically the alpha receptor. **(4)** To date no complications have occurred with the phentolamine test.

Tachycardia is a prominent effect of phentolamine administration. This can be avoided by simultaneously administering propranolol (which appears to have no effect on the pain relief evoked by phentolamine).[16] The protocol for administration of phentolamine is listed in Table 1.

Cold Hyperalgesia Test

Remarkably, all patients with SMP due to nerve injury appear to have exquisite pain following the application of mild cooling stimuli (cold hyperalgesia).[9] This can be demonstrated in a number of ways. First, patients will usually offer as their own observation that cooling

TABLE 1
Phentolamine Block Paradigm*

1. **Patient Preparation**
   Place patient in the supine position
   Monitor electrocardiogram and blood pressure
   Establish an intravenous line (screened off from the patient's view)
   Establish baseline pain level via sensory testing** every 5 min

2. **Saline Pretreatment**
   2 ml/kg/hr lactated Ringer's administration throughout the test
   Sensory testing every 5 min

3. **Reassessment of Pain Level**
   If pain level is improving, continue lactated Ringer's administration until satisfactory pain level is achieved. Do not administer phentolamine (the patient is a placebo responder!)

4. **Propranolol Pretreatment**
   1–2 mg administered intravenously over 5–10 min

5. **Reassessment of Pain Level**

6. **Phentolamine**
   Continue infusion of 36 mg (in 100-ml saline) over 20–30 min
   Continue sensory testing

7. **Postblock Assessment**
   Sensory testing every 5 min for 15–30 min
   Continue to monitor electrocardiogram and heart rate for more than 30 min
   Observe for any evidence of postural hypotension prior to discharge

*Exclusion criteria include patients suspected to be pregnant. In patients with a history of ischemic heart disease, cardiac arrhythmias, or peptic ulcer disease, use the test with caution.
**Suggested Sensory Tests.
1. Stimulus-independent (ongoing) Pain:
   10-cm visual analogue scale ranging from "no pain" to "most intense pain"
2. Stimulus-evoked Pain:
   Using a 0–10 verbal scale, a test of mechanical and cold-induced pain is undertaken
   Mechanical test (e.g. soft hair brush, blunt pressure, tuning fork)
   Cold test (e.g. small drop of acetone)

greatly exacerbates the pain. Second, patients can be shown to have cold hyperalgesia by simply comparing the effects of running cold and warm water from the tap onto the affected area. Third, one can examine the effects of placing volatile substances such as acetone on the skin. If the patient does not have cold hyperalgesia, a search for SMP will not be fruitful. It is to be noted, however, that many patients who have cold hyperalgesia do not have SMP; therefore, though the test for cold hyperalgesia is a sensitive test for SMP, it is by no means specific for SMP.

Management of SMP

Once the diagnosis of SMP is established, several treatment options are available. Since the culprit is the alpha$_1$ receptor, a major strategy of therapy is to block the activation of this receptor. This strategy has been termed *sympatholysis*.

In many situations SMP may be eliminated permanently by instituting a sustained period of sympathetic block. The length of that critical period varies from patient to patient. In other patients the duration of pain relief never outlives the interval of sympathetic blockade. Several interventional approaches that will achieve temporary sympatholysis are possible. An epidural catheter may be placed and the patient may have injection of local anesthetic through the epidural catheter for a period of hours or days. Alternately, a series of local anesthetic ganglion blocks can be performed over several days or weeks. A series of regional blocks with drugs such as guanethidine (that deplete the sympathetic terminals of norepinephrine) also may be done.

Sympathetic efferents course with the major

nerves; therefore, a sympathetic block can be achieved merely by performing a nerve block. If the patient's pain is located in the distribution of the median nerve, it might be most appropriate to simply perform a median nerve block just proximal to the painful area. It is well to remember the observations of Loh et al[14] that even if the nerve block is applied distal to the locus of nerve injury, pain relief can be obtained in patients with SMP.

Oral sympatholytic therapy may be useful in certain patients. The target, once again, is the alpha$_1$ receptor. Oral phenoxybenzamine treatment blocks both types of alpha receptors. Prazosin more specifically targets the alpha$_1$ receptor. Oral clonidine theoretically may be of some benefit. The problem with each of these drugs is that side effects may be troublesome and prohibit achieving a dosage that is adequate to block the target receptors. This is certainly not the case in all patients. Oral therapy is especially appropriate if one can use the treatment for a limited period of time, say a few weeks, and then discontinue the therapy with the acquisition of a sustained relief of the pain. Oral therapy, as a long-term treatment, is usually an untenable alternative due to side effects.

Surgical sympathectomy is an excellent treatment for SMP in situations where sympatholysis fails to achieve long-term benefit. It has been the author's experience that SMP can be eliminated with a properly performed sympathectomy. The "bad name" that surgical sympathectomy has acquired in some circles is undoubtedly due to inappropriate patient selection (a very common problem) or (in some cases) to an inadequately performed sympathectomy.

In many cases where the SMP affects the lower extremity, it is necessary to do a bilateral lumbar sympathectomy. A typical scenario is that of a patient who may have been successfully relieved of his or her pain for several weeks after an ipsilateral sympathectomy only to have a return of pain. In each case, performance of a contralateral lumbar sympathetic block has once again removed the pain. This has occasionally led to performance of a contralateral lumbar sympathectomy.

It has been the author's practice to excise approximately 8–9 cm of the sympathetic chain. This generally will include three ganglia. The lumbar sympathectomy is performed through a standard retroperitoneal approach via a flank incision (see Chapter 10; Figure 7). Patients frequently develop groin pain and pain in the proximal thigh after the operation. This usually lasts several weeks and then goes away. There has been much speculation about the cause of this proximal pain. The pain fits the distribution of the lateral femoral cutaneous, ilioinguinal, and genitofemoral nerves. It is suspected that this pain problem is a consequence of the stretching of these nerves during surgery.

The sympathectomy procedure for the hand can be performed by a variety of approaches. One such technique is to do a costotransversectomy via the posterior midline approach. The T2 ganglion is found underneath the second thoracic nerve root. Removal of the T2 ganglion generally suffices for treatment of SMP affecting the hand.

Some have advocated percutaneous techniques for the performance of a sympathectomy. Probes are placed in the region of the sympathetic ganglia. Thermal coagulation is then instituted to achieve the sympathectomy. This procedure offers the advantage of sparing the patient a major operation. In certain cases, however, this type of procedure will lead to only a temporary sympathectomy and it may be necessary to repeat the procedure.

Endoscopic T2 ganglionectomy is an alternative approach. Again, this may save the patient a major operation.

Limitations of Treatment

In some cases it is likely that the nerve injury–induced genetic signal (discussed before under Mechanism of SMP) is not susceptible to being turned off. In these cases the sympathetic block fails to induce a sustained period of pain relief that outlasts the duration of the pharmacologic action of the sympatholytic therapy. In addition, it is well to keep in mind that in some cases the injury does not go away. If, for example, the cause of the nociceptive discharge is an injury to the nerve (i.e. an entrapped nerve), sympatholytic therapy may eliminate some of the patient's pain, but will not eliminate that component of the pain that is due directly to the nerve injury (the nerve entrapment). Sympatholytic therapy only addresses that aspect of the pain that is linked to activation of the alpha₁-adrenergic receptors.

The author has encountered several patients in whom sympatholytic therapy seems to give rise only to partial pain relief. Phentolamine administration, for example, may lead to only 30% to 50% pain relief on a consistent basis. This is observed similarly with the local anesthetic sympathetic ganglion blockade. If a surgical sympathectomy is ultimately performed, it is likewise anticipated that the patient will derive only partial pain relief. If, however, the clinician is directed to the underlying disease, i.e. the nerve entrapment, perhaps both the SMP and the underlying mechanism for activation of nociceptors may be eliminated.

In many cases the diagnosis of SMP explains only part of the patient's pain. The clinician needs to keep in mind that there may be other sources of pain in patients with SMP. The phrase "sympathetically independent pain" may be used to refer to that aspect of the pain that is not maintained by sympathetic function.

Summary and Conclusions

One of the major challenges regarding chronic pain management is the establishment of the diagnosis. Nerve injury or nerve entrapment needs to be considered in the differential diagnosis when a patient has chronic and otherwise enigmatic pain. Treatment of nerve injury pain requires a detailed understanding of peripheral nervous system anatomy. The role the sympathetic nervous system plays in each case must be ascertained. Most patients can be helped if the clinician pays careful attention to detail. A multitude of therapeutic choices are available, ranging from simple disentrapment operations to spinal cord stimulation with implanted electrodes. In some cases, nerve re-

construction operations are worthy of consideration. In addition, many drugs have been documented to be useful for the treatment of nerve injury pain.

Current clinical evidence points to SMP as being a disorder linked to activation of alpha₁-adrenergic receptors. The alpha₁-adrenergic receptors, when activated, lead to stimulation of nociceptive fibers. Pain thus ensues. SMP can be diagnosed through systemic administration of phentolamine. This is a simple and well-tolerated test that lends itself to placebo controls. Once the diagnosis of SMP is established, a number of choices are available in terms of treatment. Often short-term sympatholytic therapy will lead to sustained pain relief. In these cases, that is all that is required. Short-term sympatholytic therapy can be achieved through epidural techniques, conventional nerve blocks, and oral sympatholytic therapy with drugs such as phenoxybenzamine and prazosin. Topical clonidine application to the painful area also appears to work in some patients. At times, surgical sympathectomy is necessary to remove the SMP on a permanent basis. In well-selected patients, the results of surgical sympathectomy are excellent. Many patients with SMP have pain that is independent of sympathetic function. It is also important to keep in mind that SMP may arise through an underlying disease such as a nerve entrapment which, if corrected, will also lead to the alleviation of the pain.

References

1. Abram SE, Lightfoot RW. Treatment of long-standing causalgia with prazosin. *Reg Anaesth.* 1981;6:79–81.
2. Bennett GJ, Xie Y-K. A peripheral mononeuropathy in rat that produces disorders of pain sensation like those seen in man. *Pain.* 1988;33:87–107.
3. Bonica JJ. Causalgia and other reflex sympathetic dystrophies. In: Bonica JJ, Liebeskind JC, Albe-Fessard DG, eds. *Advances in Pain Research and Therapy.* New York, NY: Raven Press; 1979;3:141–166.
4. Campbell JN, Raja SN, Cohen RH, et al. Peripheral neural mechanisms of nociception. In: Wall PD, Melzack R, eds. *Textbook of Pain.* 2nd ed. New York, NY: Churchill Livingstone; 1989:22–45.
5. Campbell JN, Raja SN, Meyer RA, et al. Myelinated afferents signal the hyperalgesia associated with nerve injury. *Pain.* 1988;32:89–94.
6. Campbell JN, Raja SN, Meyer RA. Painful sequelae of nerve injury. In: Dubner R, Gebhart GF, Bond MR,

eds. *Proceedings of the Vth World Congress on Pain.* New York, NY: Elsevier; 1988;3:135–143.

7. Campbell JN, Solomon CT, James CS. The Hopkins experience with lesions of the dorsal horn (Nashold's operation) for pain from avulsion of the brachial plexus. *Appl Neurophysiol.* 1988;51:170–174.

8. Devor M. The pathophysiology of damaged nerves. In: Wall PD, Melzack R, eds. *Textbook of Pain.* 2nd ed. New York, NY: Churchill Livingstone; 1989: 63–81.

9. Frost SA, Raja SN, Campbell JN, et al. Does hyperalgesia to cooling stimuli characterize patients with sympathetically maintained pain (reflex sympathetic dystrophy)? In: Dubner R, Gebhart GF, Bond MR, eds. *Proceedings of the Vth World Congress on Pain.* New York, NY: Elsevier; 1988;3:151–156.

10. Ghostine SY, Comair YG, Turner DM, et al. Phenoxybenzamine in the treatment of causalgia; report of 40 cases. *J Neurosurg.* 1984;60:1263–1268.

11. Hannington-Kiff JG. Intravenous regional sympathetic blocks with guanethidine. *Lancet.* 1974;1:1019–1020.

12. Jänig W. The sympathetic nervous system in pain: physiology and pathophysiology. In: Stanton-Hicks M, ed. *Pain and The Sympathetic Nervous System.* Boston, Mass: Kluwer Academic Publishers; 1990: 17–89.

13. Loh L, Nathan PW. Painful peripheral states and sympathetic blocks. *J Neurol Neurosurg Psychiatry.* 1978;41:664–671.

14. Loh L, Nathan PW, Schott GD, et al. Effects of regional guanethidine infusion in certain painful states. *J Neurol Neurosurg Psychiatry.* 1980;43:446–451.

15. Nashold BS Jr, Ostdahl RH. Dorsal root entry zone lesions for pain relief. *J Neurosurg.* 1979;51:59–69.

16. Raja SN, Treede R-D, Davis KD, et al. Systemic alpha-adrenergic blockade with phentolamine: a diagnostic test for sympathetically maintained pain. *Anesthesiology.* 1991;74:691–698.

17. Starke K. α-adrenoceptor subclassification. *Rev Physiol Biochem Pharmacol.* 1981;88:199–236.

18. Treede RD, Raja SN, Davis KD, et al. Evidence that peripheral alpha-adrenergic receptors mediate sympathetically maintained pain. In: Bond MR, Charlton JE, Woolf CJ, eds. *Proceedings of the VIth World Congress on Pain.* New York, NY: Elsevier; 1991;5:373–378.

19. Walker AE, Nulson F. Electrical stimulation of the upper thoracic portion of the sympathetic chain in man. *Arch Neurol Psychiatry.* 1948;59:559–560. Abstract.

20. Wallin G, Torebjork E, Hallin R. Preliminary observations on the pathophysiology of hyperalgesia in the causalgic pain syndrome. In: Zotterman Y, ed. *Sensory Functions of the Skin in Primates.* New York, NY: Pergamon Press; 1976:489–502.

CHAPTER 14

Peripheral Nerve Tumors

Charles L. Branch, Jr., MD

Peripheral nerve tumors are uncommon lesions. The involvement of multiple specialties in the treatment of disorders of the peripheral nerves may cause these rare lesions to be encountered infrequently by any given specialist. Peripheral nerve tumors generally are categorized into nerve sheath, primary neuronal, and non-neuronal neoplasms. Nerve sheath tumors are the most common. Peripheral nerve tumors may be malignant or benign, with the benign

TABLE 1
Classification of Peripheral Nerve Tumors

I. **Neoplasms of nerve sheath origin**
   A. Benign primary nerve sheath tumors
      1. Schwannoma
      2. Neurofibroma
   B. Malignant primary nerve sheath tumors
      1. Malignant schwannoma
      2. Nerve sheath fibrosarcoma

II. **Neoplasms of nerve cell origin**
   A. Neuroblastoma
   B. Ganglioneuroma
   C. Pheochromocytoma

III. **Tumors metastatic to peripheral nerves**

IV. **Neoplasms of non-neural origin**
   A. Lipofibromatosis of the median nerve
   B. Intraneural lipoma, hemangioma, ganglion

V. **Non-neoplasms**
   A. Traumatic neuroma
   B. Compressive "neuroma" (Morton's neuroma)

tumors more common. The spectrum of peripheral nerve tumors is presented in Table 1. This represents a modification by Mackinnon and Dellon[25] of Harkin and Reed's[17] 1968 classification of peripheral nerve tumors for the Armed Forces Institute of Pathology.

Benign Nerve Sheath Tumors

Nomenclature has been a source of confusion with regard to descriptions of nerve sheath tumors. Benign nerve sheath tumors include the *neurofibroma* and the schwannoma. The latter is occasionally referred to as a *neurilemmoma* or *neurinoma*. Electron microscopic analysis has made it evident that both of these tumors arise from a double basement membrane cell believed to be unique to the Schwann cell,[15] yet the perineural fibroblast, a nonmyelin-producing cell, has a basement membrane indistinguishable from that of the Schwann cell.[32] Lusk et al[24] have suggested that the neurofibroma is a more invasive form of the neoplasm arising from the perineural fibroblast, whereas the less invasive schwannoma arises from the Schwann cell. Pathologists tend to agree that there are distinguishing features and even subtypes of each. For example, the cellular schwannoma or plexiform schwannoma must be distinguished from its more malignant counterparts.[16] For the purpose of this discussion, the simple terminology for benign nerve sheath tumors of *schwannoma* and *neurofibroma* will be used.

Schwannoma

Schwannomas arise from the nerve sheath and generally involve one or two fascicles of the nerve. The remaining fascicles are displaced eccentrically by this well-encapsulated tumor. Schwannomas may arise from any nerve, including the peripheral portion of the cranial nerves, and are almost always solitary lesions. No known etiologic factor exists and no racial or sexual predilection is apparent.[2] The eighth cranial nerve is the most common cranial nerve involved. Schwannomas account for 10% of all primary intracranial tumors.[11] Bilateral eighth cranial nerve schwannomas may be a forme fruste of von Recklinghausen's disease or of neurofibromatosis type 2. Peripherally, schwannomas are most often found in nerves of the head and neck[7] or the flexor surfaces of the extremities. They rarely occur in the foot.[28]

Grossly, a schwannoma is oval and well circumscribed and appears to be encapsulated (Figure 1). The cut surface may reveal areas of cystic degeneration but generally has a yellow fleshy appearance. Microscopically, two distinct cell populations are usually present (Figure 2): densely packed palisading cells (Antoni A) and loosely meshed, areolar areas (Antoni B). Although both types are common, a single type may predominate. An area of densely palisading Antoni A cells is known as a *Verocay body*[11] Benign variants of the classic schwannoma include the cellular schwannoma, which may mimic a sarcoma microscopically, and the plexiform schwannoma, which should be differentiated from the plexiform neurofibroma, because the latter has a greater tendency toward malignant degeneration.[16]

Neurofibroma

Neurofibromas, although arising from the nerve sheath, involve the majority of the fascicles of the nerve either by encasement or invasion. An occasional solitary neurofibroma may be encountered, but these tumors are usually multiple and frequently occur in the patient with neurofibromatosis type 1 (von Recklinghausen's disease). Neurofibromatosis is a genetic disorder transmitted through an autosomal dominant mutant gene with full penetrance but variable expression. Features of the disease include six or more café au lait spots greater than 1.5 cm in size, in addition to few or numerous subcutaneous nodules or neurofibromas (Figure 3). Neurofibromas may be found in the central nervous system and autonomic nerves, as well as in the peripheral nerves. There is a marked tendency toward malignant degeneration in multiple tissues.[6,29]

Grossly, the neurofibroma appears as an enlargement of the nerve, either cylindric or plexiform (Figure 4). Cross-section shows a fleshy, granular tumor that microscopically (Figure 5) has fewer Schwann cells, more abundant collagen and reticulin fibers, and invariable axon cylinders. Occasional islands of what appear to be typical schwannoma cells may be identified in the background of disordered collagen and axons.

Clinical Considerations

Solitary, benign nerve sheath tumors generally are asymptomatic when small but cause pain or neurologic dysfunction as they enlarge and compress the adjacent neural elements. In the extremity, there is often the history of a well-circumscribed mass being present for months or years. The mass may be moved from side to side but is fixed in a longitudinal direction. Tinel's sign may be elicited with vigorous manipulation of the mass. Pain is seldom a presenting symptom of a benign tumor. A suspected tumor may be visualized preoperatively with ultrasound. Increased experience with and technical improvements in this technique make it a reliable modality for preoperative visualization.[18,21] In tumors of the brachial or lumbosacral plexus, the mass may become sizable before presenting clinically, but even the benign tumor in these sites may present with pain and sudden neurologic dysfunction after hemorrhage in the tumor.[1,8]

In the patient with an apparently solitary peripheral lesion and no evidence of neurofibro-

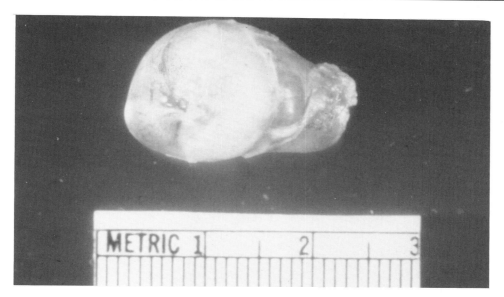

Figure 1. Totally resected schwannoma demonstrates the lobular, well-circumscribed appearance characteristic of the tumor.

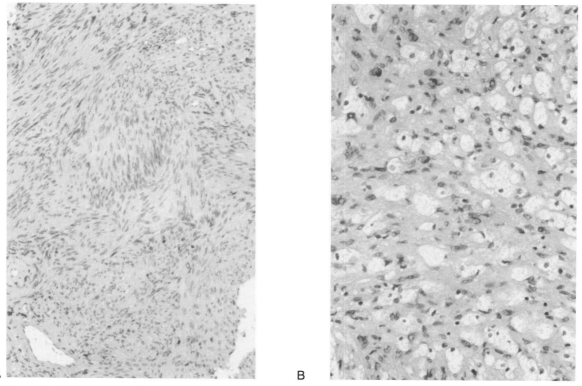

Figure 2. Schwannoma. Light microscopic pictures of a schwannoma with **(A)** densely packed Antoni A (H & E, ×83), and **(B)** loosely packed, or areolar, Antoni B cell patterns (H & E, ×200).

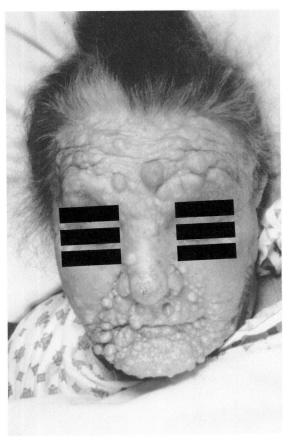

Figure 3. Neurofibromatosis type 1. Multiple sub-cutaneous nodules in addition to café au lait spots may be part of the clinical expression of neurofibromatosis type 1.

matosis, no further work-up may be necessary. Surgical excision, or biopsy if appropriate, of the symptomatic lesion is curative or becomes the basis for further diagnostic testing.

For tumors involving the brachial or lumbosacral plexus, a computed tomographic (CT) scan or magnetic resonance imaging (MRI) preoperatively provides valuable information regarding the extent of the tumor (Figure 6). It therefore aids in planning the appropriate surgical approach. The potential for extension into or from the spinal canal along a spinal root must be considered for the paramidline or proximally located tumor. Imaging of the spinal contents preoperatively is mandatory, and if

the so-called "dumbbell tumor" is present, the intraspinal component should be removed first. This prevents inadvertent traction upon and possible loss of function in the spinal cord during resection of the extraspinal component.

In the patient with known or clinically apparent neurofibromatosis, more extensive diagnostic testing may be warranted. The extent of the disease and the involvement of other systems may be determined with a CT scan of the chest and abdomen and an MRI of the central nervous system. Radioisotope bone scanning also may be of value if malignant degeneration is suspected.[8] Meticulous examination of the skin also may reveal nevi with the potential to degenerate into malignant melanoma.[2] From a practical perspective though, only the symptomatic lesion should be approached surgically for diagnostic, palliative, or cosmetic purposes.

Surgical Considerations

Schwannomas in general may be completely resected with little or no loss of neurologic function. Approaches to specific nerves or plexi are discussed elsewhere in this book. Principles to be adhered to include (1) adequate exposure of the involved nerve, both proximally and distally, (2) loupe or microscope magnification, (3) meticulous hemostasis, and (4) microsurgical dissection technique. If possible, anesthesia should be planned so that neuromuscular blockade is not present, and a nerve stimulator can be used to identify and preserve intact fascicles. Lusk et al[24] advocate the use of a stimulation/recording system that provides intraoperative identification of nerve action potentials in functional nerve fascicles (Figure 7). We have found that a disposable stimulator with variable voltage settings or a bipolar generator-based stimulator works well in the absence of neuromuscular blockade. Visualization of the extremity distal to the lesion is also mandatory to confirm responses to the stimulator. Sweeping over the surface of the tumor with the stimulator often identifies intact fascicles that may not be readily apparent visually, but whose preservation is important.

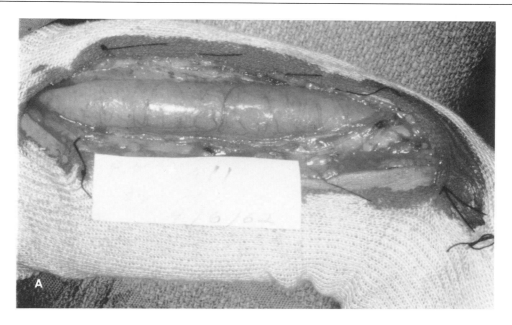

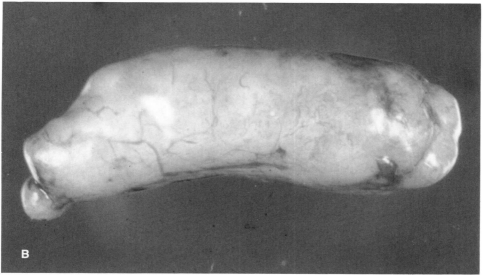

Figure 4. Plexiform neurofibroma (A) in situ and (B) after resection demonstrates the cylindric or fusiform appearance of the involved nerve.

The vascular pedicle of the tumor is usually at the proximal pole of the tumor. Dissecting and transecting this pedicle with involved fascicles allow subsequent gentle avulsion of the tumor away from the nerve. In large tumors of the brachial or lumbosacral plexus or in the pelvis, debulking the tumor with an ultrasonic aspira-tor (CUSA) may allow a more gentle avulsion of the tumor remnant from the surrounding neu-ral elements (Figure 8). Preoperative classifica-tion schemes have been developed to assist in the identification of tumors of large nerves or plexi that may not appear to be resectable.[1,4]

Solitary nonplexiform neurofibromas may

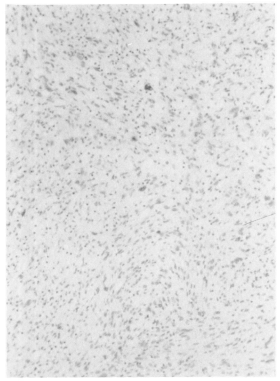

Figure 5. Neurofibroma. Light microscopic picture of a neurofibroma with more abundant collagen and few Schwann cells (H & E, ×83).

be approached surgically in a manner similar to the approach to a schwannoma. The need for more meticulous identification of functional fascicles should be anticipated.

Neurofibromas associated with neurofibromatosis or plexiform neurofibromas cannot be resected without sacrifice of the majority of the nerve fibers and the consequent loss of function. Resection of a neurofibroma on a major nerve trunk must be weighted against the deficit incurred by loss of the nerve. The major role of a surgical approach is initially to confirm the diagnosis with a biopsy. Malignant degeneration is known to occur in 10% to 13% of patients.[2,8,19] The role of biopsy in the newly symptomatic lesion is to determine whether malignant change has occurred and to plan further therapy. A benign tumor that has caused significant neurologic dysfunction in a major nerve may be considered for resection and nerve repair. This may require a cable graft, and appropriate preparation of the calf for sural nerve harvest should be made. The location of the tumor on a major nerve, the degree of dysfunction, the overall condition of the patient, and the availability of a tumor-free cable graft should all be considered seriously before this

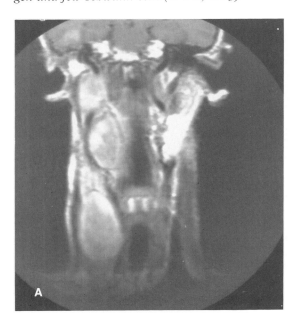

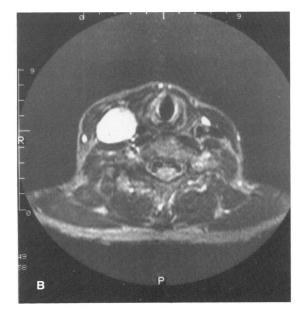

Figure 6. A. Coronal MRI of patient with neurofibromatosis shows two large neurofibromas on the right side in the cervical region. It is difficult to determine accurately the involved nerves with images in this plane. B. A gadolinium-enhanced axial view demonstrates an apparent vagal nerve tumor.

Schwannoma

Neurofibroma

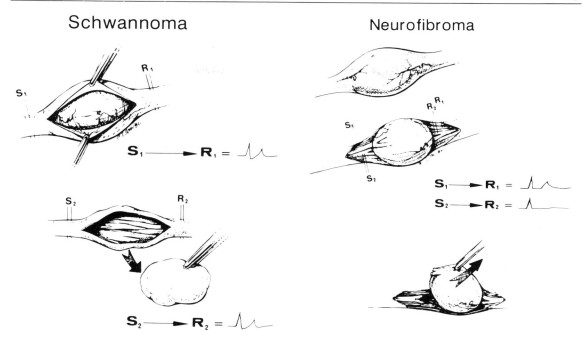

Figure 7. *Use of nerve action potentials to identify functional or nonfunctional fascicles may facilitate the safe removal of benign nerve sheath tumors. (From Lusk et al.*[24]*)*

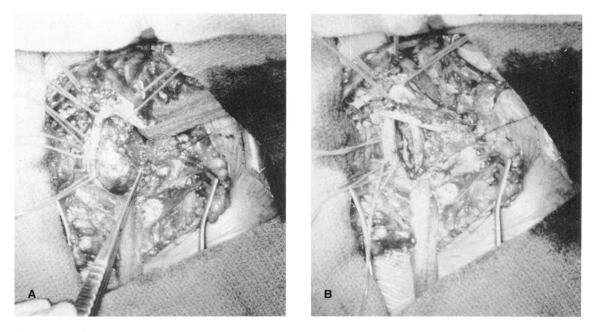

Figure 8. A 60-year-old woman presented with a painless supraclavicular mass. A biopsy under local anesthesia initiated significant pain and dysesthesia in the distribution of C5, C6, and C7 distally in the arm. The specimen was interpreted as a neurofibroma. A. A supraclavicular exposure with transection and retraction of the clavicle revealed a large, well-circumscribed tumor nestled in the plexus at the trunk and division level. B. The tumor was completely resected with preservation of neurologic function. Final pathologic diagnosis was benign schwannoma.

radical resection therapy is considered. According to Ariel,[2] other indications for surgical intervention in patients with extensive neurofibromatosis include rapid enlargement, cosmetic disfigurement, and hemorrhage into or infection of a large pachydermatocele.

Malignant Nerve Sheath Tumors

Nomenclature of malignant nerve sheath tumors also has been plagued by the use of a variety of terms that, in reality, all identify a similar or the same disease process. Malignant neurilemmoma, malignant schwannoma, malignant nerve sheath tumor, neurogenic sarcoma, and neurofibrosarcoma are all terms used to describe these malignant tumors. Some pathologists claim that at least two basic types exist: a malignant schwannoma, and a nerve sheath fibrosarcoma,[12] the cell of origin being the Schwann cell in the first and a perineural fibroblast in the second. For this discussion, *malignant nerve sheath tumor (MNST)* as an all-inclusive term will be used.

The MNST rarely, if ever, develops from the benign schwannoma, but rather from the plexiform neurofibroma. Although MNSTs may occur sporadically, their association with neurofibromatosis type 1 (von Recklinghausen's disease) is well recognized.

Grossly, the tumor may appear to be densely attached to or invading the involved nerve or plexus (Figure 9). Yet, because the malignant tumor is so similar in gross appearance to the plexiform neurofibroma, unequivocal microscopic pathologic diagnosis is mandated before proceeding with any radical surgical extirpation. Histologically (Figure 10), a reasonably reproducible and distinctive pattern exists, characterized by alternating cellular fascicular areas and more myxoid foci, striking perivascular whorling by tumor cells that often seem to extend into the vessel wall, very pale cytoplasm, and characteristically elongated and tapering nuclei.[16] The immunohistochemical demonstration of S-100 protein positivity is the best marker of neural differentiation in the context of a spindle-cell soft-tissue neoplasm,[16] although the presence of the Leu-7 antigen is helpful as well.[7] If there is apparent transforma-

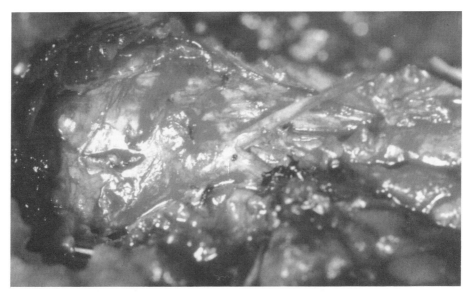

Figure 9. *Malignant schwannoma of the brachial plexus appears to demonstrate infiltration or encasement of the nerves, although it cannot be differentiated grossly from a benign plexiform neurofibroma.*

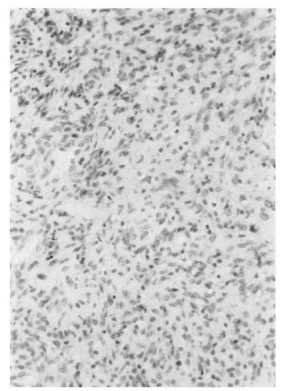

Figure 10. *Malignant schwannoma. The microscopic appearance of a malignant schwannoma shows increased cellularity and persistent whorling. S-100 positivity may help to confirm the diagnosis.*

tion into a rhabdomyosarcoma, the term *triton tumor* is used.[36]

Clinical Considerations

Initially, there may be little clinical evidence that distinguishes MNST from its benign counterpart. The mass may have been present for several months or years and only recently may have become painful or associated with a neurologic deficit. These tumors may occur more frequently in male patients (56%) if not associated with neurofibromatosis type 1. In the presence of that condition, however, an 80% male predominance has been reported.[7,13] MNSTs are also reported to occur in women at a younger age (mid-30s) as opposed to men (mid-40s). This difference, however, merely may be a manifestation of an earlier diagnosis in women

because of symptomatic changes during pregnancy.[8] The tumors tend to be located more proximally on major nerve trunks or intercostal nerves.

If an MNST is suspected preoperatively or if the diagnosis has been established by biopsy, a determination of the extent of the disease should be undertaken. CT scanning of the chest and abdomen should identify metastatic lesions. The lung is the most common site of metastasis.[11] As with neurofibromatosis type 1, central nervous system imaging also should be part of the initial staging of MNST.

Surgical Considerations

Although radical local resection or amputation is the hallmark of the treatment of MNST, the clinical and histologic ambiguities mandate a careful and positive pathologic diagnosis before a radical surgical procedure is undertaken. If the tumor is peripherally situated and there is no evidence of invasion of the surrounding tissue, a block dissection, including 5–10 cm of the nerve proximal to the lesion, may suffice.[2,8] The nerve is then anatomically reconstructed with a sural nerve cable graft.[25] Frozen-section analysis by an experienced pathologist at the time of the resection is necessary to ensure that the surrounding soft tissue and nerve are free of tumor invasion. If tumor-free margins cannot be obtained without compromise of a major muscle or limb vasculature, or if there are adjacent multiple "benign" plexiform neurofibromas in the patient with neurofibromatosis type 1, a proximal amputation should be performed.[2,8,25] If the tumor is proximally located on a major nerve without significant plexus involvement, disarticulation of the extremity (scapulohumeral or iliofemoral) appears to be appropriate. If the distal plexus is involved, interscapulothoracic (forequarter) amputation or hemipelvectomy (hindquarter amputation) probably offers the greatest potential for prolonged survival.[2,31]

Patients with proximal plexus involvement or invasion of the major vessels will not benefit from amputation. In this setting, the role of surgical exploration includes the confirmation of the diagnosis and debulking of the tumor for relief or control of symptoms. As with its benign counterpart, when a proximally placed malignant tumor is noted or suspected, preoperative evaluation of the intraspinal structures with CT myelography or MRI should be considered to evaluate the possibility of intraspinal extension along a spinal root. If such an extension is present, the intraspinal component of the tumor should be approached first and the involved root amputated to prevent traction on the spinal cord if further dissection of the extraspinal component is anticipated.

Adjuvant Therapy

Both benign and malignant nerve sheath tumors are notoriously radioresistant and chemoresistant. The role of radiation therapy is difficult to ascertain. Several have reported its use in managing incompletely resected proximal tumor for palliation of symptoms or local control of tumor growth.[2,8,12,24,31] An isolated report indicated the possibility of increased survival with postoperative radiation therapy, 52–78 Gy given in 2–Gy fractions, irrespective of how clean the surgical margins are.[3] A survival rate of 56% at 3 years is noted, but survival may not be different from other series at 5 or 10 years. The well-documented phenomenon of the induction of postradiation sarcoma must be considered when planning postoperative therapy.[12] It seems reasonable to administer a judicious dose of radiation therapy to the operative bed in the incompletely resected tumor or in the case of local recurrence. Chemotherapy has been administered according to soft tissue sarcoma protocols,[12] but, as with radiation therapy, it does not appear to affect survival.

Results of Therapy

Although the overall outlook with MNST is dismal in most cases, in certain cases, long-term, disease-free survival is possible. This potential for long-term survival appears to be related to the surgical resectability of the tumor and not to the success of adjuvant therapy. A 30% to 40% survival rate has been reported at 5 years[35] and at 10 years[2,12] in large groups with tumors in all extremities. Lusk et al[24] reported six out of seven patients with brachial plexus tumors alive from 3 months to 7 years after therapy. In a series of sciatic nerve tumors, Thomas et al[31] reported six out of twenty (30%) long-term survivors 3–28 years (mean 20.1 years) after treatment. Death is most often secondary to metastatic spread, which is most often to the lung.

Primary Neuronal Tumors

Primary neuronal tumors include neuroblastoma or malignant peripheral primitive neuroectodermal tumor, ganglioneuroma and its malignant counterparts, ganglioneuroblastoma, chemodectoma, and pheochromocytoma. These tumors tend to arise from the autonomic nerve ganglion cells along the spine or in the viscera. An extensive discussion of these tumors is not within the scope of this chapter. References providing more detailed information for neuroblastoma,[16,26] ganglioneuroma,[8] ganglioneuroblastoma,[11,14] chemodectoma,[8,22] and pheochromocytoma[8] are included here.

Tumors Metastatic to the Peripheral Nerve

Primary malignant tumors are known to metastasize to peripheral nerves, although rarely. Tumors of origin include melanoma,[8,9,24] prostate,[8] and malignant thymoma.[24] Major nerves or plexi are more likely to be affected from local invasion from breast or lung carcinoma that often already has undergone primary surgical and radiation therapy to the affected area.[24] Surgical decompression of the nerve or plexus with subtotal removal of the tumor may provide significant symptomatic relief and should be considered unless widespread disease makes the risk of further surgery prohibitive.

Tumors of Non-Neural Origin

A variety of benign neoplastic or hamartomatous conditions are known to affect peripheral nerves.

Lipoma and Lipofibromatosis

A lipoma may arise as a localized fatty mass within the nerve, simulating a schwannoma. This condition is known as an *intraneural lipoma,* and if symptomatic, its optimal treatment is surgical resection with preservation of neural elements.[10,30] A more diffuse or infiltrative form may be identified as an *intraneural lipofibroma, fibrofatty infiltration, lipomatous hamartoma,* or *lipofibromatous hamartoma.*[20,25] This form may become symptomatic slowly and usually presents early in life. If this condition involves the median nerve, decompression of the transverse carpal ligament may provide temporary symptomatic relief. Occasionally, more extensive neurolysis or even resection and grafting may be required for pain control and preservation of protective sensation to the hand.[25]

Ganglion Cysts

The ganglion cyst is one of the most common tumors of the hand. It most likely arises from extra-articular synovial remnants, and although most often found in the intertendinous spaces, it may arise totally within the nerve.[33] Symptomatic compression from an extraneural ganglion cyst occurs most often in the upper extremity, but intraneural ganglion cysts have been reported most often in the common peroneal nerve at the knee.[33] Preoperative diagnosis may be assisted with ultrasound. Treatment consists of excision of the extraneural cyst and obliteration of the connection with an adjacent synovial joint if necessary. Intraneural cysts require careful microsurgical evacuation of cyst contents and removal of the cyst wall if possible without destruction of the surrounding nerve.[33]

Vascular Lesions

The gamut of vascular malformations may present as peripheral nerve tumors. These include venous angiomas, arteriovenous malformations, and hemangiomas.[23] The hemangioma appears to be the most common of this group, although its appearance in the peripheral nerve is still rare.[5] Complete resection with preservation of the nerve using microsurgical technique has been associated with long-term recurrence-free intervals.[5]

Miscellaneous

Endometriosis has been reported with increasing frequency as a cause of sciatica.[27,34] Cyclic sciatic pain or dysfunction associated with menses is the hallmark of the clinical presentation and there is a well-documented CT and MRI appearance.[27] Although total hysterectomy with salpingo-oophorectomy is the traditional treatment, excision of the mass from the sciatic nerve with preservation of reproductive function has been reported.[34]

References

1. Abernathey CD, Onofrio BM, Scheithauer B, et al. Surgical management of giant sacral schwannomas. *J Neurosurg.* 1986;65:286-295.
2. Ariel IM. Tumors of the peripheral nerves. *Semin Surg Oncol.* 1988;4:7-12.
3. Basso-Ricci S. Therapy of malignant schwannomas: usefulness of an integrated radiologic surgical therapy. *J Neurosurg Sci.* 1989;33:253-257.
4. Benzel EC, Morris DM, Fowler MR. Nerve sheath tumors of the sciatic nerve and sacral plexus. *J Surg Oncol.* 1988;39:8-16.
5. Bilge T, Kaya A, Alatli M, et al. Hemangioma of the peroneal nerve: case report and review of the literature. *Neurosurgery.* 1989;25:649-652.
6. Bolande RP. Neurofibromatosis—the quintessential neurocristopathy: pathogenetic concepts and relationships. In: Riccardi VM, Mulvihill JJ, eds. *Advances in Neurology.* New York, NY: Raven Press; 1981; 29:67-75.
7. Bruner JM. Peripheral nerve sheath tumors of the head and neck. *Semin Diagn Pathol.* 1987;4:136-149.
8. Campbell R. Tumors of peripheral and sympathetic nerves. In: Youmans JR, ed. *Neurological Surgery,* 3rd ed. Philadelphia: WB Saunders Co; 1990:3667-3675.
9. Chason JL, Walker FB, Landers JW. Metastatic carcinoma in the central nervous system and dorsal root

ganglia: a prospective autopsy study. *Cancer.* 1963:16:781-787.

10. Chiao HC, Marks KE, Bauer TW, et al. Intraneural lipoma of the sciatic nerve. *Clin Orthop.* 1987; 221:267-271.

11. Cravioto H. Neoplasms of peripheral nerves. In: Wilkins RH, Rengachary SS, eds. *Neurosurgery.* New York, NY: McGraw Hill; 1985;2:1894-1899.

12. Ducatman BS, Scheithauer BW, Piepgras DG, et al. Malignant peripheral nerve sheath tumors: a clinicopathologic study of 120 cases. *Cancer.* 1986;57:2006-2021.

13. Enzinger FM, Weiss SW. Malignant tumors of peripheral nerves. In: *Soft Tissue Tumors.* 2nd ed. St. Louis, Mo: Mosby-Yearbook; 1988:781-815.

14. Feigin I, Cohen M. Maturation and anaplasia in neuronal tumors of the peripheral nervous system; with observations on the glial-like tissues in the ganglioneuroblastoma. *J Neuropathol Exp Neurol.* 1977;36:748-767.

15. Fisher ER, Vuzevski VD. Cytogenesis of schwannoma (neurilemoma), neurofibroma, dermatofibroma, and dermatofibrosarcoma as revealed by electron microscopy. *Am J Clin Pathol.* 1968;49:141-154.

16. Fletcher CDM. Peripheral nerve sheath tumors: a clincopathologic update. *Pathol Annu.* 1990;25 (part 1):53-74.

17. Harkin JC, Reed RJ. *Tumors of the Peripheral Nervous System.* Washington, DC: Armed Forces Institute of Pathology: 1968.

18. Hoddick WK, Callen PW, Filly RA, et al. Ultrasound evaluation of benign sciatic nerve sheath tumors. *J Ultrasound Med.* 1984;3:505-507.

19. Hosoi K. Multiple neurofibromatosis (von Recklinghausen's disease) with special reference to malignant transformation. *Arch Surg.* 1931;22:258-281.

20. Houpt P, Storm van Leeuwen JB, van den Bergen HA. Intraneural lipofibroma of the median nerve. *J Hand Surg Am.* 1989;14A:706-709.

21. Hughes DG, Wilson DJ. Ultrasound appearances of peripheral nerve tumours. *Br J Radiol.* 1986;59:1041-1043.

22. Kempe LG, VanderArk GD, Smith DR. The neurosurgical treatment of glomus jugulare tumors. *J Neurosurg.* 1971;35:59-64.

23. Kline DG. Comment on: Bilge T, Kaya A, Alatli M, et al. Hemangioma of the peroneal nerve: case report and review of the literature. *Neurosurgery.* 1989;25:652.

24. Lusk MD, Kline DG, Garcia CA. Tumors of the brachial plexus. *Neurosurgery.* 1987;21:439-453.

25. Mackinnon SE, Dellon AL. Tumors of the peripheral nerve. In: *Surgery of the Peripheral Nerve.* New York, NY: Thieme; 1988:535-548.

26. Marina NM, Etcubanas E, Parham DM, et al. Peripheral primitive neuroectodermal tumor (peripheral neuroepithelioma) in children: a review of the St. Jude experience and controversies in diagnosis and management. *Cancer.* 1989;64:1952-1960.

27. Moeser P, Donofrio PD, Karstaedt N, et al. MRI findings of sciatic endometriosis. *Clin Imaging.* 1990;14:64-66.

28. Potter GK, Feldman JS. Neoplasms of the peripheral nervous system. *Clin Podiatr Med Surg.* 1990;7:141-149.

29. Riccardi VM. Von Recklinghausen neurofibromatosis. *N Engl J Med.* 1981;305:1617-1627.

30. Rusko RA, Larsen RD. Intraneural lipoma of the median nerve: case report and literature review. *J Hand Surg.* 1981;6:388-391.

31. Thomas JE, Piepgras DG, Scheithauer B, et al. Neurogenic tumors of the sciatic nerve: a clinicopathologic study of 35 cases. *Mayo Clin Proc.* 1983;58:640-647.

32. Thomas PK, Olsson Y. Microscopic anatomy and function of the connective tissue components of peripheral nerve. In: Dyck PJ, Thomas PK, Lambert EH, eds. *Peripheral Neuropathy.* Philadelphia, Pa: WB Saunders Co; 1975:162-189.

33. Tindall SC. Ganglion cysts of peripheral nerves. In: Youmans JR, ed. *Neurological Surgery.* 3rd ed. Philadelphia, WB Saunders Co; 1990:1900.

34. Torkelson SJ, Lee RA, Hildahl DB. Endometriosis of the sciatic nerve: a report of two cases and a review of the literature. *Obstet Gynecol.* 1988;71:473-477.

35. Vieta JO, Pack GT. Malignant neurilemomas of peripheral nerves. *Am J Surg.* 1951;82:416-431.

36. Woodruff JM, Chernik NL, Smith MC, et al. Peripheral nerve tumors with rhabdomyosarcomatous differentiation (malignant "triton" tumors). *Cancer.* 1973; 32:426-439.

CHAPTER 15

Restoration of Extremity Function

Allan Friedman, MD

Modern-day surgeons are quite adept at restoring the continuity of a disrupted peripheral nerve following a peripheral nerve injury. Although restoration of neural continuity may be enough to treat some patients with a peripheral nerve injury, many patients will require additional therapy. The surgeon must be prepared to treat the patient's dysfunction, not just the injured nerve. This chapter reviews the available methods of restoring function to an extremity following nerve injury. Direct repair has been discussed in Chapters 3 and 8 and will not be discussed here.

A variety of methods are available to enhance the patient's functional recovery. During the immediate postinjury period, physical therapy and splinting must be employed to avoid skin and muscle contractures and stiff joints. Contractures limit the maximum range of motion achieved by all other forms of therapy. Muscle transfers and orthotics may improve mobility in those patients who do not achieve a full functional recovery. The surgeon treating peripheral nerve injuries must be aware of the role that these techniques can play when planning a patient's therapy.

This chapter reviews the functional deficits incurred with upper extremity peripheral nerve injuries, as well as the potential for innovative methods of therapy designed to restore lost function. The reference list provided allows the reader to pursue a more in-depth review of topics of interest. A variety of treatment schemes are presented. The merits and disadvantages of each are discussed.

Physical Therapy

The need for maintaining joint mobility cannot be overlooked by the surgeon performing a peripheral nerve repair. A reinnervated muscle or tendon transfer cannot be expected to move a joint beyond what is allowed by the joint's intrinsic limitations of motion. Passive range of motion is preserved and joint contractions avoided with the help of a physical therapist. Most patients will not need daily supervised therapy once instructed regarding the appropriate therapy. The therapy often can be carried out at home. The therapist can then monitor the patient's progress at regular intervals. Even the most compliant patient, however, will need to be monitored for early contractures.

Orthotics

Orthotics can be used to help solve two fundamental problems encountered in patients with an upper extremity nerve injury. First, the orthotic can be used to prevent or correct soft-tissue and joint contractures. The preservation of a normal range of motion will allow the patient to take full advantage of later reinnervation.[16] Both static and dynamic splints are available for this purpose. The surgeon, working with the orthotist, must choose a splint that maximizes the patient's use of the injured extremity but that is not so cumbersome or unsightly as to discourage the patient's compliance. For instance, a splint with a dynamic

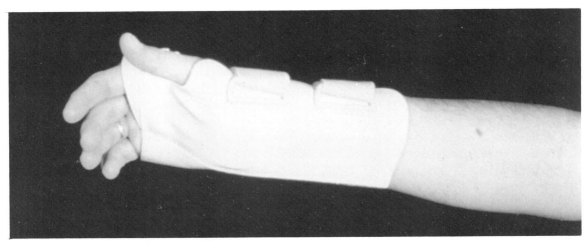

A

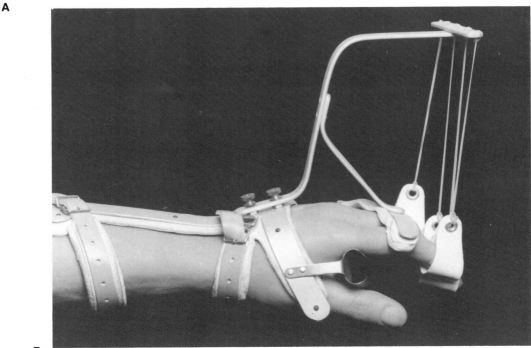

B

Figure 1. Orthotics for radial nerve palsy. *(A) Simple splint holds wrist in slight extension to strengthen grip. (B) Outriggers hold fingers in extension when not actively opposed by finger flexion.*

finger extension assembly is ideal for a secretary with a radial nerve palsy, but it most likely would be too cumbersome for a salesperson who is self-conscious about appearance (Figure 1). It is emphasized that fixed orthoses must be used with caution since they can contribute to contracture formation.

Second, an orthotic device can be used to bolster weakened movement. This can be accomplished sometimes simply by stabilizing a joint. For instance, stabilizing the wrist of a patient with radial nerve palsy in a neutral or slightly extended position will tighten the finger flexion tendons, adding strength to the patient's grip. The patient thus may benefit from the transfer of power from a forceful movement to a weakened movement.[29] In this case, the orthosis improves grasp by enhancing the normal tenodesis effect that causes the finger to flex when the wrist is extended. The patient with a severe, permanent hand paralysis may benefit from a mechanical device that is triggered by one of the patient's retained functions.[14] These devices accomplish movement with the aid of electric motors or springs. In addition, a number of prosthetic devices are available to replace a lost portion of an upper extremity.[2]

Neurotization

Despite reported success with regard to the treatment of brachial plexus lesions, the restoration of motor function following a brachial plexus avulsion remains a difficult problem.[17] Although nerve grafts placed against the spinal cord could theoretically coax anterior horn cells to sprout viable axons, this technique has not been used to treat patients with brachial plexus avulsions. Function can be restored in this group of patients by either muscle transpositions or neurotization. Neurotization is a procedure whereby intact axons are rerouted to denervated neural elements (Figure 2). Neurotization is an established technique. The spinal accessory and hypoglossal nerves long have been used for neurotization of the facial nerve.[12] In 1913 Tuttle reported his attempt at neurotization of the injured upper trunk of the brachial plexus using intact elements of the cervical plexus.[48] The duration of follow-up, however, was too short to evaluate the results of his

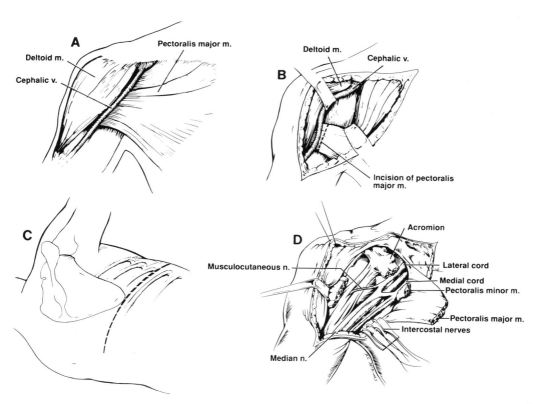

Figure 2. Technique of biceps brachialis neurotization by intercostal nerves. **(A)** Skin incision is made over the deltopectoral groove. **(B)** Deltopectoral groove is opened and the pectoralis major muscle is incised 0.5 cm from its insertion onto the humerus. **(C)** Thoracotomy incision is made over the tip of the abducted scapula. **(D)** Intercostal nerves are transposed to the anterior wound for anastomosis with the musculocutaneous nerve. (Reproduced with permission from Reference 18.)

procedure adequately. Although Tuttle's case generally is considered to be the first reported case of neurotization, Cushing cited a report of the utilization of the radial nerve to innervate the median nerve.[12,37] The first successful neurotization using intercostal nerves was reported by Yeoman[52], and the first successful neurotization using either the elements of the cervical plexus or intercostal nerve was reported by Kotani et al.[21] Intercostal nerves and elements of the cervical plexus remain the most commonly used nerves for neurotization in the upper extremity.[1,6,15,18,23,28]

The timing of the neurotization procedure is critical. Two years after the injury, muscle cells are fragmented and the muscle atrophied. At this time, restoration of innervation will not result in meaningful contraction. Since innervation of the biceps brachialis or supraspinatus will not be evident until at least 7 months following the procedure, neurotization should be performed as soon as the diagnosis of a complete avulsion is established. If the patient is evaluated at more than 1 year following the injury, or if the recipient nerve is found to be fibrotic at the time of inspection, direct neurotization has little chance for success.

Patients who have undergone a successful neurotization procedure can retrain the transposed nerves to serve a new function. Cushing noticed that as time passed, a patient with an accessory to facial nerve anastomosis could perform more and more intricate facial movements without concomitant shoulder movement.[12] Vera et al[49] further documented this plasticity by serial electromyograms performed on a 4-year-old boy who had undergone an accessory to facial nerve anastomosis. Animal experiments performed to investigate the effects of cross-neurotization indicate the ability to reeducate the transposed nerves to subserve their new job. The Duke[18] experience using intercostal nerves to reinnervate the biceps brachialis demonstrates the plasticity of the nervous system. Although initially the biceps brachialis only contracts with respiration, the patients soon learn to contract their biceps muscles independent of the respiratory cycle. Eventually biceps brachialis contraction is performed

without a conscious effort. Available donor nerves contain a relatively small number of axons as compared to potential recipient targets. Therefore, attempts at neurotization of the trunks and cords of the brachial plexus have not been successful, as the regenerating axons diffuse out along disparate paths.[1,28,43] It is best to direct available donor axons into a nerve just proximal to a single recipient muscle. Most procedures, therefore, are aimed at restoring elbow flexion or shoulder abduction.

Muscle and Tendon Transfers

Muscle transfers often are helpful in restoring function to a paretic upper extremity. A knowledge of this technique aids the surgeon in several ways. First, muscle transfers may enhance function in a patient with an irreparable nerve injury. Second, the literature on muscle transfers concentrates on the functional mechanical deficit caused by a nerve injury. It is important for the surgeon to know and document the functional evaluation of the injured nerve. A knowlege of muscle testing alone is inadequate. A knowledge of the patient's functional deficit is essential to the physician who must initiate physical therapy to avoid contractures and plan future operative procedures directed toward returning the patient to a productive life.

In this section, the general principles and the desired muscle transfers are outlined. The technical details and the merits of the variety of available procedures are not described. The interested physician therefore is directed to the literature detailing the technique of muscle transfers.[5,20,30,32]

The art of tendon and muscle transfer has evolved over the last 100 years. A review of the rules guiding successful tendon transfers will lead to an understanding of the limitations of these techniques. Each time a tendon is removed for a transfer, a joint is made less stable or a movement weakened. Therefore, each tendon transfer has a price. The surgeon must decide which transfers will be most advantageous for the needs of the individual patient. For instance, in some patients, a powerful grasp is important in carrying out work. In these patients, tendon transfers to strengthen finger flexion are important. Other patients will do perfectly well with a weakened grasp. In those patients, such transfers are superfluous.

In planning a tendon transfer, the surgeon must take into account mechanical, tissue, and rehabilitation considerations.[5] The mechanical considerations are straightforward. The muscle transferred must be of sufficient strength and have sufficient excursion to accomplish its new task. All forearm muscles do not have the same excursion. The laws of mechanical physics, especially those of vectors and levers, will determine the movement accomplished by the tendon transfer. For instance, if a tendon crosses two joints, its effect on the movement at each joint is determined by the direction of pull and length of the lever arm affecting that joint.

Tissue factors must be taken into account when planning a tendon transfer and also in planning any surgery that precedes the transfer. Muscles and tendons must have an adequate blood supply in their new position. The tendon must be routed through virgin tissue. A tendon routed through scar tissue is likely to develop adhesions that impede its excursion. This principle must be kept in mind when planning operative procedures that precede the tendon transfers. Prior to the transfer, the target joint must have a full passive range of motion. Maintaining range of motion is accomplished by preoperative physical therapy, splinting, and occasionally the surgical release of adhesions. Finally, the most perfectly planned tendon transfer procedure will not be of benefit unless the brain can be reoriented to use the muscle in its new position. The patient must have a sufficient mental capacity and interest to participate in a re-education program. This program should be coordinated by a physical therapist who has the time and experience to help the patient use the new transfer effectively. The re-education process is said to be easiest when the donor muscle's former role was synergistic with the desired motor effect of the planned transfer.

Most tendon transfers are carried out only when one is certain that there will be no further improvement in the patient's paralysis. Some authors advocate early transfers of a few tendons to help avoid contractures and to enhance function while awaiting reinnervation.[9,10] The possibility of early transfers should be considered in the patient who is severely incapacitated by a peripheral nerve injury.

Sensory Retraining

The importance of sensation in the upper extremity often goes unrecognized. In fact, loss of sensation within the hand can be quite debilitating. Even if the patient recovers good motor function, the ability of the hand to carry out fine tasks will be limited by poor sensory perception.[26]

In general, recovery of two-point discrimination in the hand is poor following the repair of an ulnar or median nerve injury.[34] The recovery of sensation following peripheral nerve repair can be improved greatly by using sensory re-education techniques. Dellon et al[13] first reported near normal sensation in four adults who had undergone a median nerve repair followed by sensory education. Several other authors have corroborated these results.[50] In sensory re-education, the patient stimulates the hypoesthetic area with progressively more intricate objects. At first, the patient looks at the object during stimulation to correlate the new sensory signal with the visual impression of the object. Then the patient blindly picks up and tries to identify the object. Using this technique, two-point discrimination is greatly improved. This improvement may persist for years.

When a nerve injury leaves a portion of the patient's palm or digit anesthetic, some sensation can be restored using neurocutaneous island pedicle flaps. With this technique, a flap of skin with a neurovascular pedicle is moved from a less vital area to a vital sensory surface. For instance, the ulnar volar surface of the ring finger can be transferred along with its neuro-

TABLE 1
Elbow Flexion

First Author	Number of points	Donor Element	Recipient Element	Results
Kotani[21] (1973)	9	Spinal accessory Intercostal nerves	Musculocutaneous Upper trunk Musculocutaneous	4 good, 1 fair 1 good 1 good, 1 fair 1 poor
Ploncard[35] (1982)	8	Intercostal	Musculocutaneous	3 good, 1 poor 4 insufficient follow up
Sedel[41] (1982)	9	Intercostal Accessory nerve	Musculocutaneous Lateral cord Lateral cord	5 fair, 2 poor 1 poor 1 fair
Dolenc[15] (1984)	55	Intercostal	Musculocutaneous	52 with functional return
Brunelli[6,7] (1984)	13	Cervical plexus	Musculocutaneous	7 good, 6 fair
Narakas[28] (1985)	13	Intercostal nerves	Musculocutaneous or lateral cord	9 good, 4 nil
Solonen[43] (1984)	9	Intercostal	Musculocutaneous or proximal elements	3 good, 6 poor
Simesen[42] (1985)	4	Intercostal nerves	Musculocutaneous	4 poor
Allieu[1] (1984)	3 15	Spinal acces. nerve Spinal acces. nerve	Upper trunk Musculocutaneous	1 fair, 2 poor, 3 good, 7 fair, 5 poor
Minami[24] (1987)	17	Intercostal nerves	Musculocutaneous	12 good, 5 fair
Yamada[51] (1991)	3	Cervical plexus	Upper trunk	2 good, 1 fair
Friedman[18] (1990)	20	Intercostal nerve	Musculocutaneous nerve Gracilis graft	7 good, 1 fair, 8 poor 2 good, 2 poor
Samardzic[39] (1990)	5 3	Spinal acces. nerve Acces. and medial pectoralis	Musculocutaneous nerve	1 good, 2 fair, 2 poor 2 good, 1 poor

vascular pedicle to the palmar surface of an insensitive thumb.[33] Some patients will gradually reorient sensation in the graft from the donor site to the thumb. Unfortunately, the transferred pedicle may develop a cold sensation and hyperesthesia.[26] Rarely, sensory nerve transpositions have been reported for restoration of sensation into the hand.

In the following section, specific nerve injuries will be discussed. The specific movements impaired and intrinsic mechanisms of compensation, or so called "trick movements" are reviewed. The more common methods used to restore lost function are outlined.

Axillary Nerve

An isolated axillary nerve injury denervates the deltoid muscle and thus greatly reduces the strength of shoulder abduction. Most patients still can raise the affected arm over the head using external rotation of the scapula as well as the supraspinatus, the long head of the biceps, and the clavicular fibers of the pectoralis major muscle.[44] Unfortunately, the movement lacks power.

Because the axillary nerve subserves motor function primarily, repair of the nerve with or without a nerve graft offers an excellent chance of restoring function.[19] This, therefore, is the preferred method of treatment.

Several ingenious muscle transfers using the trapezius, serratus anterior, levator scapulae, latissimus dorsi, and sternocleidomastoid muscles have been described to restore shoulder function.[38] These transfers seldom are necessary for patients who have suffered an isolated axillary nerve injury but should be kept in mind for treating patients who have suffered concomitant paralysis of other shoulder muscles. Patients who have paralysis of most of their shoulder musculature from a C5–6 avulsion are best treated with a fusion of the scapula to the humerus.[36] The transfer of one or two muscles will not benefit an unstable shoulder.

Neurotization of the axillary nerve only has been attempted rarely in order to restore shoulder abduction. Neurotization procedures of the supraspinatus nerve using the distal branch of the spinal accessory nerve or intercostal nerves have been described. No conclusions can be drawn from the small number of cases reported thus far (Table 1). Because of its small sensory component, neurotization of the axillary nerve should produce results at least as good as similar procedures for the musculocutaneous nerve.

Musculocutaneous Nerve

The musculocutaneous nerve rarely is injured in isolation. When such an injury occurs, some elbow flexion may be retained. The flexion in this case is carried out by the pronator teres and the brachioradialis muscles. More commonly, however, elbow flexion is lost as a part of a more extensive brachial plexus injury.

While awaiting return of elbow flexion, passive exercises should be initiated to maintain the full range of motion of the elbow. Several muscle transfers have been described to reconstitute elbow flexion.[11,45,53] The original transfers described by Steindler[45] called for a transposition of the origin of the finger flexor-pronator muscle group to a position more proximal on the humerus. Although this transfer produces only weak elbow flexion, still it is useful for treating patients who have suffered an upper brachial plexus avulsion. The latissimus dorsi, pectoralis muscle, and triceps all can be transposed to strengthen elbow flexion.

Because elbow flexion is the most vital function provided by the arm, the musculocutaneous nerve most frequently has been the target of neurotization procedures (Figure 3). In the Duke series, 16 patients had neurotization of the biceps brachialis by intercostal nerves and 4 additional patients had neurotization of a free gracilis muscle graft transposed into the position of the biceps.[18] Nine of twenty patients (45%) obtained useful antigravity strength and a full range of elbow flexion following surgery. Several other authors have reported their experiences using intercostal nerves or elements of the cervical plexus to reinnervate the biceps brachialis (Table 2).

Radial Nerve

Because the radial nerve primarily innervates muscle in the forearm and contains relatively few sensory fibers, a patient with a radial nerve injury has a good prognosis for recovery of some function following primary anastomosis or nerve grafting. A high radial nerve injury will result in weakness of the ulnar and radial wrist extensors, extension of all five digits of the metacarpophalangeal joint, abduction of the thumb, and extension of the thumb at the interphalangeal joint. Weak extension of the distal phalanx of the thumb is preserved in many patients by a slip of the abductor pollicus brevis that attaches to the extensor polliculi longus tendon. The inability to stabilize the wrist and the metacarpophalangeal joints greatly weakens the patient's grasp. This loss of wrist and finger stability is responsible for the greatest

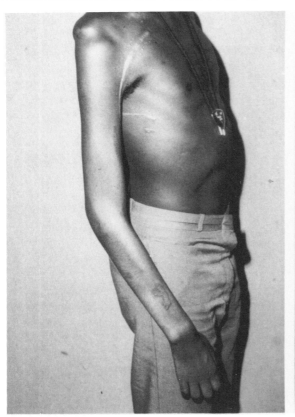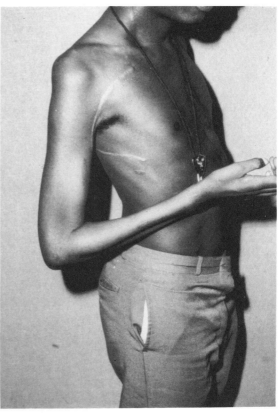

Figure 3. Intercostal to musculocutaneous nerve transposition. Twenty months following surgery this patient has good elbow flexion independent of respiration. (Reproduced with permission from Reference 18.)

TABLE 2
Shoulder Abduction

Author	Number of points	Donor Nerve	Recipient Nerve	Results
Kotani[21] (1973)	1	Spinal accessory	Upper trunk	1 good
Sedel[41] (1982)	1	Accessory	Posterior cord	1 poor
Brunelli[6,7] (1984)	13	Cervical plexus	Suprascapula	11 good, 2 fair
Narakas[28] (1985)	2 8	Spinal accessory Intercostal nerves	Suprascapula Axillary	1 good, 1 poor 4 good, 4 poor
Solonen[43] (1984)	9	Intercostal nerves	Axillary or suprascapular	1 fair, 6 poor
Yamada[51] (1991)	3	Cervical plexus	Upper trunk	3 good
Samardzic[39] (1990)	1	Spinal accessory and intercostals	Axillary	1 good

functional deficit. In some patients, sensory fibers to the dorsum of the hand travel along the antibrachial cutaneous nerve. In these patients, a radial nerve injury does not cause any loss of sensation. In any case, the sensory loss incurred by a radial nerve injury is of no functional significance unless it is accompanied by a painful neuroma.

Following radial nerve repair, the patient should be instructed in passive range of motion exercises to prevent joint adhesions and contractures of the web space between the thumb and index finger. Several types of orthoses have been described to improve the patient's function following a radial nerve palsy. A simple volar cock-up splint will hold the patient's wrist in extension, increasing the strength and accuracy of the patient's grip.[10] The patient must be instructed to continue range of motion exercises or the splint can lead to joint contractions. Dynamic finger and thumb assemblies will hold the digits in extension while the patient is at rest but will still allow the patient to flex the digits. The dynamic assemblies make the splint more complicated and cumbersome. Some authors have advocated an early tendon transfer to serve as an internal splint while awaiting the return of motor function. The most common procedure uses an end-to-side anastomosis of the pronator teres and to the extensor carpi radialis brevis. This transfer will stabilize the patient's wrist and will not interfere with the normal musculature once nerve regeneration occurs.

Muscle transfers are very successful at reducing the functional deficit that occurs following a radial nerve palsy.[4] Because all of the ulnar and median innervated extrinsic muscles of the hand are available for transfer, a large number of different transfers have been described. Wrist extension is most commonly restored by a transfer of the pronator teres to the radial wrist extensor tendons. Finger extension is achieved by a transfer of the flexor carpi radialis or a single tendon of the flexor digitorum sublimis to the extensor digitorum common. Thumb extension and abduction can be achieved by transferring the palmaris longus, flexor carpi radialis, or one tendon of the flexor digitorum sublimis to the extensor pollicus longus tendon.

Ulnar Nerve

The repair of a disrupted ulnar nerve proximal to the elbow is unlikely to result in a good return of lost motor function. Such repair still should be performed in an attempt to restore sensation to the ulnar side of the hand. A complete proximal ulnar nerve lesion will result in weakness of the flexor carpi ulnaris, flexor digitorum profundus to the small and ring finger, adduction pollicus, and several intrinsic muscles in the fingers.[22,32] Sensation will be lost over the ulnar one-and-a-half digits and adjacent hand.

Weakness of the flexor carpi ulnaris and ulnar portion of the flexor digitorum profundus muscles does not pose a significant problem to most patients. Wrist flexion is still carried out by the flexor carpi radialis and palmaris longus muscles, although there is some loss of strength and radial deviation of the wrist. Strong lateral pinch of the thumb is weakened by the loss of the adductor pollicis and the deep head of the flexor pollicis brevis muscles.[46] Some weakened thumb adduction can be carried out by the abductor pollicus brevis muscle if the thumb is held in front of the palm. If the thumb is held in the plane of the palm, weak adduction is achieved by combined actions of the extensor pollicus longus and the flexor pollicus longus muscles.[46]

The telltale flexion of the distal phalanx of the thumb with lateral pinch performed by the extensor pollicus longus results in Froment's sign. This weakened adduction diminishes the thumb's effectiveness as a stabilizer during a power grip. Interossei weakness causes loss of finger abduction and adduction. This manifests as an instability of the index finger during fine pinch. Some finger abduction is performed by the finger extensors when the fingers are allowed to flex forward away from the palm. Loss of the interossei muscles also weakens flexion of the metacarpophalangeal joint and results in a weakened "power grip" (Figure 4).[3,27]

This loss of coordinated metacarpophalangeal flexion decreases the patient's ability to wrap his or her fingers around an object. With the additional loss of the lumbricale muscles to the ring and small fingers, hyperextension of the metacarpophalangeal joints results. This hyperextension in turn decreases the patient's ability to straighten the interphalangeal joints, leading to clawing of the ulnar two fingers. Loss of the intrinsic muscles to the small finger results in flattening of the hand, which further weakens grip. A chronically abducted small finger will inhibit the patient's ability to quickly put the hand into a contained space such as a pocket or shirt sleeve. In summary, the motor deficits that occur with an ulnar nerve injury greatly weaken the patient's "power grip," i.e. the prehensile position in which the object is clamped by the flexed fingers and stabilized by the thumb.[3,27] Precision grip is much less impaired (Figure 4).

Exercise and splinting may be necessary to avoid flexion contractions of the ring and little fingers' interphalangeal joints. A splint with a metacarpophalangeal extension stop assembly will prevent metacarpophalangeal joint hyperextension and finger clawing. Some authors have advocated internal splints to coordinate the residual motor function of the hand while nerve regeneration is taking place. To this end, a single tendon from the flexor digitorum sublimis is used to stabilize the metacarpophalangeal joints of the ring and little fingers and to improve adduction of the thumb.

It is not possible to transfer enough tendons to restore each muscle lost following the loss of the ulnar nerve, so the surgeon must concentrate on restoring functions that are important to each individual patient.[30] Weakness of the flexor digitorum profundus and flexor carpi ulnaris is only of consequence if the patient's occupation requires a strong, accurate grasp across the entire palm. Grasp can be improved by attaching the flexor digitorum profundus tendons of the ring and small fingers to that of the middle finger or by attaching the extensor carpi radialis tendon to the two weakened tendons.

A number of transfers have been devised to improve flexion of metacarpophalangeal joints.

If the metacarpophalangeal joints can be kept from hyperextending, the extensor digitorum communis will adequately extend the interphalangeal joints. Most often, the extensor carpi radialis longus or flexor carpi radialis tendon is used to flex the ulnar metacarpophalangeal joints.

Thumb adduction is strengthened most often using the brachioradialis muscles, a single tendon from the flexor digitorum sublimis, or less commonly, the extensor digit proprius. A pulley is established with a fascial sling, or by passage of a tendon around the metacarpal of the long finger so that the thumb is pulled horizontally in the plane of the palm.

The strengthened thumb adductor will still pinch against the weakened index finger abductor. If the patient's occupation requires a strong lateral pinch, index finger abduction can be strengthened by a transfer from the extensor pollicis brevis and fusion of the metacarpophalangeal joint of the thumb. Cupping of the metacarpal arch and little finger adduction are accomplished by a transfer from the extensor digiti minimi or less commonly from the flexor digitorum superficialis.

These transfers are designed to increase the strength and accuracy of the patient's grip and pinch.

Some sensibility can be re-established by using a neurovascular cutaneous island graft.

Median Nerve

A high median nerve injury is a disabling condition. Denervation of the long flexors to the distal interphalangeal joint of the thumb, index, and long fingers, and the primary flexors of the proximal interphalangeal joint of all four fingers weakens the patient's power grip. Some paralysis is partially compensated for by intact muscles. The distal phalanx of the long finger usually flexes synchronously with the distal phalanx of the ring finger, as the two tendons of the flexor digitorum longus muscle share a common, ulnar innervated muscle belly. Although loss of the flexor digitorum sublimis decreases the strength of the grasp and independent finger flexion, the intact flexor di-

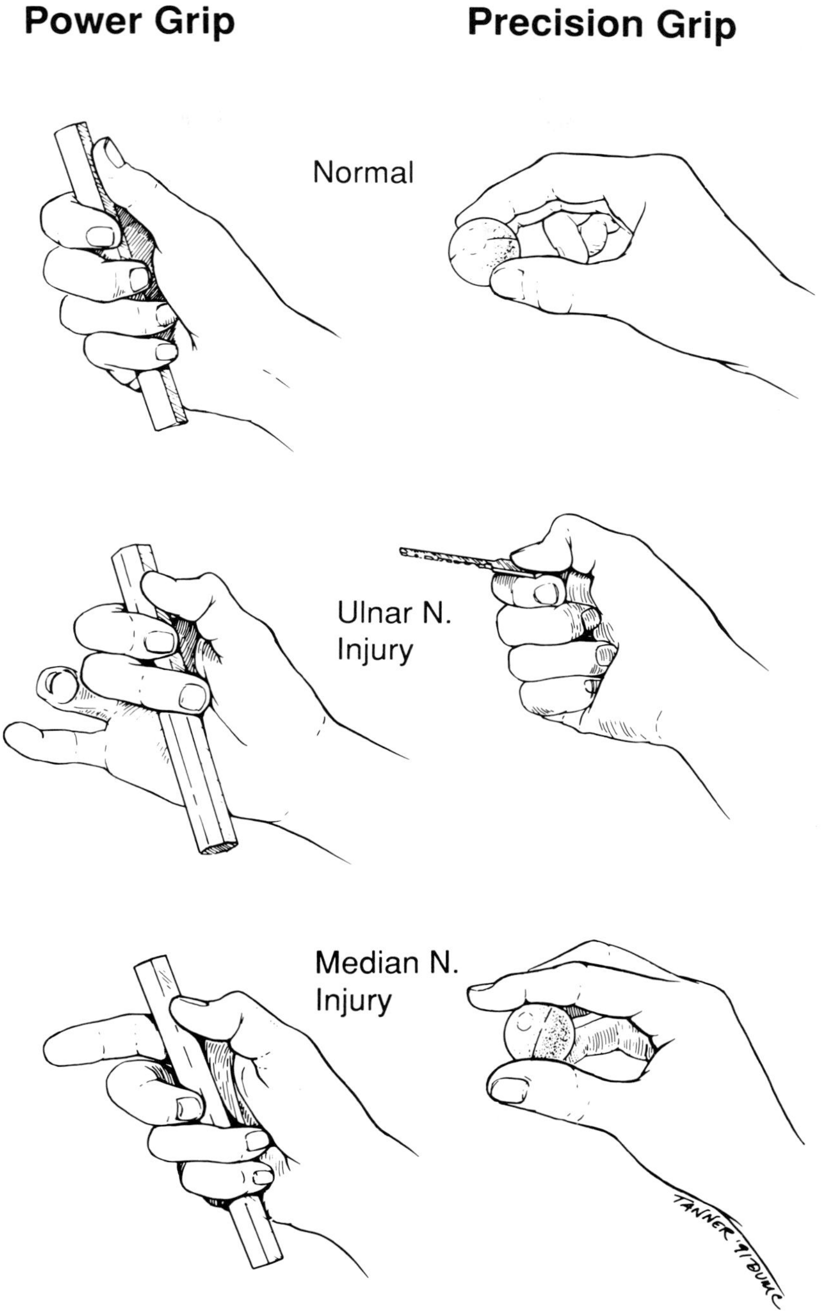

Power Grip   Precision Grip

Figure 4. With a normal power grip, the rod is clamped by the finger flexors and stabilized by the thumb. With a normal precision grip, the object is pinched between the opposing abducted thumb and the flexed index finger. Following an ulnar nerve injury, the fingers no longer wrap around the rod because of paralysis of the long ulnar finger flexors, all of the interossei, and the flexors of the metacarpophalangeal joint. The thumb loses its clamping action because of adductor pollicis muscle paralysis. Pressure grip is impaired to a lesser degree after an ulnar nerve injury by the weakness of the first dorsal interosseous and the adductor pollicis muscles (note the presence of Froment's sign). Power grip can still be performed after a median nerve injury. Precision grip, however, is greatly impaired after a median nerve injury because of loss of thenar abduction and rotation. Precision grip is also impaired by loss of sensation.

gitorum profundus to the ulnar digits flexes the proximal interphalangeal joint along with the distal interphalangeal joint. Precision pinch is impaired by loss of thenar palmar abduction (abduction perpendicular to the palm) and opposition (internal rotation) movements initiated by the opponens pollicis, abductor pollicis, and to a lesser extent, flexor pollicis brevis (Figure 4).[3,27] The flexor pollicis brevis and longus muscles add strength to the pinch.[46] Some palmar abduction and internal rotation of the thumb occur in approximately one-third of patients with a medial nerve injury as a result of a dominant ulnar innervation of the flexor pollicis brevis muscle.[22,37]

An injury to the median nerve proximal to the elbow weakens wrist pronation and flexion. Wrist flexion is still carried out in the absence of the flexor carpi radialis and digitorum flexors by the intact flexor carpi ulnaris and abductor pollicis longus muscles. This compensated motion usually occurs with concomitant ulnar wrist deviation.

It must be remembered that median nerve injury robs the patient of critical sensory perception in the tips of the thumb and index finger. Without this sensation, fine pinch is of little value.

While awaiting reinnervation of the thenar eminence following a median nerve repair, the surgeon must guard against contracture of the dorsal skin of the thenar web. This common contracture limits opposition of the thumb and, if it occurs, should be treated by splinting or even surgical release. Mobility of the interphalangeal joints of the thumb and index fingers also must be maintained. Some surgeons advocate early muscle transfers to act as internal splints.

Several orthotic devices have been developed to oppose the thumb and index fingers, stabilize the thumb, and prevent web space contractures. Accessories may be added to prevent wrist dorsiflexion. Following an irreparable injury to the hand, spring- or electrically driven devices can oppose the thumb and index fingers providing the patient has retained a useful pinch mechanism.

Several muscle transfers have been described to restore opposition of the thumb following an injury of the median nerve. The interested reader is referred to the literature that outlines the strengths and weaknesses of each of these procedures.[8] The flexor digitorum sublimis muscle is the most commonly used motor for an opponensplasty following a low median nerve injury.[47] Following a high median nerve injury that has paralyzed the long finger and wrist flexors, thumb opposition can be partially restored by a tendon graft attached to a transposed extensor muscle such as the extensor carpi ulnaris, extensor indicis proprius, or extensor digiti minimus.

Because the ulnar portion of the flexor digitorum longus is innervated by the ulnar nerve, simultaneous flexion of all of the fingers can be provided by tenodising (suturing together) the long flexor tendons of the small and ring fingers to those of the long and index fingers. This only will allow the fingers to flex in mass and may result in a "swan neck" deformity of some or all of the digits. Independent flexion of the index finger is important to the patient who depends on a precision pinch. This can be accomplished by a transfer of the extensor carpi radialis longus tendon to the flexor digitorum longus tendon of the index finger. Flexion of the thumb is accomplished by attaching the brachioradialis muscle to the tendon of the flexor pollicis longus. The ulnar deviation frequently observed in wrist flexion carried out solely by the flexor carpi ulnaris can be corrected by splitting that muscle's tendon and attaching one slip of the split tendon to the insertion of the flexor carpi radialis insertion.

Sensation can be partially restored to the ulnar volar surface of the thumb and opposing surface of the index finger by rotating a double cutaneous island with neurovascular pedicle from the opposing surfaces of the ring and small fingers.[26,31,33]

References

1. Allieu Y, Privat JM, Bonnel F. Paralysis in root avulsion of the brachial plexus: neurotization by the spinal accessory nerve. *Clin Plast Surg.* 1984;11:133–136.

2. Berger N, Burgess EM, Burkhalten WE, et al: The upper limb. In: American Academy of Orthopedic Surgeons, ed. *Atlas of Limb Prosthetics*. St. Louis Mo.: CV Mosby Co, 1981:6–218.

3. Bowden REM, Napier JR. The assessment of hand function after peripheral nerve injuries. *J Bone Joint Surg Br*. 1961;43B:481–492.

4. Boyes JH. Tendon transfers for radial palsy. *Bull Hosp J Dis*. 1960;21:97–105.

5. Brand PW. Tendon transfers in the forearm. In:Jupiter JB, ed. *Flynn's Hand Surgery*. 4th ed. Baltimore, Md: Williams & Wilkins; 1991:490–506.

6. Brunelli G. Neurotization of avulsed roots of the brachial plexus by means of anterior nerves of the cervical plexus. In:Terzis JK, ed. *Microreconstruction of Nerve Injuries*. Philadelphia, Pa: WB Saunders; 1987:435–445.

7. Brunelli G, Monini L. Neurotization of avulsed roots of brachial plexus by means of anterior nerves of cervical plexus. *Clin Plast Surg*. 1984;11:149–152.

8. Burkhalter WE. Median nerve palsy. In: Green DP, ed. *Operative Hand Surgery*. New York, NY: Churchill Livingston; 1982;2:1029–1059.

9. Burkhalter WE. Tendon transfers as internal splints. In:Omer GE, Spinner M, eds. *Management of Peripheral Nerve Problems*. Philadelphia, Pa: WB Saunders Co; 1980:798–804.

10. Burkhalter WE. Early tendon transfer in upper-extremity peripheral nerve injury. *Clin Orthop*. 1974:104:68–79.

11. Clark JMP. Reconstruction of biceps brachii by pectoral muscle transplantation. *Br J Surg*. 1946; 34:180–181.

12. Cushing H. The surgical treatment of facial paralysis by nerve anastomosis: with the report of a successful case. *Ann Surg*. 1903;37:641–659.

13. Dellon AL, Curtis RM, Edgerton MT. Reeducation of sensation in the hand after nerve injury and repair. *Plast Reconstr Surg*. 1974;53:297–305.

14. Dillner S, Georgiev G. Technical and clinical function testing of hand orthoses in Sweden. *Int J Rehabil Res*. 1979;2:47–60.

15. Dolenc VV. Intercostal neurotization of the peripheral nerves in avulsion plexus injuries. *Clin Plast Surg*. 1984;11:143–147.

16. Fishman S, Berger N, Edelstein JE, et al. Upper-limb orthoses. In:Bunch WH, Keagy R, Kritter AE, et al. *Atlas of Orthotics*. St. Louis, Mo: CV Mosby Co; 1985:163–198.

17. Friedman AH, Nashold BS Jr, Bronec PR. Dorsal root entry zone lesions for the treatment of brachial plexus avulsion injuries: a follow-up study. *Neurosurgery*. 1988;22:369–373.

18. Friedman AH, Nunley JA II, Goldner RD, et al. Nerve transposition for the restoration of elbow flexion following brachial plexus avulsion injuries. *J Neurosurg*. 1990;72:59–64.

19. Friedman AH, Nunley JA II, Urbaniak JR, et al. Repair of isolated axillary nerve lesions after infraclavicular brachial plexus injuries: case reports. *Neurosurgery*. 1990;27:403–407.

20. Goldner JL. Tendon transfers for irreparable peripheral nerve injuries of the upper extremities. *Orthop Clin North Am*. 1974;5:343–375.

21. Kotani KT, Matsuda H, Suzuki T. Trial surgical procedures of nerve transfer to avulsion injuries of plexus brachialis. In:Delchef J, de Marneffe R, Vander Elst E, eds. *Orthopaedic Surgery and Traumatology*. New York, NY: American Elsevier Publishing Co; 1973:348–350.

22. Mannerfelt L. Studies on the hand in ulnar nerve paralysis: a clinical-experimental investigation in normal and anomalous innervation. *Acta Orthop Scand Suppl*. 1966;87:11–176.

23. Millesi H. Brachial plexus injuries: management and results. *Clin Plast Surg*. 1984;11:115–120.

24. Minami M, Ishii S. Satisfactory elbow flexion in complete (preganglionic) brachial plexus injuries: produced by suture of third and fourth intercostal nerves to musculocutaneous nerve. *J Hand Surg Am*. 1987;12A:1114–1118.

25. Moberg E. Criticism and study of methods for examining sensibility in the hand. *Neurology*. 1962;12:8–19.

26. Murray JF, Ord JVR, Gavelin GE. The neurovascular island pedicle flap: an assessment of late results in sixteen cases. *J Bone Joint Surg Am*. 1967;49A:1285–1297.

27. Napier JR. The prehensile movements of the human hand. *J Bone Joint Surg Br*. 1956;38B:902–913.

28. Narakas AO. The treatment of brachial plexus injuries. *Int Orthop*. 1985;9:29–36.

29. Nickel VL, Perry J, Garrett AL. Development of useful function in the severely paralyzed hand. *J Bone Joint Surg Am*. 1963;45A:933–952.

30. Omer GE Jr. Tendon transfers for reconstruction of the forearm and hand following peripheral nerve injuries. In:Omer GE, Spinner M, eds. *Management of Peripheral Nerve Problems*. Philadelphia, Pa: WB Saunders Co; 1980;817–846.

31. Omer GE Jr. Neurovascular island flaps and fillet of finger. In Grabb WC, Myers MB, eds. *Skin Flaps*. Boston, Mass: Little Brown and Co; 1975:471–480.

32. Omer GE Jr. Evaluation and reconstruction of the forearm and hand after acute traumatic peripheral nerve injuries. *J Bone Joint Surg Am*. 1968; 50A:1454–1478.

33. Omer GE Jr, Day DJ, Ratliff H, et al. Neurovascular cutaneous island pedicles for deficient median-nerve sensibility: new technique and results of serial functional tests. *J Bone Joint Surg Am*. 1970;52A:1181–1192.

34. Önne L. Recovery of sensibility and sudomotor activity in the hand after nerve suture. *Acta Chir Scand Suppl*. 1962;300:1–69.

35. Ploncard P. A new approach to the intercosto-brachial anastomosis in the treatment of brachial plexus paralysis due to root avulsion: late results. *Acta Neurochir (wien)*. 1982;61:281–290.

36. Riggins RS. Shoulder fusion without external fixation. *J Bone Joint Surg Am*. 1976;58A:1007–1008.

37. Riordan DC. Tendon transplantations in median-nerve and ulnar-nerve paralysis. *J Bone Joint Surg Am*. 1953;35A:312–320.

38. Saha AK. Surgery of the paralysed and flail shoulder. *Acta Orthop Scand Suppl*. 1967;97:5–90.

39. Sick C, Säenger A. Heilung einer in folge traumatischen defects bedingten Lähmung des Radialis durch Vernähung des peripheren endes dieses nerven mit dem medianus. *Langenbecks Arch Klin Chir*. 1897:271–279.

40. Samardzic M, Grujicic D, Antunovic V, et al. Reinnervation of avulsed brachial plexus using the spinal accessory nerve. *Surg Neurol*. 1990;33:7–11.

41. Sedel L. The results of surgical repair of brachial plexus injuries. *J Bone Joint Surg Br*. 1982; 64B: 54–66.

42. Simesen K, Haase J. Microsurgery in brachial plexus lesions. *Acta Orthop Scand*. 1985;56:238–241.

43. Solonen KA, Vastamäki M, Ström B. Surgery of the brachial plexus. *Acta Orthop Scand*. 1984;55:436–440.

44. Staples OS, Watkins AL. Full active abduction in traumatic paralysis of the deltoid. *J Bone Joint Surg*. 1943;25:85–89.

45. Steindler A. Orthopedic reconstruction work on hand and forearm. *NY Med J*. 1918;108:1117–1119.

46. Sunderland S. Voluntary movements and deceptive action of muscles in peripheral nerve lesions. *Aust NZ J Surg*. 1944;13:160–183.

47. Thompson TC. A modified operation for opponens paralysis. *J Bone Joint Surg*. 1942;24:632–640.

48. Tuttle HK. Exposure of the brachial plexus with nerve-transplantation. *JAMA*. 1913;61:15–17.

49. Vera CL, Lewin MG, Kase JC, et al. Central functional changes after facial-spinal-accessory anastomosis in man and facial-hypoglossal anastomosis in the cat. *J Neurosurg*. 1975;43:181–190.

50. Wynn Parry CB, Salter M. Sensory re-education after median nerve lesions. *Hand*. 1976;8:250–257.

51. Yamada S, Peterson G, Solniuk AS et al. Coaption of the anterior rami of C-3 and C-4 to the upper trunk of the brachial plexus for cervical root avulsion. *J Neurosurg*. 1991;74:171–177. Abstract.

52. Yeoman P. Traction injuries of the brachial plexus. In: *Surgical Disorders of the Peripheral Nerves*. Baltimore, Md: Williams & Wilkins; 1977:184–290.

53. Zancolli E, Mitre H. Latissimus dorsi transfer to restore elbow flexion. *J Bone Joint Surg Am*. 1973;55A:1265–1275.

Index

Previously Published Books in the *Neurosurgical Topics* Series

Management of Posttraumatic Spinal Instability
  Edited by Paul R. Cooper, MD

Malignant Cerebral Glioma
  Edited by Michael L.J. Apuzzo, MD

Intracranial Vascular Malformation
  Edited by Daniel L. Barrow, MD

Neurosurgical Treatment of Disorders of the Thoracic Spine
  Edited by Edward C. Tarlov, MD

Contemporary Diagnosis and Management of Pituitary Adenomas
  Edited by Paul R. Cooper, MD

Complications of Spinal Surgery
  Edited by Edward C. Tarlov, MD

Neurosurgical Aspects of Epilepsy
  Edited by Michael L.J. Apuzzo, MD

Complications and Sequelae of Head Injury
  Edited by Daniel L. Barrow, MD

For order information call (708)692-9500.